Student Handbook
and
Solutions Manual

Concepts of Genetics

ELEVENTH EDITION

Harry Nickla
Professor Emeritus, Creighton University

William S. Klug
College of New Jersey

Michael R. Cummings
Illinois Institute of Technology

Charlotte A. Spencer
University of Alberta

Michael A. Palladino
Monmouth University

PEARSON

Boston   Columbus   Indianapolis   New York   San Francisco   Upper Saddle River
Amsterdam   Cape Town   Dubai   London   Madrid   Milan   Munich   Paris   Montréal   Toronto
Delhi   Mexico City   São Paulo   Sydney   Hong Kong   Seoul   Singapore   Taipei   Tokyo

Editor-in-Chief: Beth Wilbur

Senior Acquisitions Editor: Michael Gillespie

Executive Editorial Manager: Ginnie Simione Jutson

Program Manager Team Lead: Michael Early

Program Manager: Anna Amato

Project Editor: Chloe Veylit

Project Manager Team Lead: David Zielonka

Project Manager: Lori Newman

Production Management: Cenveo Publisher Services

Copyeditor/Proofreader: Joanna Dinsmore

Compositor: Cenveo Publisher Services

Cover Designer: Seventeenth Street Studios

Illustrators: Cenveo Publisher Services

Manufacturing Buyer: Stacey Weinberger

Cover/Interior Printer: LSC Communications

Director of Marketing: Christy Lesko

Executive Marketing Manager: Lauren Harp

Cover Photo Credit: Dr. Gopal Murti / Science Source

ISBN 10:   0-133-79680-9

ISBN 13: 978-0-133-79680-3

4 16

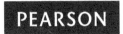

www.pearsonhighered.com

Contents

Introduction: Students, Read This Section First!

How to Increase Your Chances of Success in Genetics

1. Attend Class.
2. Read the Book.
3. Do the Assigned Problems.
4. Don't Cram.
5. Study When There Are No Tests.
6. Develop Confidence from Effort.
7. Set Disciplined Study Goals.
8. Learn Concepts.
9. Be Careful with Old Exams.
10. Don't "Second Guess" the Teacher.

A first course in genetics can be a humbling experience for many students. The intent of this book is to help you understand introductory genetics as presented in the text *Concepts of Genetics* (11th edition). It is possible that the lowest grades received in one's major, or even in one's undergraduate career, may be in genetics. It is not unusual for some students to become frustrated with their own inability to succeed in genetics. Teachers recognize this frustration as they field the following types of student comments.

"I studied all the material but failed your test."

"I must have a mental block to it. I just don't get it. I just don't understand what you are asking."

"Where did you get that question? I didn't see anything like that in the book or in my notes."

"This is the first test I have *ever* failed."

"I helped three of my friends last night and I got the lowest grade."

"I am getting a D in your course and I have never received less than a B in my whole life."

"I stayed up all night studying for your exam and I still failed."

Similar to Algebra

Think back to the first time you encountered "word problems" in your first algebra class. How many times did you ask yourself, your parents, or your teacher the following classic question?

"I hate word problems, I just can't understand them, and why do I need to learn this anyway, I'll never use it?"

At that time you had two choices: drop out and be afraid of problem solving for the rest of your life (which unfortunately happens too often) or regroup, seek help, strip away distractions, and focus on learning something new and powerful. Because you are taking genetics, you probably succeeded in algebra, perhaps with difficulty at first, and you will probably succeed in genetics.

In algebra you were forced to convert something real and dynamic (two trains leaving at different times from different stations at different speeds—when do they meet?) to a somewhat abstract formula that can be applied to an infinite number of similar problems. In genetics you will again learn something new. It will involve the conversion of something real and dynamic (genes, chromosomes, hereditary elements, gamete formation, gene splicing, and evolution) to an array of general concepts (similar to mathematical formulas), which will allow you to predict the outcome of an infinite number of presently known and yet to be discovered phenomena relating to the origin and maintenance of life.

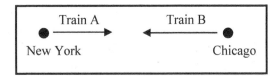

Mental Pictures and Symbols

When working almost any word problem it is often helpful to make a simple drawing that relates, in space, the primary participants. From that drawing one can often predict or estimate a likely outcome. A mathematical formula and its solution provide the precise outcome. To understand genetics, it is often helpful to make drawings of the participants, whether they be crosses ($Aa \times Aa$), gametes (A or a), or the interactions of molecules (anticodon with codon).

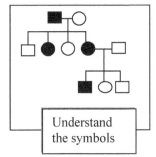

Understand the symbols

As with algebra, symbols used to represent a multitude of structures, movements, and interactions are abstract, informative, and fundamental to understanding the discipline. It is the set of symbols and their interrelationships that comprise the concepts that make up the framework of genetics. Test questions and problems exemplify the concepts and may be

Introduction: Students, Read This Section First!

completely unfamiliar to the student. Nevertheless, they refer directly to the basic concepts of genetics.

Attendance and Attention Are Mandatory

Because many professors do not take attendance in lectures, some students will likely opt to take a day off now and then. Unless those students are excellent readers and excellent students in general, continual absences will usually result in failure.

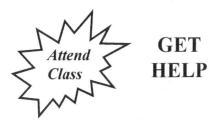

Remember how difficult it was to set up and understand the first algebra word problem on your own? It is likely that your ultimate source of understanding came from the course instructor. While using the text is important in your understanding of genetics, the teacher can walk you through the concepts and strategies much more efficiently than a text because a text is organized in a sequential manner. A good teacher can "cut and paste" an idea from here and there as needed.

To benefit from the wisdom of the instructor, the student must concentrate during the lecture session rather than sit passively taking notes, assuming that he or she can figure out the ideas at a later date. Too often the student is unable to relate to notes passively taken weeks before. In addition, the instructor will not be able to cover all the material in the text. Some parts will be emphasized and others may be omitted entirely.

There is no magic formula for understanding genetics or any other discipline of significance. Learning anything, especially at the college level, requires time, patience, and confidence. First, a student must be willing to focus on the subject matter for an hour or so each day over the entire semester (quarter, trimester, etc.). Study time must be free of distractions and framed by realistic goals.

The student must be patient and disciplined, studying even when no assignments are due and no tests are looming.

> Since it is the instructor who writes and grades the tests, who is in a better position to prepare the students for those tests?

The majority of successful students are willing to read the text ahead of the lecture material, spend time thinking about the concepts and examples, and work as many sample problems as possible. They study for a period of time, stop, and then return to review the most difficult areas. They do not try to cram information into marathon study sessions a few nights before the examinations. Although they may get away with that practice on occasion, more often than not, understanding the concepts in genetics requires more mature study habits and preparation.

Perhaps a Different Way of Thinking

Because the acquisition of problem-solving abilities requires that students rely on new and important ways of seeing things rather than memorizing the book and notes, some students find the transition more difficult than others. Some students are more able to deal in the abstract, concept-oriented framework than others. Students who have typically relied on "pure 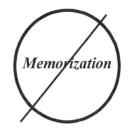 memory" for their success will find a need to focus on concepts and problem solving. They may struggle at first, just as they may have struggled with the first word problem in algebra. But the reward for their struggle is intellectual growth. That is what college is supposed to stimulate. With such growth will come an increased ability to solve a variety of problems beyond genetics. Problem solving is a process, a style, that can be applied to many disciplines. Few people are actually born with the touch of synthetic brilliance. Success comes from probing deeply into a few areas to see how problems are approached in a given discipline. Then, because problems are usually approached in a fairly consistent manner, a given problem-solving approach can often be applied to a variety of activities.

Introduction: Students, Read This Section First!

Read ahead. You have been told that it is important to read the assigned material before attending lectures. This allows you to make full use of the information provided in the lecture and to concentrate on those areas that are unclear in the readings. You are often given an opportunity to ask questions. Your questions will be received much more favorably if you can state that after reading the book and listening to the lecture a particular point is still unclear. It is very likely that your question will be quickly dealt with to your benefit and the benefit of others in the class.

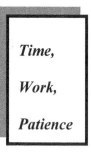

Ask Questions and Don't Tune Out!

How to Study

Genetics is a science that involves symbols (A, b, p), structures (chromosomes, ribosomes, plasmids), and processes (meiosis, replication, translation) that interact in a variety of ways. Models describe the manner in which hereditary units are made, how they function, and how they are transmitted from parent to offspring. Because many parts of the models interact in both time and space, genetics cannot be viewed as a discipline filled with facts that should be memorized. Rather, one must be, or become, comfortable with seeking to understand not only the components of the models but also the way the models work.

One can memorize the names and shapes of all the parts of an automobile engine, but without studying the interrelationships among the parts in time and space, one will have little understanding of the real nature of the engine. It takes time, work, and patience to see how an engine works, and it will take time, work, and patience to understand genetics.

Time, Work, Patience

Don't cram. A successful tennis player does not learn to play tennis overnight; similarly, you cannot expect to learn genetics under the pressure of night-long cramming. It will be necessary for you to develop and follow a realistic study schedule for genetics as well as the other courses you are taking.

Study when there are no tests

It is important that you organize your study periods into intensive, but short, sessions each day throughout the entire semester (or quarter or trimester). Because genetics tests often require you to think "on the spot," it is very important that you get a good night's sleep before each test. Avoid caffeine on the evening before the test because a clear, rested, well-prepared mind will be required.

Study goals. The instruction of genetics is often divided into large conceptual units. A test usually follows each unit. It will be necessary for you to study genetics on a routine basis long before each test. To do so, set specific study goals. Adhere to these goals and do not let examinations in one course interfere with the study goals of another course. Notice that each course being taken is handled in the same way—study ahead of time and don't cram.

Study each subject at least every other day— especially when there are no tests!

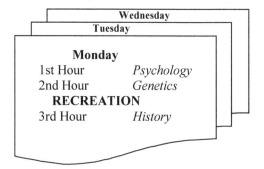

Wednesday
Tuesday
Monday
1st Hour   *Psychology*
2nd Hour   *Genetics*
RECREATION
3rd Hour   *History*

Develop a Realistic Monthly Schedule

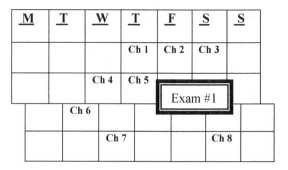

M	T	W	T	F	S	S
				Ch 1	Ch 2	Ch 3
		Ch 4	Ch 5			
			Exam #1			
	Ch 6					
		Ch 7			Ch 8	

Introduction: Students, Read This Section First!

Develop a Plan for the Semester or Quarter

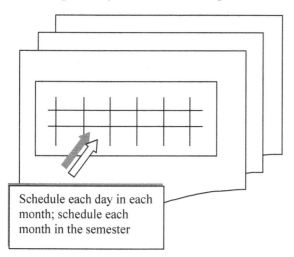

Schedule each day in each month; schedule each month in the semester

Work the assigned problems. The basic concepts of genetics are quite straightforward, but there are many examples that apply to these concepts. To help students adjust to the variety of examples and approaches to concepts, instructors often assign practice problems from the back of each chapter. If your instructor has assigned certain problems, finish working them *at least* one week before each examination. Before starting a set of problems, read the chapter carefully and consider the information presented in class.

> ## *Suggestions for working problems:*
>
> *(1) Work the problem without looking at the answer. Commit each answer to paper!*
> *(2) Check your answer in this book.*
> *(3) If incorrect, work the problem again.*
> *(4) If still incorrect, you don't understand the concept.*
> *(5) Re-read your lecture notes and the text.*
> *(6) Work the problem again.*
> *(7) If you still don't understand the solution, mark it, and go to the next problem. Return to the problem at a later date. That's why cramming won't work.*

In your next study session, return to those problems that you have marked. Expect to make mistakes and learn from those mistakes. Sometimes what is difficult to see one day may be obvious the next. If you are still having problems with a concept, schedule a meeting with your instructor. The problem can usually be cleared up in a few minutes.

You will notice that in this book, I have presented the solution to each problem. I provide different ways of looking at some of the problems. Instructors often take a problem directly from those at the end of the chapters, or they will modify an existing problem. Reversing the "direction" of a question is a common approach. Instead of giving characteristics of the parents and asking for characteristics of the offspring, the question may provide characteristics of the offspring and ask for particulars on the parents. Think as you work the problems.

Separate examples from concepts. As mentioned earlier, genetics boils down to a few (perhaps 15 to 20) basic concepts. However, many examples apply to those concepts. Too often students have trouble separating examples from the concepts. Examples allow you to picture, in concrete terms, various phenomena, but they do not exemplify each phenomenon or concept in its entirety.

Be careful when using old examinations. Often it is customary for students to request or otherwise obtain old examinations from previous students. Such a practice is loaded with pitfalls. First, students often, albeit unconsciously, find themselves "second guessing" questions on an upcoming examination. They forget that usually an examination only tests you on a subset of the available

> *Old examinations may help, but...*

information in a section. Therefore, entire conceptual areas may be available that have not appeared on recent exams.

Often the reproductions of old examinations are of poor quality (having been copied and passed around repeatedly), and it is difficult to determine whether the answer provided is correct. In addition, if a question has the same general structure as one on a previous examination but is modified, students often provide an answer for the "old" question rather than the one being asked. Granted, it is of value to see the

Introduction: Students, Read This Section First!

format of each question and the general emphasis of previous examinations, but remember that each examination is potentially a new production capable of covering areas that have not been tested before. This is especially likely in a course such as genetics where the material changes very rapidly.

> *Don't try to figure out what will be asked.*
> *Study all the material as well as possible.*

Structure of This Book

The intent of this book is to help you understand the concepts of genetics as given in the text, and most likely in the lectures, and then to apply these concepts to the solution of all problems and questions at the end of each chapter. Rather than merely provide you with the solutions to the problems, I have tried to walk you through each component of each question so that you can see where information is obtained and how it can be applied in the solution. At the beginning of each chapter is a section that relates general concept areas to particular problems. This should help you practice certain conceptual

areas as needed without having to work every single problem at the end of each chapter.

> ### *Understand the words and phrases of the discipline*

Concepts and processes checklist. Understanding the vocabulary of a discipline is essential to understanding the discipline. Throughout the text you will find terms in bold print. Those terms along with other terms of special significance are presented as checklists to make certain that you understand the meaning of each term in each chapter. Notice that the various terms are not redefined. It is important that you use the text for the original definitions.

Solved problems. Each problem at the end of each chapter is solved from a beginner's point of view. Be certain that you fully understand the solution to each of the questions suggested or assigned by your instructor. Consider also that the same concept (question) can be addressed in a variety of ways. Try to anticipate a variety of approaches to the same concept (question).

Chapter 1: Introduction to Genetics

Concept Areas	Corresponding Problems
Mendelism	1, 4, 5
Homologous Chromosomes	4, 5
Chromosome Theory of Inheritance	3
Central Dogma of Genetics	5, 6, 7
Molecular Biology	2, 8, 9, 10, 11
Genetics and Social Issues	12, 13, 14, 15, 16, 17, 18
Model Organisms	14

Concepts and Processes Checklist

(Check topic when mastered – provide examples where appropriate – understand the context of each entry)

- **Human Genome Project**
  - translational medicine
  - LDL cholesterol
  - *PCSK9*
  - familial hypercholesterolemia
  - animal domestication
  - Golden Age
  - Aristotle
  - Hippocrates
  - William Harvey
  - epigenesis
  - preformation
  - homunculus
  - cell theory
  - spontaneous generation
  - Gregor Mendel
  - Charles Darwin
  - natural selection
  - Carl Correns
- Hugo de Vries
- Erich Tschermak
- **Chromosome Theory**
  - diploid number ($2n$)
  - homologous chromosomes
  - cell division
  - mitosis
  - meiosis
  - haploid number (n)
- **Genetic Variation**
  - mutation
  - allele
  - phenotype
  - genotype
- **Chemical Nature of Genes**
  - DNA or protein
  - Avery, MacLeod, and McCarty
  - bacteriophages (phages)

Chapter 1 Introduction to Genetics

- **Molecular Genetics**
  - nucleotides (ATGC)
  - Wilkins, Watson, and Crick
  - transcription
  - messenger RNA (mRNA)
  - ribosome
  - translation
  - genetic code
  - codon
  - transfer RNA (tRNA)
  - central dogma

- **Proteins and Biological Function**
  - amino acid
  - enzymes
  - sickle-cell anemia
  - hemoglobin

- **Recombinant DNA Technology**
  - restriction enzyme
  - vector
  - clone
  - genome

- **Biotechnology**
  - herbicide resistance
  - genetically engineered crops
  - transgenic organisms
  - knock out
  - ownership
  - patents
  - medical applications
  - DNA microarrays (chips)
  - gene therapy

- **Genomics, Proteomics, and Bioinformatics**
  - Human Genome Project
  - model organisms
  - genomics
  - proteomics
  - bioinformatics
  - forward genetics
  - reverse genetics

- **Model Organisms**
- **Human Diseases**
- **Age of Genetics**
- **Nobel Prize and Genetics**
- **Genes and Society**

F1.1 Simple diagram of the relationships among major components or central dogma of molecular genetics

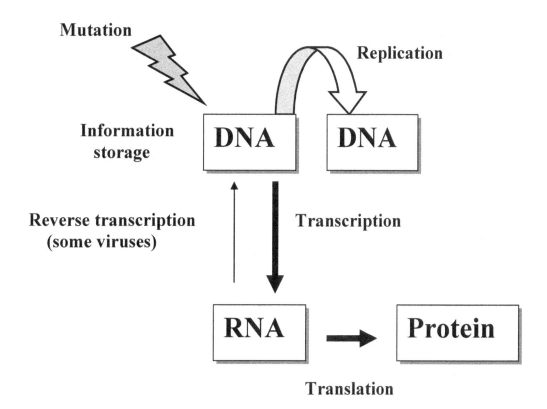

Chapter 1 Introduction to Genetics
Solutions to Problems and Discussion Questions

1. Mendel proposed that traits are passed from one generation to the next by following certain predictable patterns. He hypothesized that traits in peas are controlled by discrete units, which are now called genes. He also suggested that factors occur in pairs and that members of each gene pair separate from each other during gamete formation.

2. Your essay should include a description of the impact of recombinant DNA technology on the following: plant and animal husbandry and production, drug development, medical advances, forensics, and understanding gene function.

3. Based on the parallels between Mendel's model of heredity and the behavior of chromosomes, the chromosome theory of inheritance emerged. It states that inherited traits are controlled by genes residing on chromosomes that are transmitted by gametes.

4. The genotype of an organism is defined as the specific allelic or genetic constitution of an organism, often the allelic composition of one or a limited number of genes under investigation. The observable sum of features of those genes is called the phenotype. A gene variant is called an allele. There can be many such variants in a population, but for a diploid organism, only two such alleles can exist in any given individual.

5. Genes possess a variety of functions. Since proteins can contain up to 20 different amino acids, each being structurally unique, a vast amount of functional variation is possible. In addition, proteins can engage in a variety of enzymatic activities. DNA is made up of only six different components (sugar, phosphate, and four bases) arranged in a rather monotonous, linear fashion. It seems likely that proteins, given their cellular abundance and versatility, should be the genetic material.

6. *Genes*, linear sequences of nucleotides, usually exert their influence by producing proteins through the processes of transcription and translation. Genes are the functional units of heredity. They associate, sometimes with proteins, to form *chromosomes*. Genes are duplicated by a variety of enzymes so that

daughter cells inherit copies of the parental hereditary information.

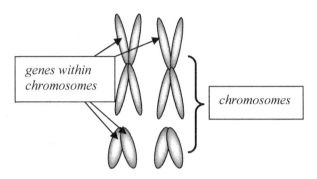

7. Genetic information is encoded in DNA by the sequence of bases. This sequence is transcribed into RNA products, which are then translated into proteins.

8. The central dogma of molecular genetics refers to the relationships among DNA, RNA, and proteins. The processes of *transcription* and *translation* are integral to understanding these relationships. See F1.1 above in this book. Because DNA and RNA are discrete chemical entities, they can be isolated, studied, and manipulated in a variety of experiments that define modern genetics.

9. If a protein chain is 5 amino acids long, at each position, there can be 20 amino acids; therefore, there would be

$$20^5$$

different possible combinations. As the length of an amino acid chain increases, the number of possible combinations becomes very large.

10. Restriction enzymes (endonucleases) cut double-stranded DNA at particular base sequences. Often, short single-stranded overhangs are generated so that ends from one fragment can anneal with ends from another (assuming the same enzyme is used). When a vector is cleaved with the same enzyme, complementary ends are created such that ends, regardless of their origin, can be combined and ligated to form intact double-stranded structures.

11. In the past 40 years, traditional transmission, cytological, and molecular genetics have provided an understanding of many aspects of both plant and animal biology, including development of pest-resistant crops and identification of hazardous organisms in our food (*E. coli,* for example). Recently, biotechnology has allowed genes to be moved in a variety of ways to generate transgenic plants. Such plants can be engineered to increase their ecological breadth, disease resistance, and/or nutrient value. Wheat, rice, corn, beans, and cassava are being modified to enhance nutritional value by increasing vitamin and mineral content.

12. Unique transgenic plants and animals can be patented, as ruled by the U.S. Supreme Court in 1980. Supporters of organismic patenting argue that it is needed to encourage innovation and allow the costs of discovery to be recovered. Capital investors assume that there is a likely chance that their investments will yield positive returns. Others argue that natural substances should not be privately owned, and that once owned by a small number of companies, free enterprise will be stifled. Individuals and companies needing vital but patented products may have limited access. Such concentration of products may reduce genetic variation as farmers are forced to grow a limited suite of crops.

13. Some mechanism should be in place to protect the investments of individuals and institutions that develop needed and useful products, such as selected stretches of human DNA. However, safeguards, both ethical and economic, need to be developed to ensure that relatively free and fair access exists when vital issues are in question. Any mechanism needs to protect investors as well as consumers.

14. Model organisms are not only useful, but also necessary for understanding genes that influence human diseases. Given that genetic/molecular systems are highly conserved across broad phylogenetic lines, what is learned in one organism is usually applied to all organisms. In addition, most model organisms have peculiarities, such as ease of growth, genetic understanding, or abundant offspring, that make them straightforward and especially informative in genetic studies.

15. This question is open to many answers depending on the individual. Although it may be difficult to put yourself in this position, consider not only what your decision would be, but also why you would make such a decision. Often, as a person ages, his or her perspective changes; for instance, how would the possibility of having children influence your decision?

16. For approximately 60 years discoveries in genetics have guided our understanding of living systems, aided rational drug design, and dominated many social discussions. Genetics provides the framework for universal biological processes and helps explain species stability and diversity. Given the central focus of genetics in so many of life's processes, it is understandable why so many genetic scientists have been awarded the Nobel Prize.

17. Safeguards should probably include tests for allergenicity, environmental impact, and likelihood of cross-pollination. In addition, concern would increase if such a crop contained antibiotic-resistant genetic markers and genes conferring toxicity to pests. Although not required in the United States, in the interest of the consumer, one might consider labeling such products as genetically modified. On a broader scale, one might reduce vulnerability by using multiple suppliers (if available) and help minimize the domination of the world food supply by a few companies.

18. Such groups seek to reclaim community involvement and decision making in governmental and industrial applications of biotechnology. They consider that profit-driven motives may compromise benefits that such technology may provide. They question the safety of genetically modified organisms to human health and ecological harmony, not to mention biotechnical applications to weapons development.

Chapter 2: Mitosis and Meiosis

Concept Areas	Corresponding Problems
Cell Structure	3
Homology of Chromosomes	1, 4, 5, 23
Cell Division	1, 2
Mitosis	1, 2, 5, 6, 7, 8, 9, 12, 14, 15, 25, 26, 32
Meiosis	9, 10, 11, 12, 14, 15, 16, 17, 18, 19, 20, 25, 27, 28, 29, 30, 31, 32, 33, 34, 35
Chromosome Structure	6, 21, 22
Gametogenesis	13, 17, 18, 24

Concepts and Processes Checklist

(Check topic when mastered – provide examples where appropriate – understand the context of each entry)

- **Genetic Continuity**
  - sexually reproducing organisms
  - mitosis
  - meiosis
  - gametes
  - spores
  - chromosome
  - chromatin
- **Cell Structure**
  - plasma membrane
  - cell wall
  - cellulose
  - glycocalyx, cell coat
  - receptor molecule
  - eukaryotic organisms
  - nucleus
  - nucleolus
  - nucleolus organizer region (NOR)
  - prokaryotic organism
  - nucleoid
  - cytoplasm
  - microtubule
  - tubulin
  - microfilament
  - actin
  - endoplasmic reticulum (ER)
  - ribosome
  - mitochondria
  - chloroplast
  - endosymbiont hypothesis
  - centriole
  - spindle fiber
- **Chromosomes**
  - centromere
  - metacentric
  - submetacentric
  - acrocentric
  - telocentric

Chapter 2 Mitosis and Meiosis

- q arm, p arm
- diploid number (*2n*)
- homologous chromosome
- karyotype
- sister chromatid
- haploid number (*n*)
- genome
- locus, loci
- biparental inheritance
- allele
- sex-determining chromosome
- **Mitosis**
  - zygote
  - karyokinesis
  - cytokinesis
- **Cell Cycle**
  - interphase
  - stages
  - S phase
  - G1 (gap I)
  - G2 (gap II)
  - G0
- **Prophase**
  - sister chromatid
  - cohesion
- **Prometaphase and Metaphase**
  - separase
  - shugoshin
  - kinetochore mictotubules
  - aligned chromosomes
- **Anaphase**
  - disjunction

- daughter chromosome
- molecular motors
- centromere division
- **Telophase**
  - cell plate
  - middle lamella
  - cell furrow
  - entry to interphase
- **Cell-Cycle Regulation and Checkpoints**
  - *cell division cycle* (*cdc*) mutations
  - kinases
  - cyclin
  - checkpoints
  - G1/S checkpoint
  - G2/M checkpoint
  - M checkpoint
- **Meiosis**
  - reduction in chromosome number
  - diploid to haploid
  - meiosis I
  - meiosis II
  - germ cells and spores
  - crossing over
  - synapsis, synapse
  - bivalent
  - tetrad
  - reductional division
  - dyads
  - equational division
  - monads

- **First Meiotic Division: Prophase I**
  - prophase I
  - homologous pairs synapse
  - leptonema (leptotene stage)
  - homology search
  - zygonema (zygotene stage)
  - synaptonemal complex
  - pachynema (pachytene stage)
  - diplonema (diplotene stage)
  - chiasma (pl. chiasmata)
  - diakinesis
  - terminalization
- **Metaphase, Anaphase, and Telophase I**
  - meiosis I, meiosis II
  - metaphase I
  - anaphase I
  - nondisjunction
  - shugoshin complex
  - telophase I
- **Second Meiotic Division**
  - meiosis II
  - prophase II
  - metaphase II
  - anaphase II
  - telophase II
- **Spermatogenesis, Oogenesis**
  - spermatogenesis

- spermatogonium
- primary spermatocyte
- secondary spermatocyte
- spermatid
- spermiogenesis
- spermatozoa, sperm
- oogenesis
- ova, ovum
- primary oocyte
- oogonium
- first polar body
- secondary oocyte
- ootid
- second polar body
- **Critical Aspects of Sexual Reproduction**
  - gamete formation and haploidy
  - independent assortment of chromosomes
  - crossing over
  - sporophyte
  - gametophyte
- **Electron Microscopy and Chromosomes**
  - folded-fiber model
  - compaction
  - 5000-fold
  - sister chromatids

F2.1 Diagram illustrating relationships among stages of interphase. Also illustrated are chromosomes, chromosome number, and structure in an organism with a diploid chromosome number of 4 ($2n = 4$). Individual chromosomes cannot be seen at interphase; therefore, the chromosomes pictured here are hypothetical. In mitosis, there is no change in chromosome number even though the DNA content doubles during the S phase. The chromosomes become doubled structures as a result of the S phase.

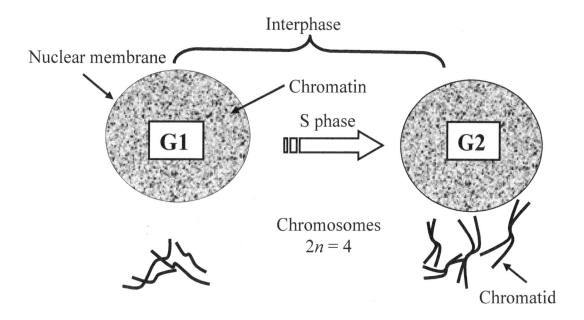

F2.2 Important nomenclature referring to chromosomes and genes in an organism where the diploid chromosome number is 4 ($2n = 4$). There are two pairs of chromosomes: one large metacentric and one small telocentric. Sister chromatids are identical to each other, whereas homologous chromosomes are similar to each other in terms of overall size, centromere location, function, and other factors described in the text.

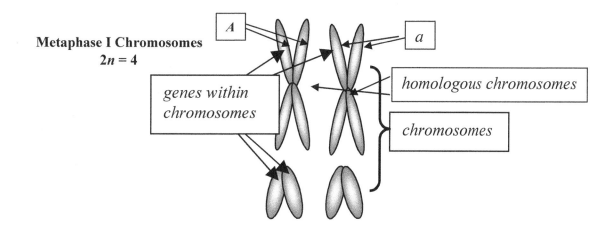

F2.3 Illustration of chromosomes of mitotic cells in an organism with a chromosome number of 4 ($2n = 4$).

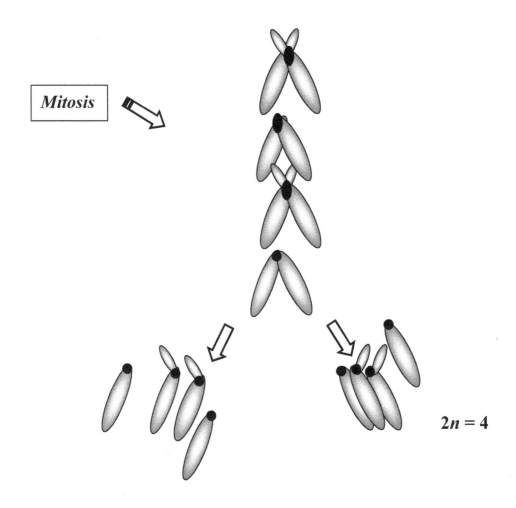

F2.4 Illustration of chromosomes of meiotic cells in an organism with a chromosome number of 4 (2*n* = 4).

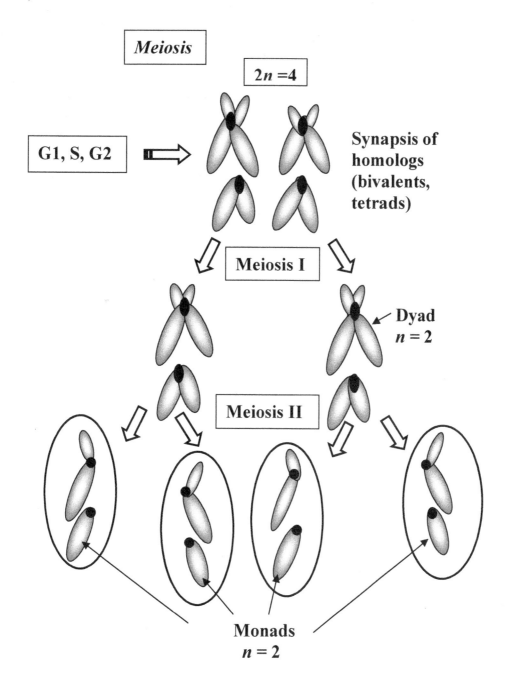

Chapter 2 Mitosis and Meiosis

Answers to Now Solve This

2-1 (a) The first sentence tells you that $2n = 16$ and it is a question about mitosis. Since each chromosome in prophase is doubled (having gone through an S phase) and is visible at the end of prophase, there should be 32 chromatids. **(b)** Because the centromeres divide and what were previously sister chromatids migrate to opposite poles during anaphase, there should be 16 chromosomes moving to each pole.

2-2 (a) If there are 16 chromosomes, there should be 8 tetrads. **(b)** Also note that, after meiosis I and in the second meiotic prophase, there are as many dyads as there are pairs of chromosomes. There will be 8 dyads. **(c)** Because the monads migrate to opposite poles during meiosis II (from the separation of dyads), there should be 8 monads migrating to *each* pole.

2-3 Not necessarily; if crossing over occurs in meiosis I, then the chromatids in the secondary oocyte are not identical. Once they separate during meiosis II, unlike chromatids reside in the ootid and the second polar body.

Chapter 2 Mitosis and Meiosis

Solutions to Problems and Discussion Questions

1. (a) When somatic cells from the same species are examined, they contain the same number of chromosomes, and the lengths and centromere placements of nearly all such chromosomes can be matched into pairs. **(b)** The initiation and completion of DNA synthesis can be detected by the incorporation of labeled precursors into DNA. DNA content in a G2 nucleus is twice that of a G1 nucleus. **(c)** If the fibers comprising the mitotic chromosomes are loosened, they reveal fibers like those of interphase chromatin. Electron microscopic observations indicate that mitotic chromosomes are in varying states of extensively folded structures derived from chromatin.

2. Compared with mitosis, which maintains chromosomal constancy, meiosis provides for a reduction in chromosome number and an opportunity for exchange of genetic material between homologous chromosomes. In mitosis there is no change in chromosome number or kind in the two daughter cells, whereas in meiosis numerous potentially different haploid (*n*) cells are produced. During oogenesis, only one of the four meiotic products is functional; however, four of the four meiotic products of spermatogenesis are potentially functional.

3. (a) During interphase of the cell cycle (mitotic and meiotic), chromosomes are not condensed and are in a genetically active, spread out form. In this condition, chromosomes are not visible as individual structures under the microscope (light or electron). See F2.1 for a sketch of what *chromatin* might look like. Chromatin contains the genetic material that is responsible for maintaining hereditary information (from one cell to daughter cells and from one generation to the next) and production of the phenotype.

(b) The *nucleolus (pl. nucleoli)* is a structure that is produced by activity of the nucleolar organizer region in eukaryotes. Composed of ribosomal DNA and protein, it is the structure for the production of ribosomes. Some nuclei have more than one nucleolus. Nucleoli are not present during mitosis or meiosis because in the condensed state of chromosomes, there is little or no RNA synthesis.

(c) The *ribosome* is the structure where various RNAs, enzymes, and other molecular species assemble the primary sequence of a protein. That is,

amino acids are placed in order as specified by messenger RNA. Ribosomes are relatively nonspecific in that virtually any ribosome can be used in the translation of any mRNA. The structure and function of the ribosome will be described in greater detail in later chapters of the text.

(d) The *mitochondrion (pl. mitochondria)* is a membrane-bound structure located in the cytoplasm of eukaryotic cells. It is the site of oxidative phosphorylation and production of relatively large amounts of ATP. It is the trapping of energy in ATP that drives many important metabolic processes in living systems.

(e) The *centriole* is a cytoplasmic structure involved (through the formation of spindle fibers) in the migration of chromosomes during mitosis and meiosis—primarily in animal cells.

(f) The *centromere* serves as an attachment point for sister chromatids (see F2.3, F2.4) and a region where spindle fibers attach to chromosomes (kinetochore). The centromere divides during mitosis and meiosis II, thus aiding in the partitioning of chromosomal material to daughter cells. Failure of centromeres or spindle fibers to function properly may result in nondisjunction.

4. One of the most important concepts to be gained from this chapter is the relationship that exists among chromosomes in a single cell. Chromosomes that are homologous share many properties, including the following:

Overall length: Look carefully at the figures above to see that each cell, prior to anaphase I, contains two chromosomes in which a homolog is of approximately the same overall length.

Position of the centromere (metacentric, submetacentric, acrocentric, telocentric): Again, look carefully at F2.2 and F2.3. Notice that if there is one metacentric chromosome, there will be another metacentric chromosome.

Banding patterns: Using various cytological techniques, bands can be induced in chromosomes. Homologous chromosomes of pair #1, for example, will have the same banding pattern. Although the overall length of chromosome pairs #16 and #17 appears to be the same, the banding patterns of these nonhomologous chromosomes will be different.

Chapter 2 Mitosis and Meiosis

Sister chromatids have identical banding patterns, as would be expected since sister chromatids are, with the exception of mutation, identical copies of each other. We would expect that homologous chromosomes would have banding patterns that are very similar (but not identical) because homologous chromosomes are genetically similar but not genetically identical.

Type and location of genes: Notice in F2.2 that a locus signifies the location of a gene along a chromosome. What that really means is that for each characteristic specified by a gene, such as blood type, eye color, and skin pigmentation, there are genes located along chromosomes. The *order* of such loci is identical in homologous chromosomes, but the genes themselves, although in the same order, may not be identical. Look carefully at the inset (box) in the upper portion of F2.2 and see that there are alternative forms of genes, *A* and *a*, at the same location along the chromosome. *A* and *a* are located at the same place and specify the same *characteristic* (eye color, for example), but they are slightly different manifestations of eye color (*brown* vs. *blue*, for example). Just as an individual may inherit gene *A* from the father and gene *a* from the mother, each zygote inherits one homolog of each pair from the father and one homolog of each pair from the mother.

Autoradiographic pattern: Homologous chromosomes tend to replicate during the same time of S phase.

Diploidy is a term often used in conjunction with the symbol 2n. It means that both members of a homologous pair of chromosomes are present. Refer to F2.1 in this book. Notice that during mitosis, the normal chromosome complement is 2n, or diploid. In humans, the diploid chromosome number is 46, whereas in *Drosophila melanogaster* it is 8. The text lists the *haploid* chromosome number for a variety of species.

Notice that in humans and flies, the haploid chromosome number is one-half the diploid number. This applies to other organisms as well. However, it is very important to realize that *haploidy* specifically refers to the fact that each haploid cell contains *one chromosome of each homologous pair of chromosomes.*

Compare the nuclear contents of a spermatid and a cell at zygonema in the text. Note that each spermatid contains one member of each of the original chromosome pairs (seen at zygonema). Haploidy is usually symbolized as *n*.

The change from a diploid (2n) to haploid (n) occurs during *reduction division* when tetrads become dyads during meiosis I. Referring to the number of human chromosomes, the primary spermatocyte (2n = 46) becomes two secondary spermatocytes each with n = 23.

5. As you examine the criteria for *homology* in question #4 above, you can see that overall length and centromere position are but two factors required for homology. Most important, genetic content in nonhomologous chromosomes is expected to be quite different. Other factors including banding pattern and time of replication during S phase would also be expected to vary among nonhomologous chromosomes.

6. Because a major section of Chapter 2 deals with mitosis, it would be best to deal with this question by reading the appropriate section in the text and examining corresponding figures. Understanding mitosis and all the related terms is essential for an understanding of genetics. There are several sample test questions at the end of this book that will help you determine your understanding of mitosis.

7. Refer to the text figures for an explanation. Notice the different anaphase shapes of chromosomes as they move to the poles: metacentric (a), submetacentric (b), acrocentric (c), telocentric (d). Your understanding of these structures will be determined by several of the sample test questions at the end of this book. Notice that the centromere is placed in the middle for a metacentric chromosome and at one end for a telocentric chromosome.

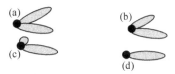

8. In plants, a cell plate that was laid down during telophase becomes the middle lamella where primary and secondary layers of the cell wall are deposited. In animals, constriction of a cell membrane produces a cell furrow of daughter cells.

9. Carefully read the section on mitosis and cell division in the text. Major divisions of the cell cycle include interphase and mitosis. Interphase is composed of four phases: G1, G0, S, and G2. During the S phase, chromosomal DNA doubles. Karyokinesis involves nuclear division, whereas cytokinesis involves division of the cytoplasm. Refer to F2.1 for information pertaining to interphase. Refer to the text figures for a diagram of mitosis. Notice that, in contrast to meiosis, there is no pairing of homologous chromosomes in mitosis and the chromosome number does not change.

10. (a) *Synapsis* is the point-by-point pairing of homologous chromosomes during prophase of meiosis I.

(b) *Bivalents* are those structures formed by the synapsis of homologous chromosomes. In other words, there are two chromosomes (and four chromatids) that make up a bivalent. If an organism has a diploid chromosome number of 46, then there will be 23 bivalents in meiosis I.

(c) *Chiasmata* is the plural form of chiasma and refers to the structure, when viewed microscopically, of crossed chromatids. Notice in figures in the text the exchange of chromatid pieces in diplonema and diakinesis.

(d) *Crossing over* is the exchange of genetic material between chromatids. Also called recombination, it is a method of providing genetic variation through the breaking and rejoining of chromatids.

(e) *Chromomeres* are bands of chromatin that look different from neighboring patches along the length of a chromosome.

(f) Examine F2.1 in this book. Notice that *sister chromatids* are "post-S phase" structures of replicated chromosomes. Sister chromatids are genetically identical (except where mutations have occurred) and are originally attached to the same centromere. Identify sister chromatids in the figures in the text. Note that sister chromatids separate from each other during anaphase of mitosis and anaphase II of meiosis.

(g) *Tetrads* are synapsed homologous chromosomes thereby composed of four chromatids. There are as many tetrads as the haploid chromosome number.

(h) Actually, each tetrad is made of two dyads that separate from each other during anaphase I of meiosis. Note that *dyads* are composed of two chromatids joined by a centromere.

(i) At anaphase II of meiosis, the centromeres divide and sister chromatids (*monads*) go to opposite poles.

11. Sister chromatids are genetically identical, except where mutations may have occurred during DNA replication. Nonsister chromatids are genetically similar if on homologous chromosomes or genetically dissimilar if on nonhomologous chromosomes. If crossing over occurs, then chromatids attached to the same centromere will no longer be identical.

12. During meiosis I, chromosome number is reduced to haploid complements. This is achieved by synapsis of homologous chromosomes and their subsequent separation. It would seem to be more mechanically difficult for genetically identical daughters to form from mitosis if homologous chromosomes paired. By having chromosomes unpaired at metaphase of mitosis, only centromere division is required for daughter cells to eventually receive identical chromosomal complements.

13. Examine appropriate figures in the text. Notice that major differences include the sex in which each occurs and that the distribution of cytoplasm is unequal in oogenesis, but considered to be equal in the products of spermatogenesis. Chromosomal behavior is the same in spermatogenesis and oogenesis except that the nuclear activity in oogenesis is "off-center," thereby producing first and second polar bodies by unequal cytoplasmic division. Each spermatogonium and primary spermatocyte produces four spermatids, whereas each oogonium and primary oocyte produces one ootid. Because early development occurs in the absence of outside nutrients, it is likely that the unequal distribution of cytoplasm in oogenesis evolved to provide sufficient information and nutrients to support development until the transcriptional activities of the zygotic nucleus begin to provide products. Polar bodies probably represent nonfunctional by-products of such evolution. (See following figures for a comparison.)

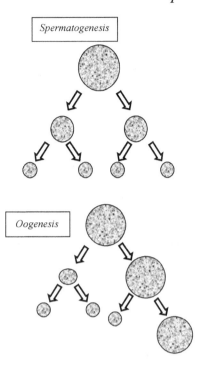

14. This answer contains several parts. First, through independent assortment of chromosomes at anaphase I of meiosis, daughter cells (secondary spermatocytes and secondary oocytes) may contain different sets of maternally and paternally derived chromosomes. Examine the diagram below. Notice that there are several ways in which the maternally and paternally derived chromosomes may align. Can you calculate the probability of all the maternally derived chromosomes going to the "right-hand" pole? Second, crossing over, which happens at a much higher frequency in meiotic cells as compared with mitotic cells, allows maternally and paternally derived chromosomes to exchange segments, thereby increasing the likelihood that daughter cells (that is, secondary spermatocytes and secondary oocytes) are genetically unique.

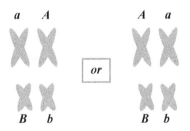

Notice that there are two different orientations of tetrads in meiosis. Independent assortment of nonhomologous chromosomes adds to genetic variability. Daughter cells resulting from the process of mitosis are usually genetically identical.

15. This question specifically tests your understanding of meiosis and the behavior of chromosomes during anaphase. In this question, you must first visualize the alignment of the three homologous chromosome pairs—C1/C2, M1/M2, and S1/S2—in mitosis where there is no synapsis of homologous chromosomes.

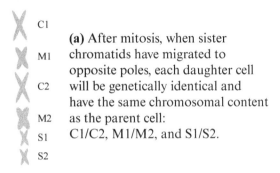

(a) After mitosis, when sister chromatids have migrated to opposite poles, each daughter cell will be genetically identical and have the same chromosomal content as the parent cell: C1/C2, M1/M2, and S1/S2.

(b) The first meiotic metaphase will have the following configuration:

Label each chromosome according to the symbols in part **(a)** above.

(c) For the haploid products of the above cell in part **(b)**, there are eight possibilities, depending on the alignment of the homologous chromosomes:

C1 **or** C2

M1 **or** M2

S1 **or** S2

16. If there are 8 combinations possible for part **(c)** in the previous problem, there would be 16 combinations with the addition of another chromosome pair.

17. As you first read this question, think about an animal with $n = 6$; therefore, there will be six tetrads. The question concerns one of these tetrads as it passes normally through meiosis I, but one dyad undergoes secondary nondisjunction. Secondary nondisjunction occurs during the second meiotic division.

(a) The mature ovum should contain $n + 1$ chromosomes: the five chromosomes from normal disjunction and two (from one dyad) from the nondisjunctional chromosome.

Chapter 2 Mitosis and Meiosis

(b) The second polar body did not receive one of the six monads it would normally receive, so it should have five monads (which are chromosomes).

(c) When the normal sperm with its n chromosome number combines with an $n + 1$ ovum, it will produce a zygote with $2n + 1$, or 13 chromosomes. This condition is termed *trisomy*.

18. One half of each tetrad will have a maternal homolog: $(1/2)^{10}$.

19. (a) Although it is likely that the molecular processes involved in crossing over occur earlier, crossing over is known to have occurred by pachynema.

(b) *Synapsis* begins at zygonema with continuation of the homology search and when homologous chromosomes align in a point-by-point fashion to form bivalents or tetrads. More intimate pairing (synapsis) is completed during pachynema.

(c) Chromosomes begin to condense at the earliest stage of prophase I, leptonema.

(d) *Chiasmata* are clearly visible at diplonema.

20. In angiosperms, meiosis results in the formation of microspores (male) and megaspores (female), which give rise to the haploid male and female gametophyte stage. Micro- and megagametophytes produce the pollen and the ovules, respectively. Following fertilization, the sporophyte is formed.

21. The transition from chromatin to individual chromosomes occurs at the beginning of mitosis (or meiosis). During this time, chromatin fibers fold up and condense into the typical mitotic chromosome. The *folded-fiber model* depicts this transition.

22. The folded-fiber model is based on each chromatid consisting of a single fiber wound like a skein of yarn. Each fiber consists of DNA and protein. A coiling process occurs during the transition of interphase chromatin into more condensed chromosomes during prophase of mitosis or meiosis. Such condensation leads to a 5000-fold contraction in the length of the DNA within each chromatid. The transition is at the end of interphase and the beginning of prophase when the chromosomes are in the condensation process. This eventually leads to the

typically shortened and "fattened" metaphase chromosome.

23. They would probably be homologous chromosomes and contain similar (but not identical) genetic information. Their centromeres would most likely be in the same position relative to chromosome arm lengths, and any physical characteristics such as secondary constrictions or bands would be similar. They would have a similar sequence of nitrogenous bases. They would most likely replicate synchronously during the S phase of the cell cycle.

24. 50, 50, 50, 100, 200

25. 0.72 picograms; 0.36 picograms; 0.72 picograms

26. Duplicated chromosomes A^m, A^p, B^m, B^p, C^m, and C^p will align at metaphase, with the centromeres dividing and sister chromatids going to opposite poles at anaphase.

27. Side-by-side alignment of A^m, A^p, B^m, B^p, C^m, and C^p will occur in various arrangements at metaphase I. Eight possible combinations of products will occur at the completion of anaphase: A^m, B^p, C^m, for example (each with sister chromatids). In other words, after meiosis I, the two product cells would be as follows: A^m or A^p, B^m or B^p, C^m or C^p.

28. As long as you have accounted for eight possible combinations in the previous problem, there would be no new ones added in this problem.

29. Eight $(2 \times 2 \times 2)$ combinations are possible.

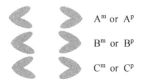

A^m or A^p

B^m or B^p

C^m or C^p

30. See the products of nondisjunction of chromosome C at the end of meiosis I as follows:

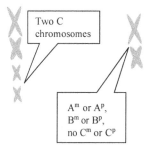

Two C chromosomes

A^m or A^p,
B^m or B^p,
no C^m or C^p

17

At the end of meiosis II, assuming that, as the problem states, the C chromosomes separate as dyads instead of monads during meiosis II, you would have monads for the A and B chromosomes, and dyads (from the cell on the left) for both C chromosomes as one possibility.

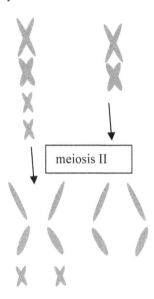

31. Taking this question exactly as it is described— nondisjunction of the C chromosome at meiosis I and dyad separation at meiosis II, you will end up, after fertilization, with the following combinations under the conditions described in Problem 30.

zygote 1:   two copies of chromosome A
                two copies of chromosome B
                three copies of chromosome C

zygote 2:   two copies of chromosome A
                two copies of chromosome B
                one copy of chromosome C

32. (a) The chromosome number in the somatic tissues of the hybrid would be the summation of the haploid numbers of each parental species: $7 + 14 = 21$.

(b) Given that no homologous chromosome pairing occurs at metaphase I, one would expect 21 univalents and random "1 × 0" separation of chromosomes at anaphase I. That is, there would be a random separation of univalents to either pole at anaphase I, usually leading to inviable haploid cells and thus sterility.

33. The following answer assumes a normal chromosomal composition of the mother. If there were two dyads of chromosome 21 in the first polar body, the secondary oocyte would completely lack chromosome 21. The resulting zygote would have one copy of chromosome 21 (from the father) and two copies of all the other chromosomes.

34. If the polar body lacked chromosome 21, the secondary oocyte would have two dyads and the resulting zygote would have three number 21 chromsomes (Down syndrome), two coming from the mother and one coming from the father.

35. The secondary oocyte would have a dyad and a monad from chromosome 21. Depending on how the monad partitioned at meiosis II, you would have either a normal chromosome 21 complement (the zygote that did not receive the monad) or a chromosome 21 trisomy in which the zygote received two number 21 chromosomes from the mother and one from the father.

Chapter 3: Mendelian Genetics

Concept Areas	Corresponding Problems
Mendel's Model	1, 2, 4, 6, 10
Monohybrid Crosses	3, 5, 14, 15, 17, 25, 26, 29, 32, 33, 34, 35
Dihybrid Crosses	7, 9, 12, 16
Other Crosses	27, 30
Homology	11, 33
Independent Assortment	13, 33
Probability	8, 23, 24, 26, 28, 31, 36
Chi-Square Analysis	1, 18, 19, 20, 32
Pedigree Analysis	1, 3, 17, 21, 22, 28

Concepts and Processes Checklist

(Check topic when mastered – provide examples where appropriate – understand the context of each entry)

- **Transmission Genetics**
  - Mendelian genetics
  - Gregor Mendel
  - Augustinian Monastery
  - 1856, 1868
  - hybridization experiments
  - peas
  - trait
  - postulates
- **Monohybrid Cross**
  - selfing
  - P_1, F_1, F_2
  - parental generation
  - first filial generation
  - second filial generation
  - 3:1 ratio
  - reciprocal cross
  - particulate unit factors

- **Mendel's First Three Postulates**
  - unit factors in pairs
  - dominance/recessiveness
  - segregation
- **Modern Genetic Terminology**
  - phenotype
  - genes
  - alleles
  - genotype
  - homozygous, homozygote
  - heterozygous, heterozygote
  - symbolism, *D*, *d*
- **Mendel's Analytical Approach**
- **Punnett Squares**
- **Testcross: One Character**
- **Dihybrid Cross**
  - unique F_2 ratio

- **Mendel's Fourth Postulate**
  - independent assortment
  - 3:1 ratio, 9:3:3:1 ratio
  - product law
  - independent events
- **Independent Assortment**
  - Mendel's 9:3:3:1 dihybrid ratio
- **A Molecular Explanation**
  - wrinkled peas
  - starch-branching enzyme
  - *SBEI*
  - transposable element
- **The Testcross: Two Characters**
  - two gene pairs
- **Trihybrid Cross**
  - multiple traits
  - forked-line method
  - branch diagram
  - 27:9:9:9:3:3:3:1
  - Rediscovery of Mendel's work
  - continuous variation
  - Charles Darwin, Alfred R. Wallace
  - discontinuous variation
- **The Chromosomal Theory of Inheritance**
  - Flemming, 1879
  - de Vries, Correns, Tschermak
  - Sutton, Boveri
  - Morgan, Sturtevant, Bridges
  - genes in chromosomes

- **Unit Factors, Genes and Homologous Chromosomes**
  - diploid number ($2n$)
  - haploid (n)
  - maternal parent
  - paternal parent
  - homolog
  - homologous pairs
  - locus (pl. loci)
- **Independent Assortment and Extensive Genetic Variation**
  - 2^n
- **Tay-Sachs Disease: The Molecular Basis**
  - hexosaminidase A (Hex-A)
  - ganglioside GM2
- **Laws of Probability**
  - product law
  - sum law
- **The Binomial Theorem**
  - binomial theorem
  - symbol !
  - $p = (n!/s!t!)a^s b^t$
- **Chi-Square Analysis**
  - evaluates the influence of chance
  - chance deviation
  - reasonable fluctuation
- **Chi-Square Calculations**
  - null hypothesis (H_0)
  - chi-square analysis
  - sample size

- $\chi^2 = \Sigma \dfrac{(o - e)^2}{e}$

- $\chi^2 = \Sigma \dfrac{d^2}{e}$

- degrees of freedom

- probability value

- p

- abscissa (horizontal or x-axis)

- ordinate (vertical or y-axis)

- **Interpreting Probability Values**

  - 0.05

  - $p = 0.05$

  - chi-square table

  - rejection of the null hypothesis

- **Pedigrees Reveal Patterns of Inheritance**

  - pedigree

  - pedigree conventions

  - consanguineous

- sibling, sib

- sibship line

- Arabic numerals

- Roman numerals

- squares, circles, diamonds

- shaded, unshaded

- diagonal line

- monozygotic twin

- dizygotic twin

- proband (p)

- **Pedigree Analysis**

  - albinism (recessive)

  - autosomal trait

  - X-linked trait

  - Huntington disease (dominant)

  - familial hypercholesterolemia

  - LDL

F3.1 Illustration of the union of maternal and paternal genes (*A* and *a*) to give two genes in the zygote. Mendelian "unit factors" occur in pairs in diploid organisms. Dominant genes are often given the uppercase letter as the symbol, while the lowercase letter is often used to symbolize the recessive gene.

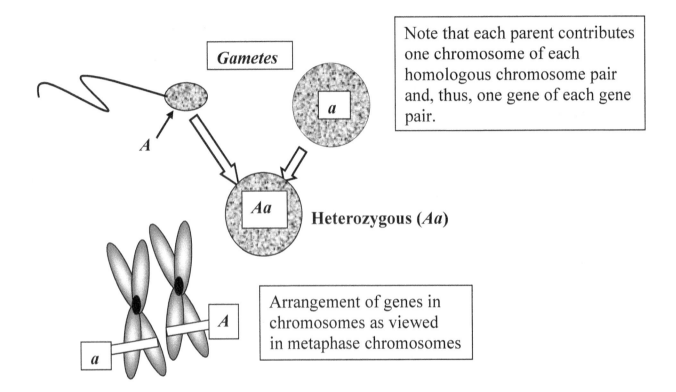

Gametes

Note that each parent contributes one chromosome of each homologous chromosome pair and, thus, one gene of each gene pair.

a

A

Aa

Heterozygous (*Aa*)

A

a

Arrangement of genes in chromosomes as viewed in metaphase chromosomes

F3.2 Critical symbolism associated with genes and chromosomes. Below two different gene pairs (*Aa* and *Bb*) are positioned on nonhomologous chromosomes. Note that with two different gene pairs, two different characteristics may be involved, such as seed shape (*A* and *a*) and seed color (*B* and *b*).

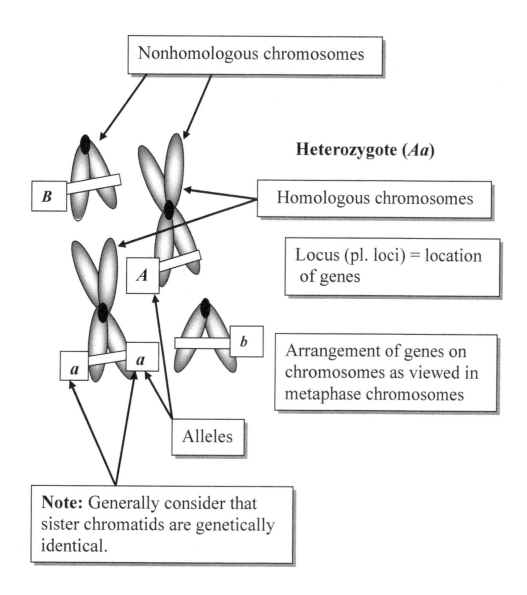

Nonhomologous chromosomes

Heterozygote (*Aa*)

B

Homologous chromosomes

A

Locus (pl. loci) = location of genes

a   *a*

b

Arrangement of genes on chromosomes as viewed in metaphase chromosomes

Alleles

Note: Generally consider that sister chromatids are genetically identical.

F3.3 One of the most important concepts is illustrated in the figure below. Two gene pairs (*W* and *B*) are presented, each representing a different characteristic: seed shape (*W* or *w*) and seed color (*B* or *b*). Different gene pairs may influence completely different characteristics (as indicated here) or the same characteristics (described in Chapter 4).

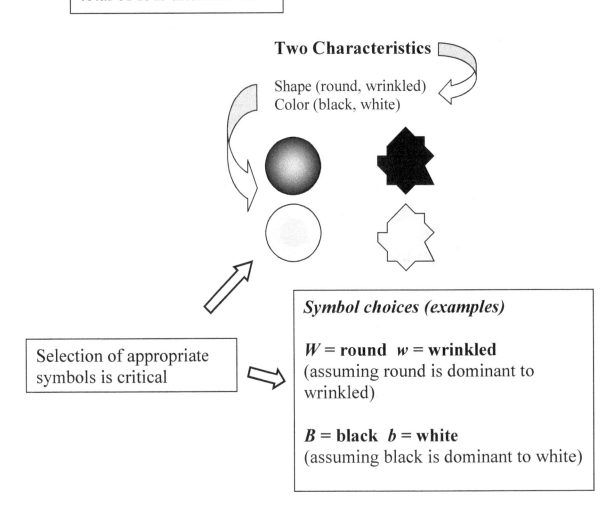

Chapter 3 *Mendelian Genetics*

Answers to Now Solve This

3-1. First, read the entire question and see that you are to determine (1) the pattern of inheritance for "checkered and plain" and (2) the gene symbols and genotypes of all the parents and offspring. Notice that there is reference to one characteristic *pattern*, with two alternatives, checkered vs. plain. We should consider this to be a monohybrid condition unless complications arise. We are to use the respective offspring from the P_1 cross (F_1 progeny a, b, and c) in a series of F_1 crosses, d through g. Approach the problem by first assigning *probable* genotypes to the P_1 crosses; then, where there is ambiguity [such as cross (a)], use the F_1 crosses for clarification.

Assignment of symbols: P = checkered; p = plain.

Checkered is tentatively assigned the dominant function because in a casual examination of the data, especially cross (b), we see that checkered types are more likely to be produced than plain types.

Cross (a):

$PP \times PP^*$ *or* $PP \times Pp$

Notice in cross (d) that the checkered offspring, when crossed to plain, produce only checkered F_2 progeny, and in cross (g), when crossed to checkered, still produce only checkered progeny. From this additional information, one can conclude that in the progeny of cross (a), there are no heterozygotes and the original cross must have been $PP \times PP^*$.

Cross (b):

$PP \times pp$

This assignment seems reasonable because among 38 offspring, no plain types are produced. In addition, we would expect all the F_1 progeny to be heterozygous and if crossed to plain, as in cross (e), to produce approximately half checkered and half plain offspring. In cross (f), we would expect such heterozygotes to produce a 3:1 ratio, which is observed.

Cross (c): Because all the offspring from this cross are plain, there is no doubt that the genotype of both parents is pp.

Genotypes of all individuals:

		Progeny	
P_1 Cross		Checkered	Plain
(a)	$PP \times PP$	PP	
(b)	$PP \times pp$	Pp	
(c)	$pp \times pp$		pp
(d)	$PP \times pp$	Pp	
(e)	$Pp \times pp$	Pp	pp
(f)	$Pp \times Pp$	PP, Pp	pp
(g)	$PP \times Pp$	PP, Pp	

3-2. Suggested symbolism:

w = wrinkled seeds g = green cotyledons

W = round seeds G = yellow cotyledons

Examine each characteristic (seed shape vs. cotyledon color) separately.

Chapter 3 Mendelian Genetics

(a) Notice a 3:1 ratio for seed shape; therefore, $Ww \times Ww$; and no green cotyledons; therefore, $GG \times GG$ or $GG \times Gg$. Putting the two characteristics together gives

$WwGG \times WwGG$

or

$WwGG \times WwGg$

(b) Notice a 1:1 ratio for seed shape (8/16 wrinkled and 8/16 round) and a 3:1 ratio for cotyledon color (12/16 yellow and 4/16 green). Therefore, the answer is

$wwGg \times WwGg$

(c) The offspring occur in a typical 9:3:3:1 ratio; therefore, the F_2 plants have the doubly heterozygous genotypes of

$WwGg \times WwGg$

(d) This is a typical 1:1:1:1 testcross (or backcross) ratio and signifies that one parent is doubly heterozygous, whereas the other is fully homozygous recessive. The answer is

$WwGg \times wwgg$

3-3. (a) When examining cross $AaBbCc \times AaBBCC$, expect there to be 8 different kinds of gametes from one parent ($AaBbCc$) and two different kinds from the other ($AaBBCC$). Therefore, there should be 16 kinds (genotypes) of offspring (8×2).

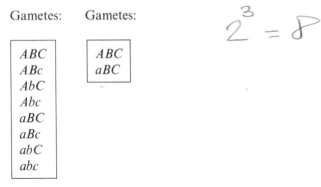

$2^3 = 8$

Gametes: Gametes:

ABC	ABC
ABc	aBC
AbC	
Abc	
aBC	
aBc	
abC	
abc	

Offspring:

Genotypes	Ratio	Phenotypes
AABBCC	(1/16)	
AABBCc	(1/16)	
AABbCC	(1/16)	
AABbCc	(1/16)	
AaBBCC	(2/16)	$A\_B\_C\_ = 12/16$
AaBBCc	(2/16)	
AaBbCC	(2/16)	
AaBbCc	(2/16)	
aaBBCC	(1/16)	
aaBBCc	(1/16)	$aaB\_C\_ = 4/16$
aaBbCC	(1/16)	
aaBbCc	(1/16)	

(b) There will be four kinds of gametes for the first parent (*AaBBCc*) and two kinds of gametes for the second parent.

Gametes: Gametes:

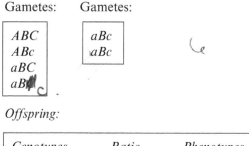

Offspring:

Genotypes	Ratio	Phenotypes
AaBBCC	1/8	*A_BBC_* = 3/8
AaBBCc	2/8	
AaBBcc	1/8	*A_BBcc* = 1/8
aaBBCC	1/8	*aaBBC_* = 3/8
aaBBCc	2/8	
aaBBcc	1/8	*aaBBcc* = 1/8

(c) There will be eight (2^n) different kinds of gametes from each of the parents and therefore a 64-box Punnett square. Doing this problem by the forked-line method helps considerably.

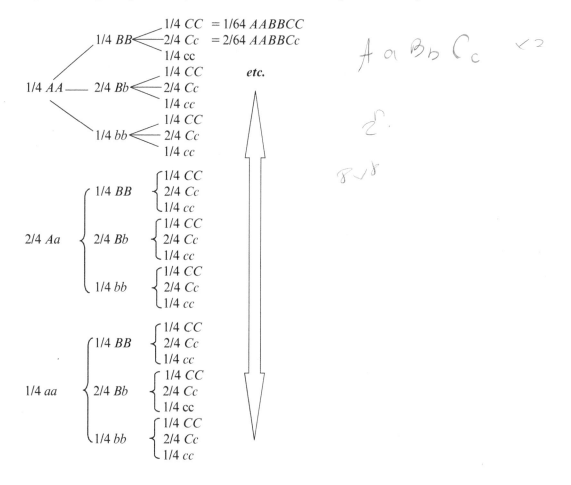

Simply multiply through each component to arrive at the final genotypic frequencies.

For the phenotypic frequencies, set up the problem in the following manner:

$$3/4\ A \overset{3/4\ B \overset{3/4\ C\_\ =\ 27/64\ A\_B\_C\_}{\underset{1/4\ cc\ =\ 9/64\ A\_B\_cc}{}}}{}$$

3/4 A—1/4 bb ⟨ 3/4 C_
                1/4 cc   *etc.*

1/4 aa—3/4 B ⟨ 3/4 C_
                1/4 cc

       1/4 bb ⟨ 3/4 C_
                1/4 cc

3-4. One must think of this problem as a dihybrid F_2 situation with the following expectations:

Expected ratio	Observed (o)	Expected (e)
9/16	315	312.75
3/16	108	104.25
3/16	101	104.25
1/16	32	34.75

$$\chi^2 = 0.47$$

Looking at the table in the text one can see that this χ^2 value is associated with a probability greater than 0.90 for 3 degrees of freedom (because there are now four classes in the χ^2 test). The observed and expected values do not deviate significantly.

To deal with parts **(b)** and **(c)** it is easier to see the observed values for the monohybrid ratios if the phenotypes are listed:

smooth, yellow	315
smooth, green	108
wrinkled, yellow	101
wrinkled, green	32

For the smooth: wrinkled *monohybrid component*, the smooth types total 423 (315 + 108), while the wrinkled types total 133 (101 + 32).

Expected ratio	Observed (o)	Expected (e)
3/4	423	417
1/4	133	139

The χ^2 value is 0.35; in examining the text for 1 degree of freedom, the *p* value is greater than 0.50 and less than 0.90. We fail to reject the null hypothesis and are confident that the observed values do not differ significantly from the expected values.

(c) For the yellow:green portion of the problem, see that there are 416 yellow plants (315 + 101) and 140 (108 + 32) green plants.

Expected ratio	Observed (o)	Expected (e)
3/4	416	417
1/4	140	139

The χ^2 value is 0.01; in examining the text for 1 degree of freedom, the *p* value is greater than 0.90. We fail to reject the null hypothesis and are confident that the observed values do not differ significantly from the expected values.

3-5. Applying the same logic as in problem #26, the gene is inherited as an autosomal recessive. Notice that two normal individuals II-3 and II-4 have produced a daughter (III-2) with myopia.

I-1 (*aa*), I-2 (*Aa* or *AA*), I-3 (*Aa*), I-4 (*Aa*)

II-1 (*Aa*), II-2 (*Aa*), II-3 (*Aa*), II-4 (*Aa*), II-5 (*aa*), II-6 (*AA* or *Aa*), II-7 (*AA* or *Aa*)

III-1 (*AA* or *Aa*), III-2 (aa), III-3 (*AA* or *Aa*)

Chapter 3 Mendelian Genetics

Solutions to Problems and Discussion Questions

1. (a) By noting that traits passed unaltered from parental to subsequent generations, Mendel not only postulated the "unit" or "particulate" nature of hereditary elements, but also described their behavior. Results of various crosses provided the basis for knowing that factors can remain hidden in some circumstances, thereby implying two participating elements, one dominating the other. Predictable ratios in crosses supported the hypothesis of two hereditary elements involved in the expression of a given trait.

(b) Typically, by conducting a testcross, one readily tests whether an organism is homozygous or heterozygous for a given trait.

(c) In general, a chi-square analysis is used to compare observed data with various genetic models.

(d) Pedigree analysis is often used to determine whether and how traits are inherited in humans. However, other methods are also used and are discussed in subsequent chapters.

2. Mendel's four postulates are related to the diagram below.

1. Factors occur in pairs. Notice A and a.
2. Some genes have dominant and recessive alleles. Notice A and a.

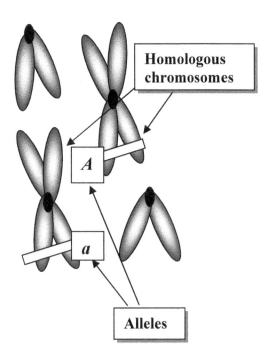

3. Alleles segregate from each other during gamete formation. When homologous chromosomes separate from each other at anaphase I, alleles will go to opposite poles of the meiotic apparatus.

4. One gene pair separates independently from other gene pairs. Different gene pairs on the same homologous pair of chromosomes (if far apart) or on nonhomologous chromosomes will separate independently from each other during meiosis.

3. Start out with the following gene symbols:

A = normal (not albino)
a = albino

Since albinism is inherited as a recessive trait, genotypes AA and Aa should produce the normal phenotype, whereas aa will give albinism.

(a) The parents are both normal; therefore, they could be either AA or Aa. The fact that they produce an albino child requires that each parent provides an a gene to the albino child; thus, the parents must both be heterozygous (Aa).

(b) To start out, the normal male could have either the AA or Aa genotype. The female must be aa. Since all the children are normal, one would consider the male to be AA instead of Aa. However, the male could be Aa. Under that circumstance, the likelihood of having six children, all normal, is 1/64.

(c) To start out, the normal male could have either the AA or Aa genotype. The female must be aa. The fact that half of the children are normal and half are albino indicates a typical "testcross" in which the Aa male is mated to the aa female.

(d)

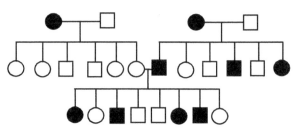

The 1:1 ratio of albino to normal in the last generation theoretically results because the mother is Aa and the father is aa.

4. *Unit Factors in Pairs*: It is important to see that each time a phenotype (normal or abnormal) is being stated, genotypes are symbolized as pairs of genes: *AA*, *Aa*, or *aa*. Review F3.2 to understand the need to assign appropriate symbols to genes.

Dominance and Recessiveness: Because the gene for normal pigmentation is completely dominant over the gene for albinism (*a* is fully recessive), it is necessary to consider, at first, whether normally pigmented individuals in the problem were homozygous normal (*AA*) or heterozygous (*Aa*). By looking at the frequency of expression of the recessive gene in the offspring (in *aa* individuals), one can often determine an *Aa* type from an *AA* type.

Segregation: During gamete formation when homologous chromosomes move to opposite poles, paired elements (genes) separate from each other.

5. Although it is very difficult, if not impossible, to know exactly how Mendel made the step from his "monohybrid results" to his postulates, he was able to develop a model with several important components or postulates. First, organisms contained **unit factors** for various traits. Second, if these **factors occurred in pairs**, there existed the possibility that some organisms would "breed true" if homozygous, whereas others would not (heterozygotes). If one "factor" of a pair had a **dominant influence** over the other, then he could explain how two organisms, looking the same, could be genetically different (homozygous or heterozygous). Third, if the **paired elements separate (segregate)** from each other during gamete formation and if gametes combine at random, he could account for the 3:1 ratios in the monohybrid crosses. The fourth postulate, independent assortment, cannot be demonstrated by a monohybrid cross because two gene pairs must be involved to do so.

Three excellent books give insight into Mendel's life and the context of his discoveries: Carlson, E. A. 1966. *The Gene: A Critical History*. Philadelphia: W. B. Saunders; Sturtevant, A. H. 1965. *A History of Genetics*. New York: Harper and Row; Voeller, B. R. 1968. *The Chromosome Theory of Inheritance*. New York: Appleton-Century-Crofts.

6. *Pisum sativum* is easy to cultivate. It is naturally self-fertilizing, but it can be crossbred. It has several visible features (e.g., tall or short, red flowers or white flowers) that are consistent under a variety of environmental conditions, yet contrast due to genetic circumstances. Seeds could be obtained from local merchants.

7. In the first sentence, you are told that there are two *characteristics* that are being studied: seed shape and cotyledon color. Expect, therefore, this to be a dihybrid situation with *two gene pairs* involved. One also sees the possible alternatives of these two characteristics: *seed shape*—wrinkled vs. round, *cotyledon color*—green vs. yellow. After reading the second sentence, you can predict that the gene for round seeds is dominant to that for wrinkled seeds and that the gene for yellow cotyledons is dominant to the gene for green cotyledons.

Symbolism:

w = wrinkled seeds g = green cotyledons

W = round seeds G = yellow cotyledons

P$_1$:

$WWGG \times wwgg$

Parents are considered to be homozygous for two reasons. First, in the introductory sentence, just after Problems and Discussion Questions, there is the statement "members of the P$_1$ generation are homozygous, unless . . .". Second, notice that the only offspring are those with round seeds and yellow cotyledons.

Gametes produced: One member of each gene pair is "segregated" to each gamete.

$WWGG$ $wwgg$
(WG)   (wg)

F$_1$: $WwGg$

F$_1$ × F$_1$: $WwGg \times WwGg$

Gametes produced: Under conditions of independent assortment, there will be four (2^n, where n = number of heterozygous gene pairs) different types of gametes produced by each parent.

Punnett Square:

	WG	Wg	wG	wg
WG	$WWGG$	$WWGg$	$WwGG$	$WwGg$
Wg	$WWGg$	$WWgg$	$WwGg$	$Wwgg$
wG	$WwGG$	$WwGg$	$wwGG$	$wwGg$
wg	$WwGg$	$Wwgg$	$wwGg$	$wwgg$

Collecting the phenotypes according to the dominance scheme presented in the previous Punnett square gives the following:

9/16 *W_G_* round seeds, yellow cotyledons

3/16 *W_gg* round seeds, green cotyledons

3/16 *wwG_* wrinkled seeds, yellow cotyledons

1/16 *wwgg* wrinkled seeds, green cotyledons

Notice that a dash (_) is used where, because of dominance, it makes no difference as to the dominant/recessive status of the allele.

Forked, or branch diagram:

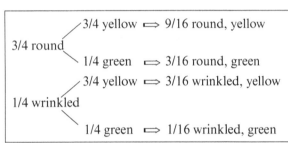

8. *WWgg* = 1/16

9. Because independent assortment may be defined as one gene pair segregating independently of another gene pair, one would need at least two gene pairs in order to demonstrate independent assortment.

10. Several points surface in the first sentence of this question. First, two alternatives (black and white) of one characteristic (coat color) are being described, therefore a monohybrid condition exists. Second, which is dominant, *black* or *white*? Note that all the offspring are black; therefore, black can be considered dominant. The second sentence of the problem verifies that a monohybrid cross is involved because of the 3/4 black and 1/4 white distribution in the offspring. Referring to appropriate figures from the text and knowing that genes occur in pairs in diploid organisms, one can write the genotypes and the phenotypes requested in part (a) as follows:

(a)

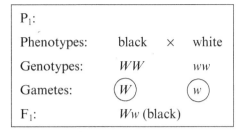

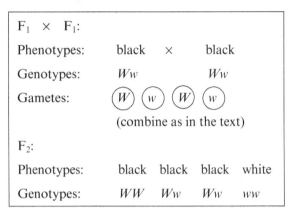

(b) Since *white* is a recessive gene (to *black*), each white guinea pig must be homozygous and a cross between two white guinea pigs must produce all white offspring.

white	×	white
ww		*ww*

(c) Recall the various possibilities of the genotypes capable of producing the black phenotype in the F$_2$ generation in part (a) above: *WW* and *Ww*. In cross 1 in the problem, all black offspring are observed and the most likely parental genotypes would be as follows:

WW	×	*WW*
	or	
WW	×	*Ww*

It is possible that black guinea pigs of the *Ww* genotype could produce all black offspring if the sample size was such that *ww* offspring were not produced. In cross 2, a typical 3:1 Mendelian ratio is observed, which indicates that two heterozygotes were crossed:

Ww	×	*Ww*

11. Briefly, the factors that specify chromosomal homology are the following:

> *overall length*
> *position of the centromere*
> *banding patterns*
> *type and location of genes**
> *autoradiographic pattern*

*functional basis for homologous chromosome designation

12. There are two characteristics presented here: body color and wing length. First, assign meaningful gene symbols.

Body color	*Wing length*
E = gray body color	V = long wings
e = ebony body color	v = vestigial wings

(a) P₁:

EEVV × *eevv*

F₁: *EeVv* (gray, long)

F₂: This will be the result of a Punnett square with 16 boxes as in the text.

Phenotypes	*Ratio*	*Genotypes*	*Ratio*
gray, long	9/16	*EEVV*	1/16
		EEVv	2/16
		EeVV	2/16
		EeVv	4/16
gray, vestigial	3/16	*EEvv*	1/16
		Eevv	2/16
ebony, long	3/16	*eeVV*	1/16
		eeVv	2/16
ebony, vestigial	1/16	*eevv*	1/16

(b) P₁:

EEvv × *eeVV*

F₁: It is important to see that the results from this cross will be exactly the same as those in part (a) above. The only difference is that the recessive genes are coming from both parents, rather than from one parent only as in (a). The F₂ ratio will be the same as (a) also. When you have genes on the autosomes (not X-linked), independent assortment, complete dominance, and no gene interaction (see later) in a cross involving double heterozygotes, the offspring ratio will be 9:3:3:1.

(c) P₁:

EEVV × *EEvv*

F1: *EEVv* (gray, long)

F₂: Notice that all the offspring will have grey bodies and you will get a 3:1 ratio of long to vestigial wings. You should see this before you even begin working through the problem. Even though this cross involves two gene pairs, it will give a "monohybrid" type of ratio because one of the gene pairs is homozygous (body color) and **one** gene pair is heterozygous (wing length).

Phenotypes	*Ratio*	*Genotypes*	*Ratio*
gray, long	3/4	*EEVV*	1/4
		EEVv	2/4
gray, vestigial	1/4	*EEvv*	1/4

NOTE: After working through this problem, it is important that you try to work similar problems without constructing the time-consuming Punnett squares, especially if each problem asks for phenotypic rather than genotypic ratios.

13. The general formula for determining the number of kinds of gametes produced by an organism is 2^n, where n = number of *heterozygous* gene pairs.

(a) 4: *AB, Ab, aB, ab*

(b) 2: *AB, aB*

(c) 8: *ABC, ABc, AbC, Abc, aBC, aBc, abC, abc*

(d) 2: *ABc, aBc*

(e) 4: *ABc, Abc, aBc, abc*

(f) $2^5 = 32$

~~ABCDE~~	*aBCDE*
~~ABCDe~~	~~aBCDe~~
~~ABCdE~~	~~aBCdE~~
~~ABCde~~	~~aBCde~~
~~ABcDE~~	~~aBcDE~~
~~ABcDe~~	~~aBcDe~~
~~ABcdE~~	*aBcdE*
~~ABcde~~	*aBcde*
~~AbCDE~~	*abCDE*
~~AbCDe~~	~~abCDe~~
~~AbCdE~~	~~abCdE~~
~~Abcde~~	~~abcde~~
~~AbcDE~~	~~abcDE~~
~~AbcDe~~	~~abcDe~~
~~AbcdE~~	~~abcdE~~
Abcde	*abcde*

Notice that there is a pattern that can be used to write these gametes so that fewer errors will occur.

14. In the first reading of this question, one should consider that there is one characteristic involved: seed color. Given that information and the F_2 progeny of 6022 yellow and 2001 green, a monohybrid condition is suspected. In addition, of the 519 self-fertilized, yellow-seeded plants, 166 bred true, whereas the others produced a 3:1 ratio of yellow to green. This is what would be expected because approximately 1/3 of the yellow F_2 plants should be homozygous, whereas 2/3 of the yellow F_2 plants should be heterozygous.

Set up the symbols as follows: G = yellow seeds, g = green seeds. We know that the gene for yellow seeds is dominant to that for green seeds because the F_1 is all yellow, not green.

Phenotypes	*Genotypes*
P_1: yellow × green	$GG \times gg$
F_1: all yellow	Gg
F_2: 6022 yellow	1/4 GG; 2/4 Gg
2001 green	1/4 gg

Of the yellow F_2 offspring, notice that 1/3 of them are GG and 2/3 are Gg. If you selfed the 1/3 GG types, then all the offspring (the 166) would breed true, whereas the others (353 that are Gg) should produce offspring in a 3:1 ratio when selfed.

GG ×	GG	= all GG
Gg ×	Gg	
		= 1/4 GG; 2/4 Gg; 1/4 gg

15. Because there is only one characteristic being dealt with in this problem (coat color) and a 3:1 ratio is mentioned in the second sentence, one can initially consider this to be a monohybrid condition. Set the gene symbols as W = black, w = white.

One hundred black animals could be all WW, all Ww, or a mixture (WW, Ww). When the WW individuals are crossed to ww, all the offspring will be black, which is what occurred in 94 of the cases. All these black offspring would be heterozygous and be expected to produce a 3:1 ratio when intercrossed. In those cases where a 1:1 ratio resulted, the parents must have been Ww.

The cross would be as follows:

P_1:	Ww × ww
F_1:	1/2 Ww, 1/2 ww

If one were to cross the black and white guinea pigs from the above cross, again the offspring would produce 1/2 black and 1/2 white as above.

16. In reading this question, notice that there are two characteristics being considered: seed color (yellow, green) and seed shape (round, wrinkled). At this point, you should be able to do this problem without writing down each of the steps. The F_1 can be considered to be a double heterozygote (with round and yellow being dominant). See the cross this way:

Symbols:

Seed shape	*Seed color*
W = round	G = yellow
w = wrinkled	g = green

P_1:	$WWgg$ × $wwGG$
F_1:	$WwGg$ cross to $wwgg$
	(which is a typical testcross)
The offspring will occur in a typical 1:1:1:1 as	
	1/4 $WwGg$ (round, yellow)
	1/4 $Wwgg$ (round, green)
	1/4 $wwGg$ (wrinkled, yellow)
	1/4 $wwgg$ (wrinkled, green)

Again, at this point, it would be very helpful if you could do such simple problems by inspection.

17. This question deals with the definition of dominance/recessiveness. Notice that there are only two alleles (one gene pair) and three phenotypes associated with the problem: normal, "minor" anemia, and "major" anemia. Under a monohybrid model, the heterozygote is distinguishable from either homozygote, and this fact does not fit the definition of dominance. One would conclude that no dominance is involved and incomplete dominance exists (see Chapter 4).

18. Since these are F_2 results from monohybrid crosses, a 3:1 ratio is expected for each. Referring to the text, one can set up the analysis easily.

(a)

Expected ratio	Observed (o)	Expected (e)
3/4	882	885.75
1/4	299	295.25

Expected values are derived by multiplying the expected ratio by the total number of organisms.

$$\chi^2 = \Sigma(o - e)^2/e = 0.064$$

By looking at the χ^2 table with 1 degree of freedom (because there were two classes and therefore $n - 1$ or 1 degree of freedom), we find a probability (p) value between 0.9 and 0.5.

We would therefore say that there is a "good fit" between the observed and expected values. Notice that as the deviations between the observed and expected values increase, the value of χ^2 increases. So the higher the χ^2 value, the more likely it is that the null hypothesis will be rejected.

(b)

Expected ratio	Observed (o)	Expected (e)
3/4	705	696.75
1/4	224	232.25

$$\chi^2 = 0.39$$

The p value in the table for 1 degree of freedom is still between 0.9 and 0.5; however, because the χ^2 value is larger in (b) we should say that the deviations from expectation are greater. The deviation in each case can be attributed to chance.

19. It would be best to set up two tables based on the two hypotheses:

Expected ratio	Observed (o)	Expected (e)
3/4	250	300
1/4	150	100

Expected ratio	Observed (o)	Expected (e)
1/2	250	200
1/2	150	200

For the test of a 3:1 ratio, the χ^2 value is 33.3 with an associated p value of less than 0.01 for 1 degree of freedom. For the test of a 1:1 ratio, the χ^2 value is 25.0, again with an associated p value of less

than 0.01 for 1 degree of freedom. Based on these probability values, both null hypotheses should be rejected.

20. Use of the $p = 0.10$ as the "critical" value for rejecting or failing to reject the null hypothesis instead of $p = 0.05$ would allow more null hypotheses to be rejected. Notice in the text that as the χ^2 values increase, there is a higher likelihood that the null hypothesis will be rejected because the higher values are more likely to be associated with a p value that is less than 0.05.

As the critical p value is increased, it takes a smaller χ^2 value to cause rejection of the null hypothesis. It would take less difference between the expected and observed values to reject the null hypothesis; therefore, the stringency of failing to reject the null hypothesis is increased.

21. Although there are many different inheritance patterns that will be described later in the text (codominance, incomplete dominance, sex-linked inheritance, etc.), the range of solutions to this question is limited to the concepts developed in the first three chapters, namely, dominance or recessiveness.

If a gene is dominant, it will not skip generations, nor will it be passed to offspring unless the parents have the gene. On the other hand, genes that are recessive can skip generations and exist in a carrier state in parents. For example, notice that II-4 and II-5 produce a female child (III-4) with the affected phenotype. Based on these criteria alone, the gene must be viewed as being recessive. Note: If a gene is recessive and X-linked (to be discussed later), the pattern will often be from affected male to carrier female to affected male.

To provide genotypes for each individual, consider that if the box or circle is shaded, the *aa* genotype is to be assigned. If offspring are affected (shaded), a recessive gene must have come from both parents.

I-1 (*Aa*), I-2 (*aa*), I-3 (*Aa*), I-4 (*Aa*)

II-1 (*aa*), II-2 (*Aa*), II-3 (*aa*), II-4 (*Aa*), II-5 (*Aa*), II-6 (*aa*), II-7 (*AA* or *Aa*), II-8 (*AA* or *Aa*)

III-1 (*AA* or *Aa*), III-2 (*AA* or *Aa*), III-3 (*AA* or *Aa*), III-4 (*aa*), III-5 (probably *AA*), III-6 (*aa*)

IV-1 through IV-7 all *Aa*.

22. (a) There are two possibilities. Either the trait is dominant, in which case I-1 is heterozygous, as are II-2 and II-3, or the trait is recessive and I-1 is homozygous and I-2 is heterozygous. Under the condition of recessiveness, both II-1 and II-4 would be heterozygous; II-2 and II-3 are homozygous.

(b) recessive: parents *Aa, Aa*

(c) recessive: parents *Aa, Aa*

(d) recessive or dominant, not sex-linked; if recessive, parents *Aa, aa*

23. (a) $p = [5!(1/2)^5(1/2)^0]/5!0! = 1/32$

(b) $p = [5!(1/2)^3(1/2)^2]/3!2! = 5/16$

(c) $p = [5!(1/2)^2(1/2)^3]/2!3! = 5/16$

(d) There are two ways of all being the same sex: all males or all females. Therefore, the final probability is the sum of the two independent probabilities:

$$1/32 + 1/32 = 1/16$$

24. $p = [8!(3/4)^6(1/4)^2]/6!2!$

25. In families where the condition is not found in parents or grandparents, a recessive gene is likely to be involved. Families in which the condition occurs in every generation suggest that a dominant gene might be involved.

26. Most likely, the attending physician misdiagnosed the syndrome of the first child by telling the parents that the birth defects were not genetic. Given the birth of the second child with Smith–Lemli–Opitz syndrome, it is highly likely that both parents were carriers for a recessive mutant gene causing Smith–Lemli–Opitz syndrome. Under that circumstance, there is a 25 percent chance that each of their children would be affected. The probability that two children of heterozygous parents would be affected would be 0.25 × 0.25 = 0.0625, or a little over 6 percent.

27. (a) First consider that each parent is homozygous (true-breeding in the question), and since in the F$_1$ only round, axial, violet, and full phenotypes were expressed, they must each be dominant.

(b) Because all genes are on nonhomologous chromosomes, independent assortment will occur. Round, axial, violet, and full would be the most frequent phenotypes:

3/4   ×   3/4   ×   3/4   ×   3/4

(c) Wrinkled, terminal, white, and constricted would be the least frequent phenotypes:

1/4   ×   1/4   ×   1/4   ×   1/4

(d)   3/4   ×   1/4   ×   3/4   ×   3/4

plus   1/4   ×   3/4   ×   1/4   ×   3/4

= 18/256

(e) There would be 16 different phenotypes in the testcross offspring, just as there are 16 different phenotypes in the F$_2$ generation.

28. (a) The first task is to draw out an accurate pedigree (one of several possibilities):

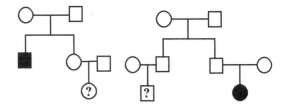

(b) The probability that the female (whose maternal uncle had TSD) is heterozygous is 1/3 because she is not TSD and her mother had a 2/3 chance of being heterozygous, and she has a 1/2 chance of passing the TSD gene to her daughter (2/3 × 1/2 = 1/3). The male (whose paternal first cousin had TSD) has a 1/4 chance of being heterozygous, assuming that either (but not both, because the gene is said to be rare) his grandmother or grandfather was heterozygous. Therefore, the probability that both the male and female are heterozygous is 1/3 × 1/4 = 1/12

(c) The probability that neither is heterozygous is 2/3   ×   3/4 = 6/12

(d) The probability that one is heterozygous is (1/3 × 3/4) + (2/3 × 1/4) = 5/12

Also, there are only three possibilities: both are heterozygous, neither is heterozygous, and at least one is heterozygous. You have already calculated the first two probabilities; the last is simply 1 − (1/12 + 6/12) = 5/12.

29. (a) Ignoring flower color for the present, notice in the first cross that a 3:1 ratio exists for the spiny to smooth phenotypes in the first cross. Thus, we would predict that the *spiny* allele is dominant to *smooth*. Applying the same reasoning to the second cross, notice that there is a 3:1 ratio of purple to white. We would also predict that the *purple* allele is dominant to *white*.

(b) One could cross a homozygous purple, spiny plant to a homozygous white, smooth plant. The purple, spiny F_1 would support the hypothesis that *purple* is dominant to *white* and *spiny* is dominant to *smooth*. In the F_2, a 9:3:3:1 ratio would not only support the above hypothesis, but also indicate the independent inheritance and expression of the two traits.

30. (a) Notice in cross 1 that the ratio of straight wings to curled wings is 3:1 and the ratio of short bristles to long bristles is also 3:1. This would indicate that straight is dominant to curled and short is dominant to long.

Possible symbols would be (using standard *Drosophila* symbolism):

straight wings $= w^+$ curled wings $= w$
short bristles $= b^+$ long bristles $= b$

(b)

Cross 1: w^+/w ; b^+/b × w^+/w ; b^+/b
Cross 2: w^+/w ; b/b × w^+/w ; b/b
Cross 3: w/w ; b/b × w^+/w ; b^+/b
Cross 4: w^+/w^+ ; b^+/b × w^+/w^+ ; b^+/b (one parent could be w^+/w)
Cross 5: w/w ; b^+/b × w^+/w ; b^+/b

31. $p = [5!(3/4)^3(1/4)^2]/3!2!$

$= 135/512$

32. (a) First, consider that the data represent a 3:1 ratio based on the information given in the problem: $Ss \times Ss$. Compute the expected quantities for each class by multiplying the totals by 3/4 and 1/4.

Set I Expected Numbers:

Tall $= 26.25$ Short $= 8.75$

Set II Expected Numbers:

Tall $= 262.5$ Short $= 87.5$

For set I the χ^2 value would be

$(30–26.25)^2/26.25 + (5–8.75)^2/8.75$
$= 2.15$ with p being between 0.2 and 0.05

so one would accept the null hypothesis of no significant difference between the expected and observed values.

For set II, the χ^2 value would be

21.43 and $p < 0.001$.

One would reject the null hypothesis and assume a significant difference between the observed and expected values.

(b) Clearly, with an increase in sample size, a different conclusion is reached. In fact, most statisticians recommend that the expected values in each class should not be less than 10. In most cases, more confidence is gained as the sample size increases; however, depending on the organism or experiment, there are practical limits on sample size.

33. (a, b) At this point, is it not possible to determine the dominant/recessive nature of the albinism in Migaloo. However, since no other albino whales have been observed, one might lean toward a recessive gene. It would be helpful to know the phenotypes of the parents of Migaloo.

34. (a) For initially rare recessive genes to become established, rare crosses between heterozygotes would have to occur at a relatively high frequency. **(b)** The likelihood of the establishment of albinism in whales with a rare dominant gene is probably higher than if the gene were recessive.

35. (a) 27/64, **(b)** 1/4, **(c)** $1/4 \times 1/2$ or 1/8

36. Given that *dentinogenesis imperfecta* is inherited as a dominant allele and the man's mother had normal teeth, the man with six children must be heterozygous. Therefore, the probability that their first child will be a male with *dentinogenesis imperfecta* would be 1/2 (passage of the allele) × 1/2 (probability of child being male) = 1/4. The probability that three of their six children will have the disease is best determined by application of the following formula.

$$p = \frac{n!}{s! \, t!} a^s b^t$$

n = total number of events (six in this case)

s = number of times outcome a happens (three in this case)

t = number of times outcome b happens (three in this case)

a = probability of being normal in this family (1/2)

b = probability of having the disease in this family (1/2)

$$p = \frac{6!}{3!3!}\ 1/2^3\ 1/2^3$$

The overall probability (p) would be 5/16, or about 0.31 (31 percent). All these types of questions are handled in the same manner. Determine the total number of events (n), then how many times one outcome will occur (s). Determine how many times the alternative outcome will occur (t). Once you know the probability (a) of the "s" outcome and the probability (b) of outcome "t," you have all the components for the equation.

Chapter 4: Extensions of Mendelian Genetics

Concept Areas	Corresponding Problems
Incomplete Dominance, Codominance	1, 3, 4, 6, 12, 13, 14, 30, 42
Multiple Alleles	1, 2, 6, 7, 8, 9, 11, 22
Lethal Alleles	1, 4, 5, 10, 38
Gene Interaction	1, 15, 19, 21, 42
Epistasis	1, 16, 17, 18, 20, 36, 37, 39, 41
X-Linkage	1, 23, 24, 25, 26, 27, 28, 29, 30, 33, 44
Sex-Limited/Sex-Influenced Inheritance	1, 31, 32, 40
Phenotypic Expression	34, 35, 43

Concepts and Processes Checklist

(Check topic when mastered – provide examples where appropriate – understand the context of each entry)

- **Alleles Alter Phenotypes in Different Ways**
  - neo-Mendelian genetics
  - wild-type allele
  - mutant allele
  - loss-of-function mutation
  - null allele
  - gain-of-function mutation
  - oncogene
  - cancerous cell
  - receptor
  - neutral mutation

- **Variety of Symbols for Alleles**
  - *D, d*
  - superscript +, e^+
  - no dominance, R^1, L^N
  - abbreviation *cdk*
  - bacteria, *leu*$^-$

- **Incomplete, or Partial, Dominance**
  - snapdragon, white, pink, red
  - 1:2:1 F_2 generation
  - R^1, R^2
  - Tay-Sachs disease
  - hexosaminidase A
  - threshold effect

- **Codominance**
  - influence of both alleles
  - MN blood group
  - 1:2:1

- **Multiple Alleles**
  - studied only in populations
  - ABO blood groups
  - antigen, antibody
  - Karl Landsteiner
  - I^A, I^B, i
  - isoagglutinogen

- ○ H substance
- ○ galactose
- ○ *N*-acetylglucosamine (AcGluNH)
- ○ **The Bombay Phenotype**
  - ○ *FUT1*, fucosyl transferase
- ○ **The *white* Locus in *Drosophila***
  - ○ Thomas H. Morgan, Calvin Bridges
  - ○ 1912
  - ○ *white* mutation
  - ○ biochemical pigments
  - ○ ommatidia
- ○ **Lethal Alleles Represent Essential Genes**
  - ○ modified ratios, 1/3, 2/3
  - ○ yellow, agouti
  - ○ Huntington disease
  - ○ late age of onset
  - ○ dominant lethal alleles rare
- ○ **Molecular Basis of Dominance and Recessiveness**
  - ○ *agouti* gene
  - ○ gain-of-function
  - ○ A^Y
  - ○ deletion
  - ○ *Merc*
- ○ **Modifications of the 9:3:3:1 Ratio**
  - ○ 3:6:3:1:2:1
  - ○ gene interaction
  - ○ epigenesis
  - ○ hereditary deafness
  - ○ heterogeneous trait

- ○ **Epistasis**
  - ○ one gene pair masks
  - ○ complement
  - ○ *FUT1* gene
  - ○ example, coat color in mice
  - ○ recessive epistasis
  - ○ dominant epistasis
  - ○ complementary gene interaction
- ○ **Novel Phenotypes**
  - ○ fruit shape, *Cucurbita pepo*
  - ○ eye color in *Drosophila*
  - ○ drosopterins
  - ○ xanthommatins
- ○ **Other Modified Dihybrid Ratios**
  - ○ 13:3
  - ○ 10:3:3
  - ○ 15:1
  - ○ 6:3:3:4
- ○ **Complementation Analysis**
  - ○ heterogeneous trait
  - ○ similar phenotypes
  - ○ same gene or different gene?
  - ○ complementation group
- ○ **Single Gene May Have Multiple Effects**
  - ○ pleiotropy
  - ○ Marfan syndrome
  - ○ Abraham Lincoln
  - ○ porphyria variegata
- ○ **X-Linkage and the X Chromosome**
  - ○ X, Y chromosomes
  - ○ X-linkage

- white eyes in *Drosophila*
- hemizygosity
- crisscross pattern of inheritance
- chromosome theory of inheritance

- **X-Linkage in Humans**
  - color blindness
  - Duchenne muscular dystrophy

- **Sex-Limited**
  - tail and neck plumage in fowl
  - cock feathering
  - hen feathering
  - milk production in dairy cattle

- **Sex-Influenced Inheritance**
  - pattern baldness in humans
  - horn formation in sheep
  - coat patterns in cattle

- **Penetrance**
  - percentage expression

- **Expressivity**
  - range of expression

- **Genetic Background**
  - position effect
  - heterochromatin
  - variegated or mottled

- **Temperature Effects**
  - conditional mutations
  - fur in rabbits
  - temperature-sensitive mutations
  - permissive condition
  - restrictive condition

- **Nutritional Effects**
  - nutritional mutations
  - auxotroph
  - *Neurospora*
  - Beadle and Tatum, 1940s
  - phenylketonuria
  - galactosemia
  - lactose intolerance

- **Onset of Genetic Expression**
  - Tay-Sachs disease
  - Lesch-Nyhan syndrome
  - HPRT
  - Duchene muscular dystrophy
  - Huntington disease

- **Genetic Anticipation**
  - progressively earlier age
  - increased severity
  - successive generations
  - Myotonic dystrophy
  - DM1, DM2

- **Genomic (Parental) Imprinting**
  - imprinting
  - insulin-like growth factor II (*Igf2*)
  - Prader-Willi syndrome
  - Angelman syndrome
  - male and female gametes
  - chromosome 15
  - epigenetics
  - DNA methylation
  - position 5 in cytosine
  - DNA methyltransferase
  - CpG islands
  - gene silencing

Chapter 4 Extensions of Mendelian Genetics

T4.1 Examples of typical monohybrid and dihybrid ratios with several modifications.

Basic Ratio	Modified Ratio	Explanation

3:1 ⟹ { 1:2:1 }
- Incomplete dominance
- Codominance

9:3:3:1 ⟹ { 9:3:4, 12:3:1, 9:7 }
- Epistasis (recessive)
- Epistasis (dominant)
- Epistasis (double recessive)

3:6:3:1:2:1 } ⟶ Dominance + incomplete dominance or codominance

1:4:6:4:1 } ⟶ Additive effects

F4.1 Illustration of gene interaction where products from more than one gene pair influence one characteristic or phenotypic trait.

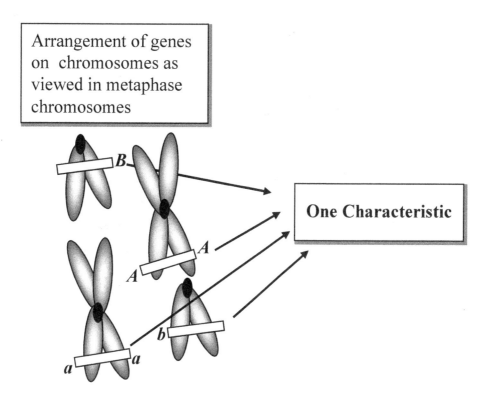

Arrangement of genes on chromosomes as viewed in metaphase chromosomes

One Characteristic

Example of gene interaction: Two gene pairs influencing the pigmentation pattern on the shark. Various gene products contribute in a variety of ways to generate a particular pigment pattern.

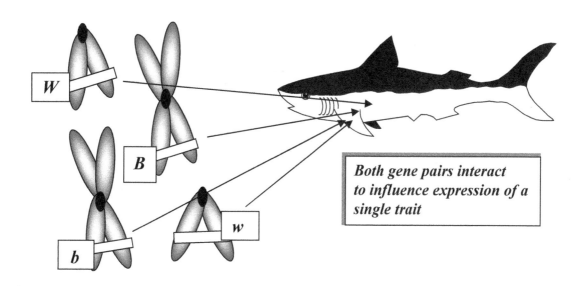

Both gene pairs interact to influence expression of a single trait

F4.2 Symbolism associated with the wild-type activity of a gene and several possible outcomes of the mutant state: **A.** wild type, **B.** too much product, **C.** too little product, **D.** no product, **E.** both products expressed, **F.** reduced product.

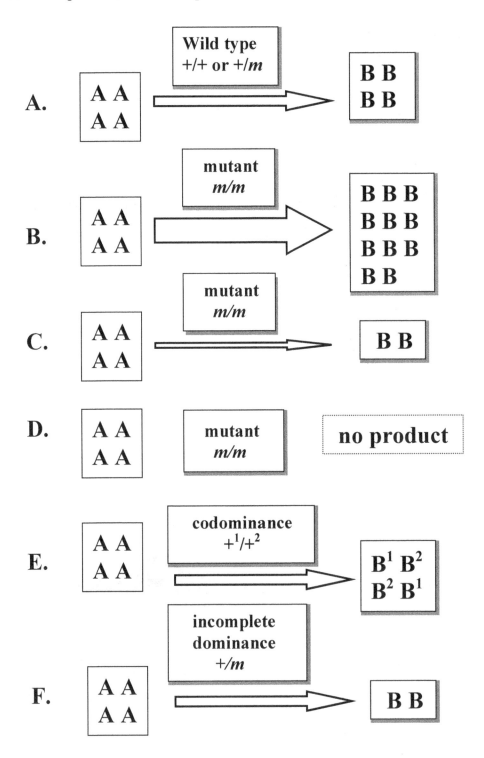

Chapter 4 Extensions of Mendelian Genetics

Answers to Now Solve This

4-1. It is important to see that this problem involves multiple alleles, meaning that monohybrid-type ratios are expected and that there is an order of dominance that will allow certain alleles to be "hidden" in various heterozygotes. As with most genetics problems, one must look at the phenotypes of the offspring to assess the genotypes of the parents.

(a) Parents: sepia × cream

Because both guinea pigs had albino parents, both are heterozygous for the c^a allele.

> Cross: $c^k c^a$ × $c^d c^a$ ⇨
>
> 2/4 sepia; 1/4 cream; 1/4 albino

(b) Parents: sepia × cream

Because the sepia parent had an albino parent, it must be $c^k c^a$. Because the cream guinea pig had two sepia parents

   ($c^k c^d$ × $c^k c^d$ or $c^k c^d$ × $c^k c^a$), the cream parent could be $c^d c^d$ or $c^d c^a$.

> Crosses: $c^k c^a$ × $c^d c^d$ ⇨
>
>   1/2 sepia; 1/2 cream*
> *(if parents are assumed to be homozygous)
>   or $c^k c^a$ × $c^d c^a$ ⇨
>
>   1/2 sepia; 1/4 cream; 1/4 albino

(c) Parents: sepia × cream

Because the sepia guinea pig had two full-color parents, which could be

   Cc^k, Cc^d,   or Cc^a

(not CC because sepia could not be produced), its genotype could be

   $c^k c^k$, $c^k c^d$,   or $c^k c^a$

Because the cream guinea pig had two sepia parents

($c^k c^d$ × $c^k c^d$ or $c^k c^d$ × $c^k c^a$), the cream parent could be $c^d c^d$ or $c^d c^a$.

> Crosses:
> $c^k c^k$ × $c^d c^d$ ⟹ all sepia
> $c^K c^k$ × $c^d c^a$ ⟹ all sepia
> $c^k c^d$ × $c^d c^d$ ⟹ 1/2 sepia; 1/2 cream
> $c^k c^d$ × $c^d c^a$ ⟹ 1/2 sepia; 1/2 cream
> $c^k c^a$ × $c^d c^d$ ⟹ 1/2 sepia; 1/2 cream
> $c^k c^a$ × $c^d c^a$ ⟹ 1/2 sepia; 1/4 cream; 1/4 albino

(d) Parents: sepia × cream

Because the sepia parent had a full-color parent and an albino parent

(Cc^k × c^ac^a), it must be c^kc^a. The cream parent had two full-color parents, which could be Cc^d or Cc^a; therefore, it could be c^dc^d or c^dc^a.

> Crosses:
>
> c^kc^a × c^dc^d ⟹ 1/2 sepia; 1/2 cream
>
> c^kc^a × c^dc^a ⟹ 1/2 sepia; 1/4 cream; 1/4 albino

4-2. Notice that the distribution of observed offspring fits a 9:3:4 ratio quite well. This suggests that two independently assorting gene pairs with epistasis are involved. Assign gene symbols in the usual manner:

A = pigment; a = pigmentless (colorless) B = purple; b = red

> $AaBb$ × $AaBb$
> ⟱
> $A\_B\_$ = purple
> A_bb = red
> $aaB\_$ = colorless
> $aabb$ = colorless

One may see this occurring in the following manner:

precursor ---+-> cyanidin ---+-> purple pigment

(colorless) aa   (red) bb

4-3. For all three pedigrees, let a represent the mutant gene and A represent its normal allele.

(a) This pedigree is consistent with an X-linked recessive trait because the male would contribute an X chromosome carrying the a mutation to the aa daughter. The mother would have to be heterozygous Aa.

(b) This pedigree is consistent with an X-linked recessive trait because the mother could be Aa and transmit her a allele to her one son (a/Y) and her A allele to her other son.

(c) This pedigree is not consistent with an X-linked recessive mode of inheritance because the aa mother has an A/Y son.

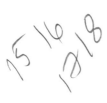

Chapter 4 Extensions of Mendelian Genetics
Solutions to Problems and Discussion Questions

1. (a) In general, they observed results of crosses that did not produce offspring in typical Mendelian ratios.

(b) Modifications of dihybrid and higher-level ratios indicated that loci were not expressed independently. A 9:3:4 ratio illustrates such a dihybrid modification. The number of gene pairs involved is often determined by the sum of the components of each ratio. For example, a 1:2:1 or 3:1 ratio adds to 4, indicating a monohybrid cross. A 9:3:4 or 15:1 ratio adds to 16, indicating a dihybrid ratio.

(c) Morgan and his colleagues observed that the sex of the parent carrying a mutant allele influenced the results of crosses when compared to a reciprocal cross. When correlated with the sex chromosome differences between males and females, a model placing a gene on the X chromosome was supported.

(d) When a gene is X-linked, ratios from crosses are influenced by which parent contributes a particular allele. When sex-limited or sex-influenced inheritance occurs, the parental source of the allele is irrelevant because the involved genes are autosomal.

2. Your essay should include a description of alleles that do not function independently of each other or reduce the viability of a class(es) of offspring. With multiple alleles, there are more than two alternatives of a gene at a given locus.

3. In the first sentence of this problem, notice that there is one characteristic (coat color) and three phenotypes mentioned: red, white, and roan. The fact that roan is intermediate between red and white suggests that this may be a case of incomplete dominance, with roan being the intermediate and, therefore, the heterozygous type. If that is the case, then we should suspect a 1:2:1 phenotypic ratio in crosses of "roan to roan."

Looking at the data given, notice that a cross of the "extremes" (red × white) gives roan, suggesting its heterozygous nature and the homozygous nature of the parents. Seeing the 1:2:1 ratio in the offspring of

$$\text{roan} \times \text{roan}$$

confirms the hypothesis of incomplete dominance as the mode of inheritance.

Symbolism:

AA = red

aa = white

Aa = roan

Crosses: It is important at this point that you not be fully dependent on writing out complete Punnett squares for each cross. Begin working these simple problems in your head.

AA	×	AA ⟹	AA
aa	×	aa ⟹	aa
AA	×	aa ⟹	Aa
Aa	×	Aa ⟶	

1/4 AA; 2/4 Aa; 1/4 aa

4. Notice that there is one typical (coat color) and one atypical (lethality) characteristic mentioned. Often under this condition of two characteristics, we must decide if the problem involves one or more than one gene pair. Because the genotypes are given here, it is obvious that lethality is associated with expression of the coat color alleles and, therefore, one gene pair is involved. This is a monohybrid condition.

Pp	×	Pp ⟶

1/4 PP (**lethal**)

2/4 Pp (platinum)

1/4 pp (silver)

Therefore, the ratio of surviving foxes is 2/3 platinum, 1/3 silver. The P allele behaves as a recessive in terms of lethality (seen only in the homozygote) but as a dominant in terms of coat color (seen in the homozygote).

5. In this problem, it would be helpful to first diagram the phenotypes of the crosses so that you can get some idea of the inheritance pattern. From those phenotypic crosses, a suggestion as to the genotypes can be made and verified.

Cross 1:

short tail × normal long tail ⟶

approximately 1/2 short, 1/2 long

This tells you that one type is heterozygous, and the other homozygous.

Cross 2:

short tail × short tail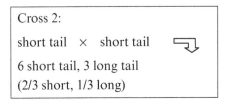

6 short tail, 3 long tail
(2/3 short, 1/3 long)

At this point, one would consider that the 2/3 *short* are heterozygotes and *long* is the homozygous class. Also, short is dominant to long. Since these ratios were repeated and verified, one can conclude that a 2:1 ratio is not a statistical artifact and that the following genotypic model would hold. Long being "normal" does not mean that it is dominant.

Symbolism: S = short, s = long

Cross 1:

Ss × ss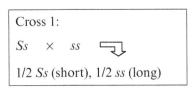

1/2 Ss (short), 1/2 ss (long)

Cross 2:

Ss × Ss

1/4 SS (lethal),
2/4 Ss (short),
1/4 ss (long)

6. In the section on multiple alleles in the text, there is a table that indicates all the genotypes requested.

Blood Group (phenotype)	Genotype(s)
A	$I^A I^A$, $I^A i$
B	$I^B I^B$, $I^B i$
AB	$I^A I^B$
O	ii

I^A and I^B are codominant (notice the AB blood group) while being dominant to i.

7. In this problem, remember that individuals with blood type B can have the genotype $I^B I^B$ or $I^B i$ and those with blood type A can have the genotype $I^A I^A$ or $I^A i$. Male Parent: must be $I^B i$ because the mother is ii and one inherits one homolog (therefore one allele) from each parent.

Female Parent: must be $I^A i$ because the father is $I^B i$ and one inherits one homolog (therefore one allele) from each parent. The father cannot be $I^B I^B$ and have a daughter of blood type A.

Offspring:

$$I^A I^o \times I^B I^o$$

	I^B	i
I^A	$I^A I^B$ (AB)	$I^A i$ (A)
i	$I^B i$ (B)	ii (O)

The ratio would be

$$1(A):1(B):1(AB):1(O).$$

8. Given that a child is blood type O (genotype ii) and the mother blood type A (she must be $I^A i$ to have had a type O child), the father could have the following genotypes: $I^B i$, $I^A i$, or ii. In other words, the father must have been able to contribute i to the child. The only *blood type* that would exclude a male from being the father would be AB, because no i allele is present. Because many individuals in a population could have genotypes with the i allele, one could not prove that a particular male was the father by this method.

9. Symbolism:

Se = secretor se = nonsecretor

$$I^A I^B \, Sese \times ii \, Sese$$

(a)

	$i \, Se$	$i \, se$
$I^A \, Se$	A, secretor	A, secretor
$I^A \, se$	A, secretor	A, nonsecretor
$I^B \, Se$	B, secretor	B, secretor
$I^B \, se$	B, secretor	B, nonsecretor

Overall ratio: 3/8 A, secretor

1/8 A, nonsecretor

3/8 B, secretor

1/8 B, nonsecretor

(b) 1/4 of all individuals will have blood type O.

10. Given that creepers never breed true and half of the offspring of a creeper crossed with a non-creeper are creepers, one would expect the creeper gene to be dominant and homozygous lethal. When creepers are interbred, two-thirds of the offspring are creepers (heterozygotes), whereas one-third are normal (homozygous recessive). The simplest explanation is that the homozygous creepers combination is lethal.

11. It is important to see that this problem involves multiple alleles, meaning that monohybrid-type ratios are expected, and that there is an order of dominance that will allow certain alleles to be "hidden" in various heterozygotes. As with most genetics problems, one must look at the phenotypes of the offspring to assess the genotypes of the parents.

(b)

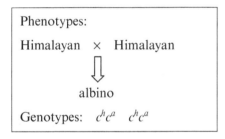

The Himalayan parents must both be heterozygous to produce an albino offspring.

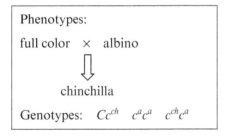

Because of the cc albino parent, the genotype of the chinchilla F_1 must be $c^{ch}c^a$. Also, in order to have a chinchilla offspring at all, the full-color parent must be heterozygous for chinchilla.

Therefore, the cross of albino with chinchilla would be as follows:

$$c^ac^a \times c^{ch}c^a$$
1/2 chinchilla; 1/2 albino

(b)

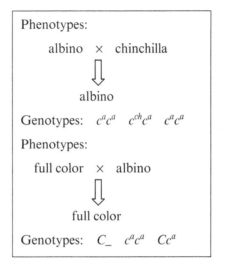

It is impossible to determine the complete genotype of the full-color parent, but the full-color offspring must be as indicated, Cc^a.

Therefore, the cross of the albino with full color would be as follows:

$$c^ac^a \times Cc^a$$
1/2 full color; 1/2 albino

(c)

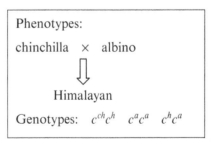

The chinchilla parent must be heterozygous for Himalayan because of the Himalayan offspring.

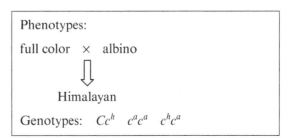

Therefore, a cross between the two Himalayan types would produce the following offpsring:

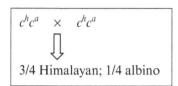

3/4 Himalayan; 1/4 albino

12. Three independently assorting characteristics are being dealt with: flower color (incomplete dominance), flower shape (dominant/recessive), and plant height (dominant/recessive).

Establish appropriate gene symbols:

Flower color:
    RR = red; Rr = pink; rr = white

Flower shape:
    P = personate; p = peloric

Plant height:
    D = tall; d = dwarf

$RRPPDD$ × $rrppdd$ ⤵
$RrPpDd$ (pink, personate, tall)

Use *components* of the forked-line method as follows:

2/4 pink × 3/4 personate × 3/4 tall
= 18/64

13. There are two characteristics: flower color and flower shape. Because pink results from a cross of red and white, one would conclude that flower color is "monohybrid" with incomplete dominance. In addition, because personate is seen in the F_1 when personate and peloric are crossed, personate must be dominant to peloric. Results from crosses (c) and (d) verify these conclusions. The appropriate symbols would be as follows:

Flower color:

    RR = red; Rr = pink; rr = white

Flower shape:

    P = personate; p = peloric

(a)
    $RRpp$ × $rrPP$ ⟹ $RrPp$
(b)
    $RRPP$ × $rrpp$ ⟹ $RrPp$
(c)
    $RrPp$ × $RRpp$ ⟹
        $RRPp$
        $RRpp$
        $RrPp$
        $Rrpp$
(d)
    $RrPp$ × $rrpp$ ⟹
        $rrPp$
        $rrpp$
        $RrPp$
        $Rrpp$

(e) In the cross of the F_1 of (a) to the F_1 of (b), both of which are double heterozygotes, one would expect the following:

$RrPp$ × $RrPp$

1/4 red
    3/4 personate → 3/16 red, personate
    1/4 peloric → 1/16 red, peloric

2/4 pink
    3/4 personate → 6/16 pink, personate
    1/4 peloric → 2/16 pink, peloric

1/4 white
    3/4 personate → 3/16 white, personate
    1/4 peloric → 1/16 white, peloric

14. (a) This is a case of incomplete dominance in which, as shown in the third cross, the heterozygote (palomino) produces a typical 1:2:1 ratio. Therefore, one can set the following symbols:

$C^{ch}C^{ch}$ = chestnut

$C^{c}C^{c}$ = cremello

$C^{ch}C^{c}$ = palomino

(b) The F_1 resulting from matings between cremello and chestnut horses would be expected to be all palomino. The F_2 would be expected to fall in a 1:2:1 ratio as in the third cross in part (a) above.

15. This is a case of gene interaction (novel phenotypes) in which the recessive, independently assorting genes *brown* and *scarlet* (both recessive) interact to give the white phenotype. Refer to the text and see that the symbolism uses a "+" superscript to indicate the wild type. For simplicity in this problem, assume that all parental crosses involve homozygotes.

(a) $bw^+/bw^+; st^+/st^+ \times bw/bw; st/st$
$$\Downarrow$$
$bw^+/bw; st^+/st$ (wild)

The F_2 would produce the expected 9:3:3:1 ratio except that gene interaction will give the white phenotype in the 1/16 class.

$bw^+/\_ ; st^+/\_$	= wild type
$bw^+/\_; st/st$	= scarlet
$bw/bw ; st^+/\_$	= brown
$bw /bw ; st /st$	= white

(b)

$bw^+/bw^+; st^+/st^+ \times bw^+/bw^+; st/st$
$\Downarrow$
$bw^+/bw^+; st^+/st$ (wild)

The F_2, resulting from a cross of
$$bw^+/bw^+; st^+/st \times bw^+/bw^+; st^+/st$$
would produce a 3:1 ratio of wild to scarlet.

(c)

$bw/bw; st^+/st^+ \times bw/bw; st/st$
$\Downarrow$
$bw/bw; st^+/st$ (brown)

The F_2, resulting from a cross of
$$bw/bw; st^+/st \times bw/bw; st^+/st$$
would produce a 3:1 ratio of brown to white. Notice that in the F_2 crosses in parts (b) and (c), one of the parents in each is homozygous; therefore, the crosses will give monohybrid types of ratios.

16. This is a case in which epistasis (from *cc*) results in a "masking" of genes at the *A* locus. In this case,

there will be modifications of typical 9:3:3:1 and 1:1:1:1 ratios because of gene interactions.

(a) In a cross of
$$AACC \times aacc$$
the offspring are all *AaCc* (agouti) because the *C* allele allows pigment to be deposited in the hair and when it is, it will be agouti.

F_2 offspring would have the following "simplified" genotypes with the corresponding phenotypes:

$A\_C\_$	= 9/16 (agouti)
A_cc	= 3/16 (colorless because *cc* is epistatic to *A*)
$aaC\_$	= 3/16 (black)
$aacc$	= 1/16 (colorless because *cc* is epistatic to *aa*)

The two colorless classes are phenotyically indistinguishable; therefore, the final ratio is 9:3:4.

(b) Results of crosses of female agouti
$$(A\_C\_) \times aacc \text{ (males)}$$
are given in three groups:

(1) To produce an even number of agouti and colorless offspring, the female parent must have been *AACc* so that half of the offspring are able to deposit pigment because of *C*, and when they do, they are all agouti (having received only *A* from the female parent).

(2) To produce an even number of agouti and black offspring, the mother must have been *Aa*, and so that no colorless offspring were produced, the female must have been *CC*. Her genotype must have been *AaCC*.

(3) Notice that half of the offspring are colorless; therefore, the female must have been *Cc*. Half of the pigmented offspring are black and half are agouti; therefore, the female must have been *Aa*. Overall, the *AaCc* genotype seems appropriate.

17. This is a case of gene interaction (novel phenotypes) where the yellow and black types (double mutants) interact to give the cream phenotype and epistasis where the *cc* genotype produces albino.

(a) *AaBbCc* ⟹ gray (*C* allows pigment)

(b) *A_B_Cc* ⟹ gray (*C* allows pigment)

(c) Use the forked-line method for this portion.

Combining the phenotypes gives (always count the proportions to see that they add up to 1.0):

16/32	albino
9/32	gray
3/32	yellow
3/32	black
1/32	cream

(d) Use the forked-line method for this portion.

Combining the phenotypes gives (always count the proportions to see that they add up to 1.0):

9/16	(gray)
3/16	(black)
4/16	(albino)

(e) Use the forked-line method for this portion.

The final ratio would be

3/8	(gray)
1/8	(yellow)
4/8	(albino)

18. Treat each of the crosses as a series of monohybrid crosses, remembering that albino is epistatic to color, and black and yellow interact to give cream.

(a) Since this is a 9:3:3:1 ratio with no albino phenotypes, the parents must each have been double heterozygotes and incapable of producing the *cc* genotype.

Genotypes:
AaBbCC × *AaBbCC*
or
AaBbCC × *AaBbCc*
Phenotypes:
gray × gray

(b) Since there are no black offspring, there are no combinations in the parents that can produce *aa*. The 4/16 proportion indicates that the *C* locus is heterozygous in both parents.

If the parents are

AABbCc × *AaBbCc*
or
AABbCc × *AABbCc*

then the results would follow the pattern given.

Phenotypes: gray × gray

(c) Notice that 16/64 or 1/4 of the offspring are albino; therefore, the parents are both heterozygous at the *C* locus. Second, notice that without considering the *C* locus, there is a 27:9:9:3 ratio that reduces to a 9:3:3:1 ratio.

Given this information, the genotypes must be

AaBbCc × *AaBbCc*
Phenotypes: gray × gray

(d) Notice that 2/8 or 1/4 of the offspring are albino, which indicates that both parents are *Cc*. Also notice that the ratio of black to cream is 1:1, suggesting that the parents are *Bb* and *bb*. Because there are no gray or yellow offspring, there can be no *A* alleles.

Genotypes:

$aaBbCc \times aabbCc$

Phenotypes: black $\times$ cream

(e) Notice that half of the offspring are albino, indicating that for the *C* locus, the genotypes are *Cc* and *cc*. There is a 3:1 ratio of black to cream, indicating heterozygosity for the *B* locus in each parent. Because there are no gray or yellow offspring, there can be no *A* alleles.

Genotypes:

$aaBbCc \times aaBbcc$

Phenotypes: black $\times$ albino

19. After reading the problem, glance at the kinds of F_1 and F_2 ratios. Notice that the first two, (A) and (B), appear as monohybrid ratios, and (C) is clearly dihybrid. You need to see this combination of crosses as being solved with one set of gene symbols. The fact that cross (C) yields a 9:3:3:1 ratio gives you a start.

(a) Going back to the basics, set up the relationship that you know holds for a 9:3:3:1 ratio as follows:

$A\_B\_ = 9/16$
$A\_bb = 3/16$
$aaB\_ = 3/16$
$aabb\_ = 1/16$

Then assign the phenotypes from cross (C) as indicated:

$A\_B\_ = 9/16$ (green)
$A\_bb = 3/16$ (brown)
$aaB\_ = 3/16$ (gray)
$aabb = 1/16$ (blue)

Now it should become clear that blue results from interaction of the *aa* and *bb* genotypes and brown and gray result from homozygosity of either of the two genes as shown above. From this model, see if crosses (A), (B), and (C) and the resulting progeny make sense.

Cross A:

P_1: $AABB \times aaBB$

F_1: $AaBB$

F_2:   3/4 A_BB: 1/4 $aaBB$

Cross B:

P_1: $AABB \times AAbb$

F_1: $AABb$

F_2:   3/4 $AAB\_$: 1/4 $AAbb$

Cross C:

P_1: $aaBB \times AAbb$

F_1: $AaBb$

F_2:   9/16 $A\_B\_$: 3/16 A_bb:

3/16 $aaB\_$: 1/16 $aabb$

(b) This question is exactly as that in cross (C). The genotype of the unknown P_1 individual would be *AAbb* (brown), whereas the F_1 would be *AaBb* (green).

20. First, see in this problem that a 9:7 ratio is involved, which implies a dihybrid condition with epistasis. Going back to a basic 9:3:3:1 ratio, one can see that if the 3:3:1 groups were lumped together, the 9:7 ratio would result. Assign tall to any plant with both *A* and *B*, and any dwarf plant that is homozygous for either or both the recessive alleles. The initial cross must have been

$AABB \times aabb$

There are two gene pairs involved.

(a)
$A\_B\_ = 9/16$ (tall)
$A\_bb = 3/16$ (dwarf)
$aaB\_ = 3/16$ (dwarf)
$aabb = 1/16$ (dwarf)

(b) There are three different classes of dwarf plants. Within each of the 3/16 classes, there are two types:

$A\_bb = 3/16$ (dwarf)
$= 1/3 \, AAbb$ and $2/3 \, Aabb$
and
$aaB\_ = 3/16$ (dwarf)
$= 1/3 \, aaBB$ and $2/3 \, aaBb$

Therefore, the true breeding dwarf plants would be the following:

$AAbb, aaBB,$ and *aabb*

and they would constitute 3/7 of the dwarf group.

Chapter 4 Extensions of Mendelian Genetics

21. Problems of this type often pose difficulties for students. It is important for students to go back to basic patterns of inheritance when getting started. First, see that a 9:3:3:1 ratio is involved as indicated below:

$$A\_B\_ = 9/16$$
$$A\_bb = 3/16$$
$$aaB\_ = 3/16$$
$$aabb = 1/16$$

(a) Assign the phenotypes as given; then see if patterns emerge.

$$A\_B\_ = 9/16 \text{ (yellow)}$$
$$A\_bb = 3/16 \text{ (blue)}$$
$$aaB\_ = 3/16 \text{ (red)}$$
$$aabb = 1/16 \text{ (mauve)}$$

From this information, the genotypes for the various phenotypes and the solution to the problem become clear. As stated in the problem, all colors *may* be true breeding. See that each type can exist as a full homozygote. If plants with blue flowers (homozygotes) are crossed to red-flowered homozygotes, the F_1 plants would have yellow flowers. Also, as stated in the problem, if yellow-flowered plants are crossed with mauve-flowered plants, the F_1 plants are yellow and the F_2 will occur in a 9:3:3:1 ratio. All of the observations fit the model as proposed.

(b) If one crosses a true-breeding red plant ($aaBB$) with a mauve plant ($aabb$), the F_1 should be red ($aaBb$). The F_2 would be as follows:

$$aaBb \times aaBb$$
3/4 $aaB\_$ (red); 1/4 $aabb$ (mauve)

22. First, make certain that you understand the genetics of all the gene pairs being described in the problem. The ABO system involves multiple alleles, codominance, and dominance. The MN system is codominant. The easiest way to approach these types of problems is to consider those gene pairs that produce a low number of options in the offspring. Notice in cross 1 that there are two options in the offspring for the ABO system (types A and O), but only one option for the MN system (type MN). By looking at the most restrictive classes, one can see that option (c) is the only one

that is both MN and O. The remainder of the combinations can be determined using the same logic.

Cross 1 = (c)
Cross 2 = (d)
Cross 3 = (b)
Cross 4 = (e)
Cross 5 = (a)

Given that each parental/offspring grouping can be used only once, there are no other combinations.

23. In order to solve this problem, one must first see the possible genotypes of the parents and the grandfathers. Since the gene is X-linked, the cross will be symbolized with the X chromosomes.

RG = normal vision; rg = color-blind
Mother's father: X^{rg}/Y
Father's father: X^{rg}/Y
Mother: $X^{RG}X^{rg}$
Father: X^{RG}/Y

Notice that the mother must be heterozygous for the rg allele (being normal-visioned and having inherited an X^{rg} from her father) and the father, because he has normal vision, must be X^{RG}. The fact that the father's father is color-blind does not mean that the father will be color-blind. On the contrary, the father will inherit his X chromosome from his mother.

$X^{RG}X^{rg} \times X^{RG}/Y$
$X^{RG}X^{RG}$ = 1/4 daughter normal
$X^{RG}X^{rg}$ = 1/4 daughter normal
X^{RG}/Y = 1/4 son normal
X^{rg}/Y = 1/4 son color-blind

Looking at the distribution of offspring:

(a) 1/4
(b) 1/2
(c) 1/4
(d) zero

24. The mating is $X^{RG}X^{rg}$; $I^A i$ × $X^{RG}Y$; $I^A i$

Based on the son who is color-blind and blood type O, the mother must have been heterozygous for the RG locus, and both parents must have had one copy of the *i* gene. The probability of having a female child is 1/2, that she has normal vision is 1 (because the father's X is normal), and that she has type O blood is 1/4. The final product of the independent probabilities is

$$1/2 \ \times \ 1 \ \times \ 1/4 \ = \ 1/8$$

25. Symbolism: Normal wing margins = sd^+; scalloped = sd

(a)

P_1:	$X^{sd}X^{sd}$ × X^+/Y
F_1:	1/2 X^+X^{sd} (female, normal)
	1/2 X^{sd}/Y (male, scalloped)
F_2:	1/4 X^+X^{sd} (female, normal)
	1/4 $X^{sd}X^{sd}$ (female, scalloped)
	1/4 X^+/Y (male, normal)
	1/4 X^{sd}/Y (male, scalloped)

(b)

P_1:	X^+/X^+ × X^{sd}/Y
F_1:	1/2 X^+X^{sd} (female, normal)
	1/2 X^+/Y (male, normal)
F_2:	1/4 X^+X^+ (female, normal)
	1/4 X^+X^{sd} (female, normal)
	1/4 X^+/Y (male, normal)
	1/4 X^{sd}/Y (male, scalloped)

If the *scalloped* gene were not X-linked, then all of the F_1 offspring would be wild (phenotypically) and a 3:1 ratio of normal to scalloped would occur in the F_2.

26. Assuming that the parents are homozygous, the crosses would be as follows. Notice that the *X* symbol may remain to remind us that the *sd* gene is on the X chromosome. It is extremely important that one account for both the mutant genes and each of their wild-type alleles.

P_1:	$X^{sd}X^{sd}$; e^+/e^+ × X^+/Y; e/e
F_1:	1/2 X^+X^{sd}; e^+/e (female, normal)
	1/2 X^{sd}/Y; e^+/e (male, scalloped)

F_2:

	X^+e^+	X^+e	$X^{sd}e^+$	$X^{sd}e$
$X^{sd}e^+$				
$X^{sd}e$		Fill in box on your own.		
Ye^+				
Ye				

Phenotypes:

3/16 normal females

3/16 normal males

1/16 ebony females

1/16 ebony males

3/16 scalloped females

3/16 scalloped males

1/16 scalloped, ebony females

1/16 scalloped, ebony males

Forked-line method:

P_1:	$X^{sd}X^{sd}$; e^+/e^+ × X^+/Y; e/e

F_1:	1/2 X^+X^{sd}; e^+/e (female, normal)
	1/2 X^{sd}/Y; e^+/e (*male*, scalloped)

F_2:

	Wings	Color	
1/4	females, normal	3/4 normal	3/16
		1/4 ebony	1/16
1/4	females, scalloped	3/4 normal	3/16
		1/4 ebony	1/16
1/4	males, normal	3/4 normal	3/16
		1/4 ebony	1/16
1/4	males, scalloped	3/4 normal	3/16
		1/4 ebony	1/16

27. Set up the symbolism and the cross in the following manner:

P_1:	X^+X^+; su-v/su-v × X^v/Y; su-v^+/su-v^+
F_1:	1/2 X^+X^v; su-v^+/su-v (female, normal)
	1/2 X^+/Y; su-v^+/su-v (male, normal)

F$_2$: 2/4 females, —— 3/4 *su-v*$^+$/_
    X$^+$/_   —— 1/4 *su-v/su-v*

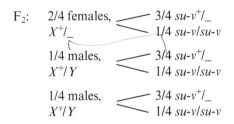

    1/4 males, —— 3/4 *su-v*$^+$/_
    X$^+$/Y   —— 1/4 *su-v/su-v*

    1/4 males, —— 3/4 *su-v*$^+$/_
    X^v/Y   —— 1/4 *su-v/su-v*

8/16 are wild-type females (none of the females are homozygous for the *vermilion* gene).

5/16 are wild-type males (4/16 because they have no *vermilion* gene and 1/16 because the X-linked, hemizygous *vermilion* gene is suppressed by *su-v/su-v*).

3/16 are vermilion males (no suppression of the *vermilion* gene).

28. It is extremely important that one account for both the mutant genes and each of their wild-type alleles.

(a)

P$_1$:   X^{v}X^v; +/+ × X$^+$/Y; *b^r/b^r*

F$_1$:   1/2 X$^+$X^v; +/*b^r* (female, normal)

        1/2 X^v/Y; +/*b^r* (male, vermilion)

F$_2$:

Eye color (X)	Eye color	(autosomal)
1/4 females, normal	3/4 normal	3/16
	1/4 brown	1/16
1/4 females, vermilion	3/4 normal	3/16
	1/4 brown	1/16
1/4 males, normal	3/4 normal	3/16
	1/4 brown	1/16
1/4 males, vermilion	3/4 normal	3/16
	1/4 brown	1/16

3/16 = females, normal

1/16 = females, brown eyes

3/16 = females, vermilion eyes

1/16 = females, white eyes

3/16 = males, normal

1/16 = males, brown eyes

3/16 = males, vermilion eyes

1/16 = males, white eyes

(b)

P$_1$: X$^+$X$^+$; *b^r/b^r* × X^v/Y; +/+

F$_1$:

1/2 X$^+$X^v; +/*b^r* (female, normal)

1/2 X$^+$/Y; +/*b^r* (male, normal)

F$_2$:

Eye color (X)	Eye color (autosomal)
2/4 females, normal	3/4 normal
	1/4 brown
1/4 males, normal	3/4 normal
	1/4 brown
1/4 males, vermilion	3/4 normal
	1/4 brown

6/16 = females, normal

2/16 = females, brown eyes

3/16 = males, normal

1/16 = males, brown eyes

3/16 = males, vermilion eyes

1/16 = males, white eyes

(c)

P$_1$: X^{v}X^v; *b^r/b^r* × X +/Y; +/+

F$_1$: 1/2 X$^+$X^v; +/*b^r* (female, normal)

     1/2 X^v/Y; +/*b^r* (male, vermilion)

F$_2$:

Eye color (X)	Eye color (autosomal)
1/4 females, normal	3/4 normal
	1/4 brown
1/4 females, vermilion	3/4 normal
	1/4 brown
1/4 males, normal	3/4 normal
	1/4 brown
1/4 males, vermilion	3/4 normal
	1/4 brown

3/16 = females, normal

1/16 = females, brown eyes

3/16 = females, vermilion eyes

1/16 = females, white eyes

3/16 = males, normal

1/16 = males, brown eyes

3/16 = males, vermilion eyes

1/16 = males, white eyes

29. (a)

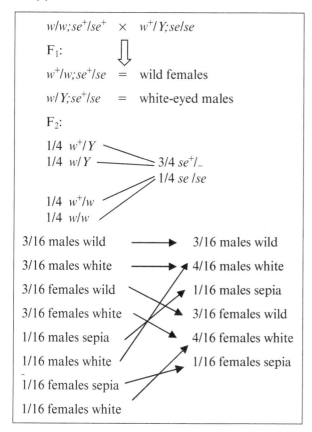

(b)

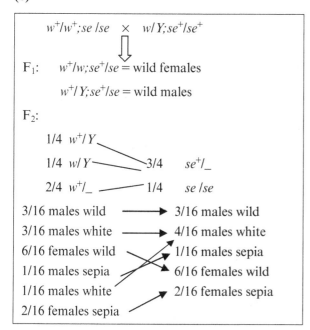

30. (a, b) In looking at the pedigrees, one can see that the condition cannot be dominant because it appears in the offspring (II-3 and II-4) and not the parents in the first two cases. The condition is, therefore, *recessive*. In the second cross, note that the father is not shaded, yet the daughter (II-4) is. If the condition is recessive, then it must also be *autosomal*.

(c)   II-1 = *AA* or *Aa*

II-6 = *AA* or *Aa*

II-9 = *Aa*

31. Seeing the different distribution between males and females, one might consider sex-influenced inheritance as a model and have males more likely to express bearded and females more likely to express beardless in the heterozygote. This situation is similar to pattern baldness in humans. Consider two alleles that are autosomal and let

BB = beardless in both sexes

Bb = beardless in females

Bb = bearded in males

bb = bearded in both sexes

P$_1$: female: *bb* (bearded) × male: *BB* (beardless)

F$_1$: *Bb* = females beardless; males bearded

Because half of the offspring are males and half are females, one could, for clarity, rewrite the F$_2$ as

	1/2 *females*	1/2 *males*
1/4 *BB*	1/8 beardless	1/8 beardless
2/4 *Bb*	2/8 beardless	2/8 bearded
1/4 *bb*	1/8 bearded	1/8 bearded

One could test this model by crossing F$_1$ (heterozygous) beardless females with bearded (homozygous) males.Comparing these results with the reciprocal cross would support the model if the distributions of sexes with phenotypes were the same in both crosses.

32. In looking at the information provided in the text, notice that the only genotype that gives cock-feathering in males is *hh*, whereas three genotypes give hen-feathering in females:

HH, *Hh*, and *hh*

Remember that these genes are sex-limited and autosomal.

P$_1$:   female: *HH*   ×   male: *hh*

F$_1$:   all hen-feathering

F$_2$:

	1/2 females	1/2 males
1/4 *HH*	hen-feathering	hen-feathering
2/4 *Hh*	hen-feathering	hen-feathering
1/4 *hh*	hen-feathering	cock-feathering

All of the offspring would be hen-feathered except for 1/8 of the males, which are cock-feathered.

33. Passage of X-linked genes typically occurs from carrier mother to affected son. The fact that the father in couple 2 has hemophilia would not predispose his son to hemophilia. The first couple has no valid claim.

34. Phenotypic expression is dependent on the genome of the organism, the immediate molecular and cellular environment of the genome, and numerous interactions among a genome, the organism, and the environment.

35. *Penetrance* refers to the percentage of individuals that expresses the mutant phenotype, whereas *expressivity* refers to the range of expression of a given phenotype.

36. First, look for familiar ratios that will inform you as to the general mode of inheritance. Notice that the last cross (h) gives a 9:4:3 ratio, which is typical of epistasis. From this information, one can develop a model to account for the results given.

Symbolism:

$$A\_B\_ = black$$
$$A\_bb = golden$$
$$aabb = golden$$
$$aaB\_ = brown$$

The combination of *bb* is epistatic to the *A* locus.

(a) *AAB_* × *aaBB* (other configurations are possible, but each must give all offspring with *A* and *B* dominant alleles)

(b) *AaB_* × *aaBB* (other configurations are possible, but no *bb* genotypes can be produced)

(c) *AABb* × *aaBb*

(d) *AABB* × *aabb*

(e) *AaBb* × *Aabb*

(f) *AaBb* × *aabb*

(g) *aaBb* × *aaBb*

(h) *AaBb* × *AaBb*

Those genotypes that will breed true will be as follows:

black   = *AABB*

golden   = all genotypes that are *bb*

brown   = *aaBB*

37. A first glance would seem to favor a 9:7 ratio; however, the phenotypes would have to be reversed for such a result to fit. Therefore, one must consider an alternative explanation. A 27:9:9:9:3:3:3:1 ratio fits very well with *A_B_C_* being purple and any homozygous recessive combination giving white. Thus, a 27 (purple):37 (white) ratio fits well. To test this hypothesis, one might take the purple F$_1$s and cross them to the pure breeding (*aabbcc*) white type. Such a cross should give a 1 (purple):7 (white) ratio.

38. The clue to the solution comes from the description of the Dexters as not true breeding and of low fertility. This indicates that Dexters are heterozygous and the Kerry breed is homozygous recessive. The homozygous dominant type is lethal. Polled is caused by an independently assorting dominant allele, whereas horned is caused by the recessive allele to polled.

39. (a) Because the denominator in the ratios is 64, one would begin to consider that there are three independently assorting gene pairs operating in this problem. Because there are only two characteristics (eye color and croaking), however, one might hypothesize that two gene pairs are involved in the inheritance of one trait, whereas one gene pair is involved in the other.

(b) Notice that there is a 48:16 (or 3:1) ratio of rib-it to knee-deep and a 36:16:12 (or 9:4:3) ratio of blue to green to purple eye color. Because of these relationships, one would conclude that croaking is due to one (dominant/recessive) gene pair, whereas eye color is due to two gene pairs. Because there is a 9:4:3 ratio regarding eye color, some gene interaction (epistasis) is indicated.

(c, d) Symbolism:

Croaking: $R\_$ = rib-it; rr = knee-deep

Eye color: Since the most frequent phenotype is blue eye, let $A\_B\_$ represent the genotypes. For the purple class, "a 3/16 group" uses the A_bb genotypes. The "4/16" class (green) would be the $aaB\_$ and the $aabb$ groups.

(e) The cross involving a blue-eyed, knee-deep frog and a purple-eyed, rib-it frog would have the genotypes

$$AABBrr \quad \times \quad AAbbRR$$

which would produce an F_1 of $AABbRr$ that would be blue-eyed and rib-it. The F_2 will follow a pattern of a 9:3:3:1 ratio because of homozygosity for the A locus and heterozygosity for both the B and R loci.

9/16 $AAB\_R\_$ = blue-eyed, rib-it

3/16 AAB_rr = blue-eyed, knee-deep

3/16 $AAbbR\_$ = purple-eyed, rib-it

1/16 $AAbbrr$ = purple-eyed, knee-deep

(f) The different results can arise because of the genetic variety possible in producing the green-eyed frogs. Since there is no dependence on the B locus, the following genotypes can define the green phenotype:

aaBB, aaBb, aabb

(g) In doing these types of problems, take each characteristic individually and then build the complete genotypes. Notice that the ratio of purple-eyed to green-eyed frogs is 3:1; therefore, expect the parents to be heterozygous for the A locus. Because the ratio of rib-it to knee-deep is also 3:1, expect both parents to be heterozygous at the R locus. The B locus would have the bb genotype because both parents are purple-eyed as given in the problem. Both parents would therefore be $AabbRr$.

40. In looking at the pedigree, one can see that the typical carrier mother-to-son X-linked pattern is not present. One cannot default to a Y-linked pattern because of sons (II-1, IV-1) not having precocious puberty. We might then consider a sex-limited form of inheritance whereby the gene(s) is(are) autosomal, but expression is limited to one sex, male in this case. Because of the relatively high frequency of occurrence of precocious puberty in the pedigree, one might consider a dominant gene to be involved. Indeed, there is no skipping of generations typical of recessive traits. Notice, however, that there is an apparent skipping of generations in giving rise to the IV-5 son. The reason is that females are not capable of expressing the gene. Given the degree of outcrossing, that the gene is probably quite rare and, therefore, heterozygotes are uncommon, and that the frequency of transmission is high, it is likely that this form of male precocious puberty is caused by an autosomal dominant, sex-limited gene.

41. (a) The reduced ratio is 12 white, 3 orange, and 1 brown, and in a dihybrid cross ($AaBb \times AaBb$) the following would occur:

12 white	$A\_B\_$ or $aaB\_$
3 orange	A_bb
1 brown	$aabb$

(b, c) The following model would also hold for a trihybrid set of crosses:

white = $A\_B\_C\_$ or $aaB\_C\_$

orange = A_bbcc

brown = $aabbcc$

42. Given the following genotypes of the parents:

$Aabb$ = crimson

$AABB$ = white

the F_1 consists of $AaBb$ genotypes with a rose phenotype.

In the F_2, the following genotypes correspond to the given phenotypes:

$AAB\_$ = white	4/16
$AaBB$ = magenta	2/16
$AaBb$ = rose	4/16

Aabb = orange	2/16
aaBB = yellow	1/16
aaBb = pale yellow	2/16
aabb = crimson	1/16

Notice that different phenotypes result from heterozygous versus homozygous dominant states. *AaBB* gives magenta, whereas *AaBb* gives rose. However, in the presence of *AA*, the same phenotype is found regardless of *Bb* or *BB* genotypes. Gene interaction is occurring along with the absence of complete dominance.

43. Since proto-oncogenes stimulate a cell to progress through a cell cycle, loss of function of such genes should inhibit such cellular progress. In this case, the gene would likely function as a recessive.

However, if overproduction of a proto-oncogene should occur, then the cell would be stimulated to undergo more rapid cycles (perhaps), which would lead to an expressed phenotype such as a tumor or cancer. Under this condition (gain of function), the gene would behave as a dominant.

If the regulatory region of a proto-oncogene is mutated such that loss of control occurs and the proto-oncogene is overexpressed, then it would "gain function" and be dominant. If the proto-oncogene product is defective, there would be a loss of function and it would more than likely behave as a recessive.

44. Beatrice, Alice of Hesse, and Alice of Athlone are carriers. There is a 1/2 chance that Princess Irene is a carrier.

Chapter 5: Chromosome Mapping in Eukaryotes

Concept Areas	Corresponding Problems
Linkage vs. Independent Assortment	1, 17, 22, 29, 33
Chromosome Mapping	1, 2, 4, 8, 9, 10, 11, 12, 18, 19, 22, 23, 26, 27, 30, 31, 32
Multiple Crossovers and Three-Point Mapping	6, 13, 14, 15, 16
Determining Gene Sequence	9, 14, 15, 16
Interference and Coefficient of Coincidence	7, 15
Crossing Over in the Four-Strand Stage	1, 3, 5
Mechanism of Crossing Over	3, 4, 21
Mitotic Recombination	20
Somatic Cell Hybridization and Human Maps	1, 24, 25, 28, 33, 34

Concepts and Processes Checklist

(Check topic when mastered – provide examples where appropriate – understand the context of each entry)

- **Linkage**
  - Sutton, Boveri
  - 1903
  - genes linked
  - absence of independent assortment
  - crossing over
  - recombination
  - interlocus distance
  - chromosome map

- **Genes Linked on the Same Chromosome**
  - linkage, no linkage
  - complete linkage
  - parental gametes
  - noncrossover gametes
  - recombinant gametes

  - crossover gametes
  - 50 percent
  - 1:1:1:1 ratio

- **The Linkage Ratio**
  - genes in close proximity
  - horizontal line designation
  - linkage group
  - 1:2:1 ratio

- **Crossing Over Serves . . . Mapping Genes**
  - Morgan, Sturtevant
  - 1911
  - recombinant offspring
  - X-linked genes
  - white eyes, yellow body
  - Janssens

- chiasmata (sing. chiasma)
- linear sequence
- crossing over
- physical exchange
- recombination
- **Sturtevant and Mapping**
  - strength of linkage
  - spatial separation of genes
  - linear dimension
  - frequencies additive
  - chromosome
  - Calvin Bridges
  - autosomal linkage
  - 1910, chromosomal theory
  - centiMorgan (cM)
- **Single Crossovers**
  - nonsister chromatids
  - tetrad
  - theoretical limit 50 percent
- **Analysis of Multiple Crossovers**
  - multiple exchanges
  - double crossovers (DCOs)
  - relationship to distance
  - product law
- **Three-Point Mapping**
  - heterozygosity at all loci
  - distinguishable genotypes
  - adequate sample size
  - representative sample size
  - hemizygosity
  - reciprocal classes
  - double crossovers

- least frequent numbers (DCOs)
- map unit (mu)
- **Determining the Gene Sequence**
  - Method I
  - arrangement of alleles
  - Method II
- **Mapping Problem in Maize**
  - reciprocal phenotypic classes
  - four reciprocal classes
  - no crossover class (NCO)
  - single crossover class (SCO)
- **As the Distance…Estimate …Inaccurate**
- **Interference and the Coefficient of Coincidence**
  - Interference (I)
  - coefficient of coincidence (C)
  - positive interference
  - negative interference
  - physical constraints
- ***Drosophila* Genes…Extensively Mapped**
  - linkage groups
  - cytological map
- **Lod Score Analysis**
- **Somatic Cell Hybridization**
  - segregate together
  - Rh antigens
  - elliptocytosis
  - lod score method
  - Haldane and Smith, 1947
  - Barsky

- heterokaryon
- synkaryon
- synteny testing
- **Chromosome Mapping…DNA Markers**
  - restriction fragment length polymorphism
  - RFLP
  - microsatellite
  - DNA markers
  - single nucleotide polymorphism
  - SNP
  - cystic fibrosis
  - sequence maps
  - Human Genome Project
  - bioinformatics
  - physical map
- **Crossing Over Involves Physical Exchange…**
  - Creighton, McClintock
  - 1930s
  - physical exchange
  - translocated chromosome
- **Exchanges Also Occur between Sister Chromatids**
  - sister chromatid exchange (SCEs)
  - thymidine analog
  - bromodeoxyuridine (BrdU)
  - harlequin chromosomes
  - Bloom syndrome
  - *BLM*, chromosome 15
  - German and colleagues
  - DNA helicase
- **Did Mendel Encounter Linkage?**

F5.1 Illustration of critical arrangements of linked genes. Notice that there are two possible arrangements for an *AaBb* double heterozygote. In order to do linkage problems correctly, such arrangements must be understood.

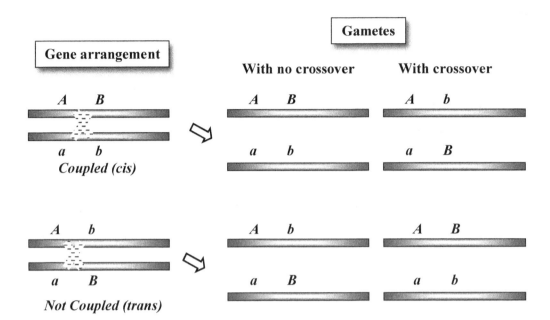

Answers to Now Solve This

5-1. The initial cross for this problem would be *AaBb* × *aabb*.

(a) If the two loci are on different chromosomes, independent assortment would occur and the following distribution (1:1:1:1) is expected:

1/4	*AaBb*
1/4	*Aabb*
1/4	*aaBb*
1/4	*aabb*

(b) Even though the two loci are linked and on the same chromosome, the frequency of crossing over is so high that crossovers always occur. Under that condition, independent assortment would occur and the following distribution (1:1:1:1) is expected:

1/4	*AaBb*
1/4	*Aabb*
1/4	*aaBb*
1/4	*aabb*

(c) If crossovers never occur, then all of the gametes from the heterozygous parent are *parental*. If the arrangement is *AB/ab* × *ab/ab*

then the two types of offspring will be

1/2	*AB/ab*
1/2	*ab/ab*

Under this condition, *AB* are *coupled*. If, however, *A* and *B* are not coupled, then the symbolism would be *Ab/aB* × *ab/ab*.

The offspring would occur as follows:

1/2	*Ab/ab*
1/2	*aB/ab*

5-2. Since there is no indication as to the configuration of the *P* and *Z* genes (*coupled or not coupled*) in the parent, one must look at the percentages in the offspring. Notice that the most frequent classes are *PZ* and *pz*. These classes represent the parental (noncrossover) groups, which indicate that the original parental arrangement in the testcross was *PZ/pz* × *pz/pz*. Adding the crossover percentages together (6.9 + 7.1) gives 14 percent, which would be the map distance between the two genes.

5-3. In typical trihybrid crosses, one expects eight kinds of offspring. In this example, only six are listed, and one can assume that since the double crossover class is the least frequent, it is the double crossovers that are not listed. To work this type of problem, examine the list to see which types are not present in the offspring. In this case, the double crossover classes are the following:

++ *c*   and   *a b* +

(a, b) Notice that if you compare the parental classes (most frequent) with the double crossover classes (zero in this case), you can, by using the logic of the methods described in the text, determine that the gene b is in the middle and the arrangement is as follows. Note: For consistency, the zeros (double crossovers) are included in the calculations.

$$+ b \, c \, / \, a + +$$

$$a - b = \frac{32 + 38 + 0 + 0}{1000} \times 100 = 7 \text{ map units}$$

$$b - c = \frac{11 + 9 + 0 + 0}{1000} \times 100 = 2 \text{ map units}$$

(c) The progeny phenotypes that are missing are $+ + c$ and $a \, b +$, which, of 1000 offspring, 1.4 ($0.07 \times 0.02 \times 1000$) would be expected. Perhaps by chance or some other unknown selective factor, they were not observed.

$$0.0014 \ \%$$

$$\frac{0.0014}{100} = \frac{x}{1000}$$

$$.14$$

Solutions to Problems and Discussion Questions

1. (a) Morgan and his students, especially Alfred Sturtevant, correlated chiasma frequency with the distance between linked genes. The farther apart two genes, the higher the chiasma and, therefore, crossover frequency. The most important hint was that recombination frequency between genes *a* and *c* could be equal to the recombination frequency between *a* and *b* plus the recombination frequency between *b* and *c*.

(b) The discovery of linkage, genes segregating together during gamete formation, indicated a physical association among genes.

(c) Two experimental lines, one using maize (Creighton and McClintock) and the other using *Drosophila*, showed that each time a crossover occurred, an actual physical exchange of chromosomes also occurred. Each experiment demonstrated a switch in chromosomal markers when genetic markers exchanged.

(d) Even when sister chromatid exchanges do not produce new allelic combinations, they can be demonstrated using molecular markers such as bromodeoxyuridine.

(e) Linkage analysis in humans was historically accomplished by lod score analysis, somatic cell hybridization (synteny testing), and pedigree analysis. Modern methods combine these historical approaches with database analyses often employing a variety of physical markers (microsatellites, minisatellites, RFLPs, and SNPs).

2. Your essay should include methods of detection through crosses with appropriate, distinguishable markers and that in most cases, the frequency of crossing over is directly related to the distance between genes.

3. First, in order for chromosomes to engage in crossing over, they must be in proximity. It is likely that the side-by-side pairing that occurs during synapsis is the earliest time during the cell cycle that chromosomes achieve that necessary proximity. Second, chiasmata are visible during prophase I of meiosis, and it is likely that these structures are intimately associated with the genetic event of crossing over.

4. With some qualification, especially around the centromeres and telomeres, one can say that crossing over is somewhat randomly distributed over the length of the chromosome. Two loci that are far apart are more likely to have a crossover between them than two loci that are close together.

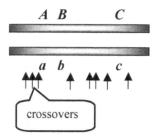

5. Crossing over occurs at the four-strand stage of the cell cycle (that is, after S phase) such that each single crossover involves only two of the four chromatids.

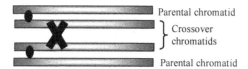

6. As mentioned in an earlier answer (#4), with some qualifications, crossovers occur randomly along the lengths of chromosomes. Within any region, the occurrence of two events is less likely than the occurrence of one event. If the probability of one event is

$$1/X$$

then the probability of two events occurring at the same time will be

$$1/X^2$$

7. Positive interference occurs when a crossover in one region of a chromosome interferes with crossovers in nearby regions. Such interference ranges from zero (no interference) to 1.0 (complete interference). Interference is often explained by a physical rigidity of chromatids such that they are unlikely to make sufficiently sharp bends to allow crossovers to be close together.

8. Each cross must be set up in such a way as to reveal crossovers because it is on the basis of crossover frequency that genetic maps are developed. It is necessary that genetic heterogeneity exist so that

Chapter 5 Chromosome Mapping in Eukaryotes

different arrangements of genes, generated by crossing over, can be distinguished.

The organism that is heterozygous must be the sex in which crossing over occurs. In other words, it would be useless to map genes in *Drosophila* if the male parent is the heterozygote since crossing over is not typical in *Drosophila* males.

Lastly, the cross must be set up so that the phenotypes of the offspring readily reveal their genotypes. The best arrangement is one in which a fully heterozygous organism is crossed with an organism that is fully recessive for the genes being mapped.

9. Since the distance between *dp* and *ap* is greatest when compared to the distances, they must be on the "outside" and *cl* must be in the middle. The genetic map would be as follows:

dp--- cl-----------------------ap

3 *mu*   39 *mu*

10. In looking at this problem, one can immediately conclude that the two loci (kernel color and plant color) are linked because the testcross progeny occur in a ratio other than 1:1:1:1 (and epistasis does not appear because all phenotypes expected are present). The question is whether the arrangement in the parents is *coupled*

$$RY/ry \quad \times \quad ry/ry$$

or *not coupled*

$$Ry/rY \quad \times \quad ry/ry$$

Notice that the most frequent phenotypes in the offspring, the parentals, are colored, green (88) and colorless, yellow (92). This indicates that the heterozygous parent in the testcross is coupled

$$RY/ry \quad \times \quad ry/ry$$

with the two dominant genes on one chromosome and the two recessives on the homolog (F5.1). Seeing that there are 20 crossover progeny among the 200, or 20/200, the map distance would be 10 map units (20/200 × 100 to convert to percentages) between the *R* and *Y* loci.

11. Start this problem by working through the expected offspring under two models: one with no crossing over and the second with 30 percent crossing over in the female.

No *crossing* over:

Female gametes: Male gametes:

1/2 e ca⁺   1/2 e ca⁺

1/2 e⁺ ca   1/2 e⁺ ca

Offspring:

1/4   "e" phenotype

2/4   wild

1/4   "ca" phenotype

With 30% crossing over:

Female gametes: Male gametes:

35% e ca⁺   1/2 e ca⁺

35% e⁺ ca   1/2 e⁺ ca

15% e⁺ ca⁺

15% e ca

Offspring: (obtained by combining gametes and phenotypes)

"e" phenotype = 17.5% + 7.5% = **25%**

wild phenotype =
17.5% + 7.5% + 17.5% + 7.5% = **50%**

"ca" phenotype = 17.5% + 7.5% = **25%**

Notice that the distribution of phenotypes is the same, regardless of the contribution of the crossover classes.

12. This problem can be approached by looking for the most distant loci (*adp* and *b*) and then filling in the intermediate loci. In this case, the map for parts **(a)** and **(b)** is the following:

d....	......b....	......pr....	......vg....	.......c....	......adp
31	48	54	67	75	83

Map Units

The expected map units between *d* and *c* would be 44, *d* and *vg* would be 36, and *d* and *adp* 52. However, because there is a theoretical maximum of 50 map units possible between two loci in any one cross, that distance would be below the 52 determined by simple subtraction.

13.

	female A:	female B:	Frequency:
NCO	3, 4	7, 8	first
SCO	1, 2	3, 4	second
SCO	7, 8	5, 6	third
DCO	5, 6	1, 2	fourth

The single crossover classes that represent crossovers between the genes that are closer together (*d-b*) would occur less frequently than the classes of crossovers between more distant genes (*b-c*).

14. For two reasons, it is clear that the genes are in the *coupled* configuration in the F_1 female. First, a completely homozygous female was mated to a wild-type male and second, the phenotypes of the offspring indicate the following parental classes:

$$sc\ s\ v \text{ and } +++$$

(a)

$$P_1: \quad sc\ s\ v\ /sc\ s\ v \quad \times \quad +++/Y$$
$$F_1: \quad +++/sc\ s\ v \quad \times \quad sc\ s\ v/Y$$

(b) Using method I or II for determining the sequence of genes, examine the parental classes and compare the arrangement with the double crossover (least frequent) classes. Notice that the *v* gene "switches places" between the two groups (parentals and double crossovers). The gene that switches places is in the middle.

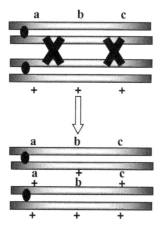

The map distances are determined by first writing the proper arrangement and sequence of genes, then computing the distances between each set of genes.

$$\frac{sc\ v\ s}{+\ +\ +}$$

$$sc - v = \frac{150 + 156 + 10 + 14}{1000} \times 100$$

$$= 33\% \text{ (map units)}$$
$$v - s = \frac{46 + 30 + 10 + 14}{1000} \times 100$$
$$= 10\% \text{ (map units)}$$

Double crossovers are always added into each crossover group because they represent a crossover in each region.

$$\underbrace{sc\text{-------}}_{33}\underbrace{v\text{-------}s}_{10}$$

(c, d) The coefficient of coincidence =

$$\frac{\text{observed freq. DCO}}{\text{expected freq. DCO}}$$
$$= \frac{(14 + 10)/1000}{0.33 \times 0.1}$$
$$= \frac{0.024}{0.033}$$
$$= 0.727$$

which indicates that there were fewer double crossovers than expected; therefore, positive chromosomal interference is present.

15. This setup involves an F_1 in which the fully heterozygous female has the genes *y* and *w* in *coupled* and *ct not coupled*. The arrangement for the cross is therefore:

(a) $y\ w\ +/++ ct \quad \times \quad y\ w\ +/Y$

It is important at this point to determine the gene sequence. Using method I or II, examine the parental classes and compare the arrangement with the double crossover (least frequent) classes. Notice that the *w* gene "switches places" between the two groups (parentals and double crossovers). The gene that switches places is in the middle.

Therefore, the arrangement as written above is correct.

(b)

$$y - w = \frac{9 + 6 + 0 + 0}{1000} \times 100$$
$$= 1.5 \text{ map units}$$
$$w - ct = \frac{90 + 95 + 0 + 0}{1000} \times 100$$
$$= 18.5 \text{ map units}$$

$$y\text{-----------------}w\text{-----------------------------}ct$$
$$0.0 \qquad\qquad 1.5 \qquad\qquad\qquad\qquad 20.0$$

(c) There were

$$0.185 \times 0.015 \times 1000 = 2.775$$
double crossovers expected.

(d) Because the cross to the F_1 males included the normal (wild-type) gene for *cut wings,* it would not be possible to unequivocally determine the genotypes from the F_2 phenotypes for all classes.

16. (a) The cross will be as follows. Represent the *Dichaete* gene as an uppercase letter because it is dominant.

P_1:	$D++/+++$	$\times$	$+e\,p/+e\,p$
F_1:	$D++/+e\,p$	$\times$	$+e\,p/+e\,p$
F_2:	$D++/+e\,p$	Dichaete
	$+e\,p/+e\,p$	ebony, pink
	$D\,e+/+e\,p$	Dichaete, ebony
	$++p/+e\,p$	pink
	$D+p/+e\,p$	Dichaete, pink
	$+e+/+e\,p$	ebony
	$D\,e\,p/+e\,p$	Dichaete, ebony, pink
	$+++/+e\,p$	wild type

(b) Determine which gene is in the middle by comparing the parental classes with the double crossover classes. Notice that the *pink* gene "switches places" between the two groups (parentals and double crossovers). The gene that switches places is in the middle. So rewriting the sequence of genes with the correct arrangement gives the following:

F_1: $D++/+p\,e \times +p\,e/+p\,e$

Distances: Remember to add in the double crossover classes.

$$D - p = \frac{12 + 13 + 2 + 3}{1000} \times 100$$
$$= 3.0 \text{ map units}$$

$$p - e = \frac{84 + 96 + 2 + 3}{1000} \times 100$$
$$= 18.5 \text{ map units}$$

17. Because two of the genes are linked and are 20 map units apart on the third chromosome, and one is on the second chromosome, the problem is a combination of linkage and independent assortment. First, provide the genotypes of the

parents in the original cross and the reciprocal. Use a semicolon to indicate that two different chromosome pairs are involved.

P_1: females: $+/+$; $p\,e/p\,e$
$\times$
males: dp/dp; $++/++$

F_1: females: $+/dp$; $++/p\,e$
$\times$
males: dp/dp; $p\,e/p\,e$

Female gametes: Use a modification of the forked-line method for determining the types of gametes to be produced. The *dumpy* locus will give $0.5\ +$ and $0.5\ dp$ to the gametes because of independent assortment (on a different chromosome), and the other two loci will segregate with 20 percent (map units) being the recombinants and 80 percent being the parentals.

$0.5 +$	$0.4 +$	$+$ (parental)	$= 0.20 +++$
	$0.1 +$	e (crossover)	$= 0.05 ++e$
	$0.1\ p$	$+$ (crossover)	$= 0.05 +p+$
	$0.4\ p$	e (parental)	$= 0.20 +p\,e$

$0.5\ dp$	$0.4 +$	$+$ (parental)	$= 0.20\ dp ++$
	$0.1 +$	e (crossover)	$= 0.05\ dp + e$
	$0.1\ p$	$+$ (crossover)	$= 0.05\ dp\ p +$
	$0.4\ p$	e (parental)	$= 0.20\ dp\ p\,e$

Crossing with $dp\ p\ e$ from the male gives the following offspring:

0.20 wild type
0.05 ebony
0.05 pink
0.20 pink, ebony
0.20 dumpy
0.05 dumpy, ebony
0.05 dumpy, pink
0.20 dumpy, pink, ebony

For the reciprocal cross:

F_1: males: $+/dp$; $++/p\,e$
$\times$
females: dp/dp; $p\,e/p\,e$

there would be no crossover classes.

$$0.5 + \diagup \begin{array}{l} 0.5 + \\ 0.5\,p \end{array}$$
+ (parental) = 0.25 + + +
e (parental) = 0.25 + p e

$$0.5\,dp \diagup \begin{array}{l} 0.5 + \\ 0.5\,p \end{array}$$
+ (parental) = 0.25 dp + +
e (parental) = 0.25 dp p e

Crossing with *dp p e* from the female gives the following offspring:

  0.25 wild type
  0.25 pink, ebony
  0.25 dumpy
  0.25 dumpy, pink, ebony

The results would change because of no crossing over in males.

18. Since *stubble* is a dominant mutation (and homozygous lethal), one can determine whether it is heterozygous (*Sb/+*) or homozygous wild type (*+/+*). One would use the typical testcross arrangement with the *curled* gene, so the arrangement would be

  + *cu/* + *cu*

19. You can set up the cross in the following manner:

  Females: *Sb cu/+ +* × + *cu/* + *cu*

With 8.2 map units between the *Sb* and *cu* loci, there would be the following distribution of female gametes:

  45.9 % *Sb* *cu*
  4.1 % *Sb* +
  4.1 % + *cu*
  45.9 % + +

Which, when crossed with + *cu* gametes from the male, would give the following offspring phenotypes and numbers:

  459 = Sb cu
  41 = Sb
  41 = cu
  459 = wild

20. Because sister chromatids are genetically identical (with the exception of rare new mutations), crossing over between sisters provides no increase in genetic variability. Individual genetic variability could be generated by somatic crossing over because certain patches on the individual would be genetically different from those in other regions. This variability would be of only minor consequence

in all likelihood. Somatic crossing over would have no influence on the offspring produced.

21. These observations, as well as the results of other experiments, indicate that the synaptonemal complex is required for crossing over.

22. (a) There would be $2^n = 8$ genotypic and phenotypic classes, and they would occur in a 1:1:1:1:1:1:1:1 ratio.

(b) There would be two classes, and they would occur in a 1:1 ratio.

(c) There are 20 map units between the *A* and *B* loci, and locus *C* assorts independently from both *A* and *B* loci.

23. Since the genetic map is more accurate when relatively small distances are covered and when large numbers of offspring are scored, this map would probably not be too accurate with such a small sample size.

24. In contrast to the other organisms mentioned, a single human mating pair produces relatively few offspring, and the haploid number of chromosomes is relatively high (23), so there are rather small numbers of identifiable genes per chromosome. In addition, accurate medical records are often difficult to obtain, and the life cycle is relatively long.

25. DNA markers are unique DNA sequences whose sequence and chromosomal location are known. They serve as landmarks for the mapping of genes. Typical markers include restriction fragment length polymorphisms (RFLPs), microsatellites, and single nucleotide polymorphisms (SNPs). Because the number of DNA markers in an individual may be in the tens of thousands, they can "mark" small intervals of each of the 23 human chromosomes.

26. Assign the following symbols:

  R = red r = yellow
  O = oval o = long

  Progeny A: *Ro/rO* × *rroo* = 10 map units
  Progeny B: *RO/ro* × *rroo* = 10 map units

27. The easiest way to approach this problem is to set up fractions representing the proportions of gametes, with the frequency of the recombinant gametes adding up to 25 percent. For each, the gamete proportions would be the following:

3/8 *Ab*; 3/8 *aB*; 1/8 *AB*; 1/8 *ab*

Now, combine the gametes from each parent (they are the same) and arrive at the following frequency:

$A_B_$ 33/64; A_bb 15/64; $aaB_$ 15/64; *aabb* 1/64

28. Look for overlap between chromosome number in given clones and genes expressed. Note that *ENO1* is expressed in clones B, D, and E; chromosomes 1 and 5 are common to these clones. However, since *ENO1* is not expressed in clone C, which is missing chromosome 1 (and has chromosome 5), *ENO1* must be on chromosome 1.

MDH1: chromosome 2
PEPS: chromosome 4
PGM1: chromosome 1

29. First make a drawing with the genes placed on the homologous chromosomes as follows:

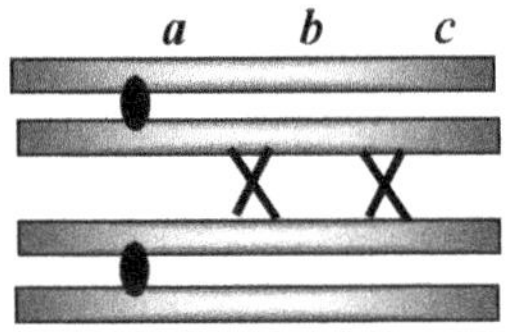

Realize that there are four chromatids in each tetrad and a single crossover involves only two of the four chromatids. Noninvolved chromatids must be added to the noncrossover classes. Do all the crossover classes first; then add up the noncrossover chromatids. For example, in the first crossover class (20 between *a* and *b*), notice that there will be 40 chromatids that were not involved in the crossover. These 40 must be added to the *abc* and +++ classes.

a b c	= 168
+ + +	= 168
a + +	= 20
+ *b c*	= 20
+ + *c*	= 10
a b +	= 10
+ *b* +	= 2
a + *c*	= 2

The map distances would be computed as follows:

$$a - b = \frac{20 + 20 + 2 + 2}{400} \times 100$$
$$= 11 \text{ map units}$$
$$b - c = \frac{10 + 10 + 2 + 2}{400} \times 100$$
$$= 6 \text{ map units}$$

30. It is important to remember that there is no crossing over in males and that if two genes are on the same chromosome, there will be complete linkage of the genes in the male gametes. In females, crossing over will produce parental and crossover gametes. What you will have is the following gametes from the females (left) and males (right):

$bw^+ st^+$	1/4	$bw^+ st^+$	1/2
$bw^+ st$	1/4	$bw\ st$	1/2
$bw\ st^+$	1/4		
$bw\ st$	1/4		

Combining these gametes will give the ratio presented in the table of results.

31. (a) There are several ways to think through this problem. Remember that there is no crossing over in *Drosophila* males. Therefore, any gene on the same chromosome will be completely linked to any other gene on the same chromosome. Since you can get *pink* by itself, *short* cannot be completely linked to it. This leaves linkage to *black* on the second chromosome, the fourth chromosome, or the X chromosome. Since the distribution of phenotypes in males and females is essentially the same, the gene cannot be X-linked. In addition, the F_1 males were wild, and if the *short* gene is on the X, the F_1 males would be short.

It is also reasonable to state that the gene cannot be on the fourth chromosome because there would be eight phenotypic classes (independent assortment of three genes) instead of the four observed. Through these insights, one could conclude that the *short* gene is on chromosome 2 with the *black* gene.

Another way to approach this problem is to make three chromosomal configurations possible in the F_1 male. By producing gametes from this male, the answer becomes obvious.

Case A		Case B		Case C	
$\frac{p\ b}{+\ +}$	$\frac{sh}{+}$	$\frac{p\ sh}{+\ +}$	$\frac{b}{+}$	$\frac{b\ sh}{+\ +}$	$\frac{p}{+}$

Develop the gametes from case C and cross them out to the completely recessive triple mutant. You will get the results in the table.

(b) The parental cross is now the following:

Females: $\underline{b\ sh}$	p	×	Males: $\underline{b\ sh}$	p
$+\ +$	$+$		$b\ sh$	p

The new gametes resulting from crossing over in the female would be $b\ +$ and $+\ sh$. Since the gene p is assorting independently, it is not important in this discussion. Because 15 percent of the offspring now contain these recombinant chromatids, the map distance between the two genes must be 15.

32. Notice that in the description of the genotype of the female, no mention is made of the *cis-trans* (coupling-repulsion) arrangement of the genes. The data will supply that information. Begin with a set of symbols as indicated below:

B^+ = wild eye shape
B = Bar eye shape

m^+ = wild wings
m = miniature wings

e^+ = wild body color
e = ebony body color

Superficially, the cross would be as follows: $B^+B\ m^+m\ e^+e\ \times\ B^+?\ m?\ e?$ (The *?* is used at this point to indicate that we have no information allowing us to decide whether any of the alleles in the male are X-linked.)

Notice from the data that there are approximately as many ebony offspring (282) as those with wild body color (283). Therefore, we can conclude that the *ebony* locus is not linked to B or m. Notice also that the most frequent offspring regarding eye shape and wing size are wild-miniature and Bar-wild. This suggests that the arrangement is "trans" or "repulsion" as indicated below:

$$B\ m^+/B^+m;\ e^+/e$$

Notice that a semicolon is used to indicate that the *ebony* locus is on a different chromosome.

At this point and without prior knowledge, we still do not know whether any of the genes are X-linked; however, it is of no consequence to the

solution of the problem. (In actuality, both B and m loci are X-linked.)

To determine the map distances (again, *ebony* is out of the mapping picture at this point because it is not linked to either B or m):

$111 + 115 = 226$	= wild miniature = parental
$117 + 101 = 218$	= Bar wild = parental
$26 + 31 = 57$	= Bar miniature = crossover
$29 + 35 = 64$	= wild wild = crossover

Mapping the distance between B and m would be as follows:

$$(57 + 64)/(226 + 218 + 57 + 64) \times 100 =$$
$$121/565 \times 100 = 21.4 \text{ map units.}$$

We would conclude that the *ebony* locus is either far away from B and m (50 map units or more) or that it is on a different chromosome. In fact, *ebony* is on a different chromosome.

33. Once the pedigree is established as requested in part (a), one can address part (b) by detailing the genotypes of each daughter and her husband. To symbolize the two alleles at the EMWX locus, a "+" superscript is used for the normal allele and a "−" superscript is used for the mutant allele.

Daughter 1:

$$EMWX^+\ Xg^+/EMWX^-\ Xg^- \ \times\ Xg^+/Y$$

Daughter 2:

$$EMWX^+\ Xg^+/EMWX^-\ Xg^- \ \times\ Xg^-/Y$$

Daughter 3:

$$EMWX^+\ Xg^+/EMWX^-\ Xg^- \ \times\ Xg^-/Y$$

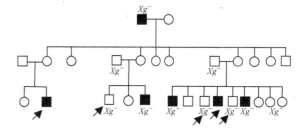

By examining the chromosomal configurations in the three daughters along with their husbands, one can determine, at least for the male offspring, whether a crossover was required to produce the given phenotypes. Crossover offspring are noted by an arrow.

34. (a) A number of studies have suggested a relationship between maternal chromosome nondisjunction and crossover frequency and/or chromosomal location of crossovers. Data presented in this table show an inverse correlation between recombination frequency and live-born children having various trisomies. As the frequency of crossing over decreases, the frequency of trisomy increases. Although these data indicate a correlation, other factors such as intrauterine survival are also likely to play a role in determining trisomy live-born frequencies.

(b) If positive interference does spread out crossovers among and within chromosomes, then ensuring that crossovers are distributed among all the chromosomes (and all portions of chromosomes) may reduce nondisjunction and therefore be of selective advantage. This model assumes that the total number of crossovers per oocyte is limiting.

Chapter 6 : Genetic Analysis and Mapping in Bacteria and Bacteriophages

Concept Areas	Corresponding Problems
Media and Growth Characteristics	1, 25
Genetic Recombination in Bacteria	1, 2, 27
Conjugation	3, 4, 5, 6, 7, 8, 25, 30
Chromosome Mapping	25, 26
Transformation	9, 10, 24, 27, 28, 29
Bacteriophages	1, 2, 12, 15, 16, 17
Transduction	11, 13
Mutation and Recombination in Viruses	1, 14, 18, 19, 20, 21, 22, 23, 26, 31
Intragenic Recombination in Phages	1

Concepts and Processes Checklist

(Check topic when mastered – provide examples where appropriate – understand the context of each entry)

- **Bacteria Mutate Spontaneously**
- **Grow at an Exponential Rate**
  - adaptation hypothesis
  - lysis
  - *E. coli*
  - spontaneous mutation
  - fluctuation test
  - Luria and Delbruck
  - minimal medium
  - carbon source
  - inorganic ions
  - minimal medium
  - prototroph
  - auxotroph
  - complete medium
  - lag phase
  - logarithmic (log) phase
  - petri dish

- 20-minute doubling
- colony
- **Genetic Recombination Occurs in Bacteria**
  - conjugation
  - transformation
  - transduction
  - vertical gene transfer
  - horizontal gene transfer
- **Conjugation in Bacteria F^+ and F^- Strains**
  - *E. coli* strain K12
  - Lederberg, Tatum
  - 1946
  - F^+, F^-
  - sintered glass filter
  - pore size
  - Davis U-tube

- o physical contact
- o F pilus (sex pilus, pl. pili)
- o fertility factor (F factor)
- o Hayes, Cavalli-Sforza
- o genetic recombination
- o recipient cell

- o **Hfr Bacteria and Chromosome Mapping**
  - o Cavalli-Sforza
  - o 1950
  - o nitrogen mustard
  - o Hayes
  - o 1953
  - o Hfr, high-frequency recombination
  - o recipients remain F⁻
  - o nonrandom gene transfer
  - o Wollman, Jacob
  - o mid-1950s
  - o antibiotic-resistance F⁻
  - o blender
  - o interrupted mating technique
  - o time-dependent transfer
  - o ordered transfer of genes
  - o time mapping
  - o minutes of transfer
  - o *O* site transferred first
  - o F transferred last

- o **Recombination in F⁺ × F⁻ Matings**
  - o excision
  - o no genetic recombination
  - o low frequency of Hfr cells

- o **The F′ State and Merozygotes**
  - o Adelberg
  - o 1959
  - o F factor carries bacterial genes
  - o merozygote
  - o partial diploid cell

- o **Rec Proteins Are Essential**
  - o *recA, recB, recC, recD*
  - o RecA protein
  - o single-strand displacement
  - o RecBCD protein

- o **The F Factor Is an Example of a Plasmid**
  - o plasmid
  - o episome
  - o R plasmid
  - o resistance transfer factor (RTG)
  - o r-determinants
  - o multiple antibiotic resistance
  - o Japan 1950s
  - o *Shigella*
  - o hospital bacteria
  - o Col plasmid
  - o colicins
  - o colicinogenic
  - o recombinant DNA research

- o **Transformation…Genetic Recombination**
  - o transformation
  - o extracellular
  - o exogenous
  - o electroporation

Chapter 6 Genetic Analysis and Mapping in Bacteria and Bacteriophages

- **The Transformation Process**
  - competence
  - heteroduplex

- **Transformation and Linked Genes**
  - 1/200
  - 10,000 to 20,000 nucleotide pairs
  - cotransformation
  - linkage

- **Bacteriophages Are Bacterial Viruses**
  - bacteriophage (phage)
  - transduction

- **Phage T4: Structure and Life Cycle**
  - T-even phage
  - lytic cycle
  - lysozyme
  - self-assembly
  - enzyme-directed processes

- **The Plaque Assay**
  - plaque
  - serial dilution

- **Lysogeny**
  - no lysis
  - prophage
  - temperate phage
  - virulent phage
  - lysogenized
  - lysogenic
  - episome

- **Transduction Is Virus-Mediated Bacterial DNA Transfer**
  - Zinder, Lederberg
  - 1952
  - transduction
  - *Salmonella*

- **The Lederberg-Zinder Experiment**
  - strains LA-22, LA-2
  - auxotrophic
  - prototrophic
  - Davis U-tube
  - filterable agene
  - P22

- **The Nature of Transduction**
  - P1, SPO1, F116
  - lysogenized bacterium
  - transducing phage
  - abortive transduction
  - complete transduction
  - generalized transduction

- **Transduction and Mapping**
  - cotransduction
  - simultaneous recombination
  - linkage

- **Bacteriophages Undergo Intergenic Recombination**

- **Bacteriophage Mutations**
  - Hershey
  - 1946
  - unusual T2 plaques
  - *E. coli* strain B
  - halo
  - rapid lysis
  - replating
  - host range
  - *E. coli* strain B-2

Chapter 6 Genetic Analysis and Mapping in Bacteria and Bacteriophages

- **Mapping in Bacteriophages**
  - mixed infection experiments
  - intergenic recombination
  - three or more chromosomes involved
- **Intragenic Recombination Occurs in Phage T4**
  - Benzer
  - 1950s
  - *rII*
- **The *rII* Locus of Phage T4**
  - *E. coli* K12(λ)
  - *E. coli* B
  - complementation assay
- **Complementation by *rII* Mutations**
  - complementation group
- A, B
- cistron
- **Recombinational Analysis**
  - *rII A*
  - *rII B*
  - mapping
- **Deletion Testing of the *rII* Locus**
  - deletion testing
- **The *rII* Gene Map**
  - 307 distinct sites
  - hot spots
  - 200 recombinational units
  - mutational units
- **Evolving Concept of a Gene**

F6.1 Simple illustration comparing *abortive* and *complete* transduction.

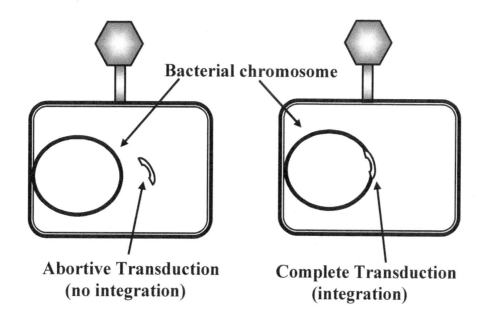

Bacterial chromosome

Abortive Transduction
(no integration)

Complete Transduction
(integration)

Answers to Now Solve This

6-1. One can approach this problem by lining up the data from the various crosses in the following order:

Hfr Strain	*Order*
1	*T C H R O*
2	*H R O M B*
3	*<< C H R O M*
4	*M B A K T >>*
5	*< < B A K T C*

Overall: *T C H R O M B A K*

Notice that all of the genes can be linked together to give a consistent map and that the ends overlap, indicating that the map is circular. The order is reversed in two of the crosses, indicating that the orientation of transfer is reversed.

6-2. In the first data set, the transformation of each locus, a^+ or b^+, occurs at a frequency of 0.031 and 0.012, respectively. To determine if there is linkage, one would determine whether the frequency of double transformants a^+b^+ is greater than that expected by a multiplication of the two independent events. Multiplying 0.031×0.012 gives 0.00037, or approximately 0.04 percent. From this information, one would consider no linkage between these two loci. Notice that this frequency is approximately the same as the frequency in the second experiment, in which the loci are transformed independently.

6-3. The approach for determining the complementation groupings and the results of the missing data is to recall that if lysis occurs, different complementation groups (genes) exist. If no lysis occurs, then the two mutations are in the same complementation group. For group A, *d* and *f* are in the same complementation group (gene), whereas *e* is in a different one. Therefore,

$e \times f =$ lysis

For group B, all three mutations are in the same gene; hence

$b \times i =$ no lysis

In group C, *j* and *k* are in different complementation groups than *j* and *l*. It would be impossible to determine whether *l* and *k* are in the same or different complementation group if the *rII* region had more than two cistrons. However, because only two complementation regions exist, and both are not in the same one as *j*, *k* and *l* must both be in the other.

Chapter 6 Genetic Analysis and Mapping in Bacteria and Bacteriophages

Solutions to Problems and Discussion Questions

1. (a) Genetic variants of bacteria were discovered by their resistance to infection by bacteriophage and their dependence on certain media. Mutant strains could be established that provided the raw material for the discovery of a variety of recombinant strategies. Mutant bacteriophages were discovered by variations in their plaque morphology and host range.

(b) A variety of experiments involving transformation, conjugation, and transduction showed that genetic elements from one bacterial strain can be transferred to another strain. Historically, transformation set the stage for the discovery that DNA is the genetic material in bacteria.

(c) The general strategy for determining the dependence of cell-to-cell contact in one form of bacterial recombination involved a Davis U-tube and a filter. When the filter separated two auxotrophic strains, no genetic recombination occurred.

(d) A filterable agent was discovered such that when two auxotrophic strains were placed on opposite sides of a Davis U-tube apparatus, there was a one-way passage of genetic material. The filterable agent was insensitive to DNase treatment and was therefore not naked DNA.

(e) Intergenic recombination in bacteria was demonstrated by mixed infections that yielded recombinants. Such recombinants can be used in mapping of genes.

(f) Early experiments by Benzer showed that in certain pair-wise combinations of *rII* mutant strains, wild-type function could be restored. Such complementation experiments demonstrated the presence of functional domains (cistrons) within certain complex genes.

2. Your essay should include a description of the following: conjugation, transformation, transduction in bacteria, and how infection of bacteria by bacteriophages brings about recombination.

3. (a) The requirement for physical contact between bacterial cells during conjugation was established by placing a filter in a U-tube such that the medium can be exchanged, but the bacteria cannot come in contact. Under this condition, conjugation does not occur.

(b) By treating cells with streptomycin, an antibiotic, it was shown that recombination would not occur if one of the two bacterial strains was inactivated. However, if the other was similarly treated, recombination would occur. Thus, directionality was suggested, with one strain being a donor strain and the other being the recipient. Additional experimentation revealed that each donor strain contained a fertility factor (F factor) that confers the ability to donate part of its chromosome.

(c) An F^+ bacterium contains a circular, double-stranded, structurally independent DNA molecule that can direct recombination.

4. (a) In an $F^+ \times F^-$ cross, the transfer of the F factor produces a recipient bacterium, which is F^+. Any gene may be transferred on an F′, and the frequency of transfer is relatively low. Crosses that are Hfr $\times$ F^- produce recombinants at a higher frequency than the $F^+ \times F^-$ cross. The transfer is oriented (non-random) and the recipient cell remains F^-.

(b) Bacteria that are F^+ possess the F factor, whereas those that are F^- lack the F factor. In Hfr cells, the F factor is integrated into the bacterial chromosome; in F′ bacteria, the F factor is free of the bacterial chromosome, yet it possesses a piece of the bacterial chromosome.

5. Mapping the chromosome in an Hfr $\times$ F^- cross takes advantage of the oriented transfer of the bacterial chromosome through the conjugation tube. For each F type, the point of insertion and the direction of transfer are fixed; therefore, breaking the conjugation tube at different times produces partial diploids with corresponding portions of the donor chromosome being transferred. The length of the chromosome being transferred is contingent on the duration of conjugation; thus, mapping of genes is based on time.

6. Participating bacteria typically consist of two types, prototrophs and auxotrophs. If a minimal medium is used first, the auxotrophs would be unable to grow. The transfer to a minimal medium allows the detection of recombinant bacteria. Mutant bacteria would not be identifiable if participating bacteria were transferred to a complete medium.

7. In an Hfr × F⁻ cross, the F factor is directing the transfer of the donor chromosome. It takes more than 90 minutes to transfer the entire chromosome. Because the major portion of the F factor is the last element to be transferred and the conjugation tube is fragile, the likelihood for complete transfer is low.

8. As shown in the text, the F⁺ element can enter the host bacterial chromosome, and upon returning to its independent state, it may pick up a piece of a bacterial chromosome. When combined with a bacterium with a complete chromosome, a partial diploid, or merozygote, is formed.

9. Notice that the incorporation of loci a^+ and b^+ occurs much more frequently than the incorporation of b^+ and c^+ together (210 to 1), and the incorporation of all three genes $a^+b^+c^+$ occurs relatively infrequently. If a and b loci are close together and both are far from locus c, then fewer crossovers would be required to incorporate the two linked loci compared to all three loci (see diagram).

If all three loci were close together, then the frequency of incorporation of all three would be similar to the frequency of incorporation of any two contiguous loci, which is not the case.

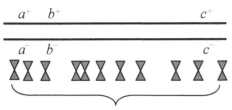

sites of crossing over

10. During transformation, incoming DNA forms a complex with the host chromosome leading to a double helix that contains one host DNA strand and one incoming DNA strand. Since these two single strands are different in base sequence (otherwise genetic recombination would not occur), the term *heteroduplex* seems appropriate. After one round of replication, the heteroduplex DNA is resolved into a double-stranded structure identical to the host's original DNA and one double-stranded mutant DNA.

11. In their experiment, a filter was placed between the two auxotrophic strains; this would not allow contact. F-mediated conjugation requires contact; without that contact, such conjugation cannot occur. The treatment with DNase showed that the filterable agent was not naked DNA.

12. A *plaque* results when bacteria in a "lawn" are infected by a phage and the progeny of the phage destroy (lyse) the bacteria. A somewhat clear region is produced that is called a plaque.

Lysogeny is a complex process whereby certain temperate phages can enter a bacterial cell and, instead of following a lytic developmental path, integrate their DNA into the bacterial chromosome. In doing so, the bacterial cell becomes lysogenic. The latent, integrated phage chromosome is called a *prophage*.

13. In *generalized* transduction, virtually any genetic element from a host strain may be included in the phage coat and thereby be transduced. In *specialized (restricted)* transduction, only those genetic elements of the host that are closely linked to the insertion point of the phage can be transduced. Specialized transduction involves the process of lysogeny. Because only certain genetic elements are involved in specialized transduction, it is not useful in determining linkage relationships. Cotransduction of genes in generalized transduction allows linkage relationships to be determined.

14. The first problem to be solved is the gene order. Clearly, the parental types are

$$a^+b^+c^+ \text{ and } a^-b^-c^-$$

because they are the most frequent. The double crossover types are the least frequent,

$$a^-b^-c^+ \text{ and } a^+b^+c^-$$

Because it is the gene in the middle that switches places when one compares the parental and double crossover classes, the c gene must be in the middle. The map distances are as follows:

$$a \text{ to } c = (740 + 670 + 90 + 110)/10,000$$
$$= 16.1 \text{ map units}$$
$$c \text{ to } b = (160 + 140 + 90 + 110)/10,000$$
$$= 5 \text{ map units}$$

To determine the type of interference, first determine the *expected* frequency of double crossovers ($0.161 \times 0.05 = 0.000805$), which when multiplied by 10,000 gives approximately 80. The *observed* number of double crossovers is $90 + 110$, or 200. Since many more double crossovers are observed than expected, negative interference is occurring.

15. The translation machinery of the infected bacterium provides the necessary materials for protein synthesis.

16. Starting with a single bacteriophage, one lytic cycle produces 200 progeny phages; three more lytic cycles would produce $(200)^4$, or 1,600,000,000 phages.

17. (a) Remembering that 0.1 mL is typically used in the plaque assay, the initial concentration of phage per mL is greater than 10^5.

(b) Remembering that 0.1 mL is typically used in the plaque assay, the initial concentration of phage per mL is around 140×10^5 or 1.4×10^7.

(c) Remembering that 0.1 mL is typically used in the plaque assay, the initial concentration of phage is less than 10^7. Coupling this information with the calculations in part (b) above, it would appear that the initial concentration of phage is around 1×10^7 and the failure to obtain plaques in this portion of the experiment is expected and due to sampling error.

18. Both mutant (*rII*) and wild-type strains of phage T4 can grow on *E. coli* B; however, only wild-type T4 can grow on K12. Therefore, the degree of recombination between various *rII* strains can be determined by examining the number of plaques on K12 because only recombinant, wild-type strains can grow. A greater number of T4 phage can grow on *E. coli* B.

19. Because there are only two complementation groups in the *rII* region, one would have the following groupings:

Group A: *1, 4, 5 Group* B: *2, 3*

(a) Therefore, the result of testing is

$2 \times 3 = $ no lysis
$2 \times 4 = $ lysis
$3 \times 4 = $ lysis

20. Because mutant *5* failed to complement with mutations in either cistron, it probably represents a major alteration in the gene such that both cistrons are altered. A deletion that overlaps both cistrons could cause such a major alteration.

21. (a) The recombination frequency is given by the following formula. Recall that only one of the two recombinant types is recovered in this type of experiment when the assay of growth on *E. coli* K12 is used. Remember to include the dilution factor in the setting of the observed values.

General formula:

$$\frac{2(\text{number of recombinant types})}{\text{total number of progeny}}$$

$$= 2(5 \times 10^1)/(2 \times 10^5) = 5 \times 10^{-4}$$

(b) Because mutant *6* complemented mutations *2* and *3*, it is likely to be in the cistron with mutants *1*, *4*, and *5*. A lack of recombinants with mutant *4* indicates that mutant *6* is a deletion that overlaps mutation *4* or it is extremely close to mutant *4*. Recombinants with *1* and *5* indicate that the deletion does not overlap these mutations.

22. (a)

Combination	Complementation
1, 2	−
1, 3	+
2, 4	+
4, 5	−

23 (a) Because mutants can lyse *E. coli* B but not K12, one can determine the total number of plaque-forming units (phages) as 4×10^7. The number of recombinants (those that grow on K12) would be 8×10^2. The recombination frequency would therefore be

$$2(8 \times 10^2/4 \times 10^7) = 4 \times 10^{-5}$$

(b) The dilution would be 10^{-3} and the colony number would be 8×10^3.

(c) Mutant *7* might well be a deletion spanning parts of both A and B cistrons.

24. Because the frequency of double transformants is quite high (compare the *trp⁺tyr⁺* transformants in A and B experiments), one may conclude that the genes are quite closely linked together. Part B in the experiment gives one the frequencies of transformations of the individual genes and the frequency of transformants receiving two pieces of DNA (2 in the data table). One must know these numbers in order to estimate the actual number of *trp⁺tyr⁺* cotransformations.

25. (a) Rifampicin eliminates the donor strain, which is *rif* ˢ.

(b) <u>*b a*   *c*   F</u>

(c) To determine the location of the *rif* gene, one could use a donor strain, which was *rif^r* but sensitive to another antibiotic (ampicillin, for example). The interrupted mating experiment is conducted as usual on an ampicillin-containing medium, but the recombinants must be replated on a rifampicin medium to determine which ones are sensitive.

26. Because 1/10 mL of a 10^{-6} dilution is used to add to the bacterial suspension, the concentration of the original phage suspension would be

$$10 \times 10^6 \times 17 = 1.7 \times 10^8$$

plaque-forming units per mL or pfu/mL.

27. The basis for answering this question rests in the fact that it is easier to transform two genes that are close together (that is, cotransform) than if the same two genes are far apart. If two genes are cotransforming at a relatively high rate, they are said to be "linked" in the sense that they are closer together than two genes that do not cotransform. The data indicate that *a* and *d* are linked; *b* and *c* are linked; and since *f* cotransforms with *b*, *b*, *c*, and *f* are likely to be linked. However, if the arrangement is <u>*c b f*</u>, or the reverse, there is a possibility that whereas both *c* and *f* are "linked" to *b*, *c* and *f* may not be strongly linked enough to cotransform. Gene *e* does not cotransform with any gene so it must be independent of the other linkage groups.

28. Since *g* cotransforms with *f*, it is likely to be in the *c b f* "linkage group" and would be expected to cotransform with each. One would not expect transformation with *a*, *d*, or *e*.

29. (a) Some strains, *E. fergusonii* for example, undergo relatively low transfer as a donor strain, whereas others, *E. chrysanthemi*, undergo relatively frequent transfer as a donor strain. Within-species transfer is not necessarily more frequent than between-species transfer. The direction of transfer (which are the donor and recipient strains) in some cases influences the frequency of transfer; for example, notice the frequencies of transfer when *E. chrysanthemi* is the donor and *E. coli* is the recipient (−1.7), compared with when *E. coli* is the donor and *E. chrysanthemi* is the recipient (−3.7).

(b) *E. chrysanthemi* (−2.4); *E. coli*-*E. chrysanthemi* (−1.7)

(c) Conjugative plasmids can share genes when bacteria are in proximity, and since such plasmids may contain either pathological genes or genes that compromise the use of antibiotics, any harmful variant that develops in one species may be spread to others. Although a particular gene may be harmless in one bacterium, it may confer pathogenicity or drug resistance to a different species.

30. (a) No, all functional groups do not impact similarly on conjugative transfer of R27. Regions 1, 2, and 4 appear to be least influenced by mutation because transfer is at 100 percent.

(b) Regions 3, 5, 6, 8, 9, 10, 12, 13, and 14 appear to have the most impact on conjugation because when mutant, conjugation is abolished.

(c) Regions 7 and 11, when mutant, only partially abolish conjugation; therefore, they probably have less impact on conjugation than those listed in part (b).

(d) The data in this problem provide some insight into the complexity of the genetic processes involved in bacterial conjugation. The regions that have the most impact on conjugation fall into three different functional groups. In addition, notice that regions 1, 2, 4, 7, and 11, those that appear to have little, if any, impact on conjugation, are functionally related, as indicated by their shading.

31. (a) Each process, mutation, recombination, and reassortment provides genetic diversity upon which sustained infectivity is dependent. As host defenses adapt, viral diversity provides for viral survival.

(b) Because of its relatively volatile genome, the influenza virus is able to present a variety of unique surface elements that are foreign to the human immune system. As the immune system responds to viral uniqueness, new variants are generated that again evade the immune system.

(c) A successful vaccine is one that stimulates a response in the immune system to a specific antigen or array of antigens presented by a pathogen or toxin. Since the influenza virus alters its surface antigens at a relatively rapid pace, by the time a vaccine is developed, new strains have evolved. Recently, researchers have become more successful at developing useful short-term vaccines for variants of influenza viruses that evolve relatively rapidly.

Chapter 7: Sex Determination and Sex Chromosomes

Concept Areas	Corresponding Problems
Sex Chromosomes	1, 2, 6, 11, 12, 14, 15, 16, 18, 27, 28, 31
Nondisjunction	18
Life Cycles	3, 4
Sex Ratios	1, 25, 26, 34
Sex Determination	1, 5, 7, 9, 10, 30, 31, 32, 34
Sexual Differentiation	1, 5, 9, 10, 13, 29, 35, 36
Dosage Compensation	1, 8, 17, 19, 20, 21, 22, 23, 24, 33

Concepts and Processes Checklist

(Check topic when mastered – provide examples where appropriate – understand the context of each entry)

- **Overview**
  - heteromorphic chromosomes
  - sex chromosomes
  - sex determination
  - *Chlamydomonas*
  - *Zea mays*
  - *Caenorhabditis elegans*
  - *Drosophila*
- **Life Cycles Depend on Sexual Differentiation**
  - primary sexual differentiation
  - gonads, gametes
  - secondary sexual differentiation
  - mammary glands
  - external genitalia
  - unisexual
  - dioecious
  - gonochoric
  - bisexual
  - monoecious
  - hermaphroditic
  - intersex
- ***Chlamydomonas***
  - isogametes
  - isogamous
  - two mating types
  - zoospores
  - mt^+, mt^-
  - *mt* locus
  - chromosome VI
  - nitrogen depletion
- ***Zea mays***
  - haploid gametophyte
  - diploid sporophyte
  - monoecious seed plant
  - stamen

- tassel
- diploid microspore mother cells
- haploid microspores
- male microgametophyte
- pollen grain
- two haploid sperm nuclei
- megaspore mother cell
- pistil
- sporophyte
- four haploid megaspores
- three mitotic divisions
- endosperm nuclei
- micropyle
- two synergids
- antipodal nuclei
- pollination
- pollen grain
- silk (stigma)
- two sperm nuclei
- double fertilization
- diploid zygote nucleus
- triploid endosperm nucleus
- kernel
- florets
- tassel seed (*ts1, ts2*)
- silkless (*sk*)
- barren stalk (*ba*)
- sexual determination
- sexual differentiation

- ***Caenorhabditis elegans***
  - approximately 1000 cells
    - precise lineage
    - two sexual phenotypes
    - males
    - hermaphrodites
    - testes, ovaries
    - self-fertilization
    - genes on X and autosomes
    - ratio of X/autosomal sets
    - absence of heteromorphic Y

- **X and Y Chromosomes Linked to Sex Determination…Early Twentieth Century**
  - Henking, 1891
  - X-body
  - McClung
  - heterochromosome
  - Wilson, 1906
  - *Protenor*, 14 chromosomes
  - two X chromosomes
  - males, 13 chromosomes
  - X = sex determination
  - XX/XO mode of sex determination
  - *Lygaeus turcicus*
  - 14 chromosomes both sexes
  - autosomes
  - X chromosome
  - Y chromosome
  - XX/XY mode of sex determination
  - heterogametic sex
  - homogametic sex

- males homogametic sex in some species
- moths and butterflies
- some fish
- reptiles
- amphibians
- some plants
- birds

- **Y Chromosome Determines Maleness in Humans**
  - von Winiwarter, 1912
  - Painter, 1920s
  - Tjio and Levan
  - 1956
  - 46 chromosomes
  - Ford, Hamerton
  - 23 pairs of chromosomes
  - X, Y chromosomes

- **Klinefelter and Turner Syndromes**
  - Klinefelter syndrome (46,XXY)
  - Turner syndrome (45,X)
  - nondisjunction
  - 48,XXXY
  - 48,XXYY
  - 49,XXXXY
  - 49,XXXYY
  - mosaics
  - 45,X/46,XY
  - 45,X/46,XX
  - 47,XXX syndrome
  - triplo-X

- 48,XXXX
- 49,XXXXX
- 47,XYY condition
- Jacobs, 1965
- antisocial criminal acts
- tall
- Walzer and Gerald, 1974

- **Sexual Differentiation in Humans**
  - gonadal (genital ridges)
  - primordial germ cells
  - outer cortex
  - inner medulla form
  - Wolffian ducts
  - Müllerian ducts
  - ovaries
  - testes
  - bipotential gonad

- **Y Chromosome and Male Development**
  - Y fewer genes than X
  - 75 genes
  - X chromosome 900–1400 genes
  - pseudoautosomal regions (PARs)
  - nonrecombinant region of the Y (*NRY*)
  - male-specific region of the Y (MSY)
  - heterochromatic regions
  - *sex-determining region* Y (*SRY*)
  - testis-determining factor (TDF)
  - transgenic mice
  - transcription factor

- Müllerian inhibiting substance (MIS)
- MIH
- anti-Müllerian hormone
- cascade of genetic expression
- *SOX9*
- seminiferous tubules
- fibroblast growth factor 9 (*Fgf9*)
- *SF1*
- *Foxl2*
- transdifferentiation
- downregulation
- 23 Mb
- X-transposed region
- Page
- 2010
- palindromes
- human/chimpanzee comparisons
- X-degenerative region
- pseudogenes
- ampliconic retion
- amplicon
- wasteland

- **The Ratio of Males to Females in Humans Is Not 1.0**
  - heteromorphic sex chromosomes
  - X/Y, Z/W
  - sex ratio
  - primary sex ratio
  - secondary sex ratio

- **Dosage Compensation Prevents Excessive Expression of X-linked Genes in Humans and Other Mammals**
  - dosage compensation
  - X-linked genes

- **Barr Bodies**
  - Barr, Bertram
  - Feulgen reaction
  - sex chromatin body
  - $N - 1$ rule

- **The Lyon Hypothesis**
  - mammalian females
  - random inactivation
  - Lyon, Russell
  - 1961
  - blastocyst stage
  - Lyon hypothesis
  - X-linked coat color genes
  - hemizygous
  - clone
  - *G6PD*
  - electrophoretic field
  - Davidson
  - 1963
  - lyonization
  - red-green color blindness

- **The Mechanism of Inactivation**
  - imprinting
  - epigenetics
  - X inactivation center (*Xic*)
  - X-inactive specific transcript (*XIST*)

- *Tsix*
- Penny
- 1996
- transgenes
- blockage of X–X pairing

- **The Ratio of X Chromosomes to Sets of Autosomes Determines Sex in *Drosophila***

  - *Drosophila melanogaster*
  - Bridges, 1916
  - nondisjunction
  - XXY/XO flies
  - metafemales
  - metamales
  - ratio of X chromosomes to haploid sets of autosomes
  - 2X:2A, etc.
  - intersex
  - genic balance theory
  - *transformer* (*tra*)
  - *Sex-lethal* (*Sxl*)
  - Sturtevant
  - Muller
  - *doublesex* (*dsx*)

- RNA splicing
- alternative splicing

- **Dosage Compensation in *Drosophila***

  - *maleless* (*mle*)
  - dosage compensation complex (DCC)

- ***Drosophila* Mosaics**

  - bilateral gynandromorph
  - XX/XO

- **Temperature Variation Controls Sex Determination in Reptiles**

  - genotypic sex determination (GSD)
  - temperature-dependent sex determination (TSD)
  - lizards, boas, pythons
  - crocodiles, most turtles, some lizards
  - T_p (pivotal temperature)
  - aromatase
  - androgen
  - testosterone
  - estrogens
  - thermosensitive factor

Chapter 7 Sex Determination and Sex Chromosomes

Answers to Now Solve This

7-1. In mammals, the scheme of sex determination is dependent on the presence of a piece of the Y chromosome. If present, a male is produced. In *Bonellia viridis*, the female proboscis produces some substance that triggers a morphological, physiological, and behavioral developmental pattern that produces males. To elucidate the mechanism, one could attempt to isolate and characterize the active substance by testing different chemical fractions of the proboscis. Second, mutant analysis usually provides critical approaches into developmental processes. Depending on characteristics of the organism, one could attempt to isolate mutants that lead to changes in male or female development. Third, by using micro-tissue transplantations, one could attempt to determine which anatomical "centers" of the embryo respond to the chemical cues of the female.

7-2. (a) Something is missing from the male-determining system of sex determination at the level of the genes, gene products, or receptors, etc. **(b)** The *SOX9* gene, or its product, is probably involved in male development. Perhaps it is activated by *SRY*. **(c)** There is probably some evolutionary relationship between the *SOX9* gene and *SRY*. There is considerable evidence that many other genes and pseudogenes are also homologous to *SRY*. **(d)** Normal female sexual development does not require the *SOX9* gene or gene product(s).

7-3. Different cells manage X chromosome inactivation in different ways. The absence of orange patches is due to the fact that in gonadal tissue, whereas oogonia have a single active X chromosome, the inactive X chromosome is reactivated at, or more likely, shortly before, entry into meiotic prophase (Kratzer and Chapman, 1981). Thus, X chromosome inactivation does not remain in certain ovarian cells as in somatic tissue. However, since the timing of reactivation is variable in different cell lines, there is some uncertainty as to which cell is in which state of inactivation. The actual result was a kitten (CC) with black spots on a white background. If one assumes that the ovarian cell was engaging in X chromosome inactivation, the ovarian cell that Rainbow donated to create CC contained an activated *black* gene and an inactivated *orange* gene (from X-inactivation). This would mean that as CC developed, her cells did not change that inactivation pattern. Therefore, unlike Rainbow, CC developed without any cells that specified orange coat color. The result is CC's black and white tiger-tabby coat. Had the inactivation pattern been reversed such that both the *black* and *orange* alleles were originally active and subsequently inactivated randomly, CC would still not have appeared identical to Rainbow because the pattern of inactivation is random and the distribution of white patches is variable.

Chapter 7 Sex Determination and Sex Chromosomes
Solutions to Problems and Discussion Questions

1. (a) Mutations such as *tassel seed* (*ts*), *silkless* (*sk*), and *barren stalk* (*ba*) have provided insight into sex determination in a monoecious plant such as *Zea mays*. Studies on such mutations indicate that many genes are responsible for sex differentiation in maize.

(b) The Y chromosome has been shown to play a crucial role in sex determination in mammals and some insects because its presence or absence determines sex. In others, such as *Drosophila*, presence of certain X chromosome complements, as a ratio to the autosomes, determines sex.

(c) Supported by the discovery of sex chromosome aneuploids (XO, XXY, for example), presence or absence of a Y chromosome has been shown to be fundamental in sex determination in humans.

(d) Based on consensus data of the sex of embryos and fetuses recovered from miscarriages and abortions, showing that fetal mortality is higher in males than females, it is estimated that the primary sex ratio favors males.

(e) Calvin Bridges studied a number of chromosomal compositions in *Drosophila* and determined that the critical factor in sex determination is the ratio of X chromosomes to the number of haploid sets of autosomes. Given two haploid sets, XO is male and XXY is female.

(f) The most direct evidence in support of random inactivation of either X chromosome in an XX cell came from experiments using electrophoretic variants of the *G6PD* locus. Such studies, coupled with mosaic coat patterns in mammals, support the random inactivation hypothesis.

2. Your essay should include various aspects of sex chromosomes that contain genes responsible for sex determination. Mention should also be made to those organisms in which autosomes play a role in concert with the sex chromosomes.

3. Maize (*Zea mays*) is a monoecious seed plant in which the sporophyte phase predominates during the life cycle. Both male and female structures are present on the adult plant. The stamens produce diploid microspore mother cells, which undergo meiosis to produce four haploid microspores. Each haploid microspore develops into a microgametophyte that contains two sperm nuclei.

Female diploid cells, megaspore mother cells, are located in the pistil of the sporophyte. Following meiosis, only one of the four haploid megaspores survives and divides mitotically three times, producing a total of eight haploid nuclei. Two of these nuclei unite to become the endosperm nuclei. At the end of the sac where the sperm enters, three nuclei remain: the oocyte nucleus and two synergids. The other three antipodal nuclei cluster at the opposite end of the embryo sac.

When pollen grains make contact with the stigma and successfully develop, two sperm nuclei enter the embryo sac: one sperm nucleus unites with the haploid oocyte nucleus and the other sperm nucleus unites with two endosperm nuclei.

In *Caenorhabditis elegans*, there are two sexual phenotypes: males, which have only testes, and hermaphrodites, which contain both testes and ovaries. While in the larval stage of development of hermaphrodites, testes produce sperm, which is stored. Oogenesis does not occur until the adult stage is reached. The eggs are fertilized (self-fertilized) by the stored sperm. The majority of the offspring are hermaphrodites, whereas less than 1 percent of the offspring is male. As adults, males can mate with hermaphrodites, producing about half male and half hermaphrodite offspring.

4. (a) The term *homomorphic* refers to the situation in which both the sex chromosomes have the same form. The term *heteromorphic* refers to the condition in many organisms in which there are two different forms (morphs) of chromosomes such as X and Y.

(b) In *isogamous* species, there is little visible difference between the haploid vegetative cells that reproduce asexually and the haploid gametes that are involved in sexual reproduction. The two gametes that fuse during mating are morphologically indistinguishable and are called *isogametes*. An organism that is *heterogamous* is one in which there are two morphologically distinct gametes.

5. Sexual differentiation is the response of cells, tissues, and organs to signals provided by the genetic mechanisms of sex determination. In other words, genes are present that signal developmental pathways whereby the sexes are generated. Sexual differentiation is the complex set of responses to those genetic signals.

6. In the XX/XO form of sex determination, sex is determined by the presence or absence of a chromosome, whereas in the XX/XY scheme, the Y chromosome may be sex determining. However, in some cases the autosomes play a role in sex determination. The *Protenor* form of sex determination involves the XX/XO condition, whereas the *Lygaeus* mode involves the XX/XY condition.

7. Calvin Bridges (1916) studied nondisjunctional *Drosophila*, which had a variety of sex chromosome complements. He noted that XO produced sterile males, whereas XXY produced fertile females. Other investigators have determined that the Y chromosome is male determining in humans. Individuals with the 47,XXY complement are males, whereas those with 45,XO are females.

In *Drosophila,* it is the balance between the number of X chromosomes and the number of haploid sets of autosomes that determines sex. In humans, there is a small region on the Y chromosome that determines maleness.

8. Mammals possess a system of X chromosome inactivation whereby one of the two X chromosomes in females becomes a chromatin body or Barr body. If one of the two X chromosomes is randomly inactivated, the dosage of genetic information is more or less equivalent in males (XY) and females (XX).

9. Whereas a specific region on the Y chromosome specifies the eventual cellular fate as male in humans, sexual differentiation of the genital ridge does not occur until around the seventh week of development. In the absence of the Y chromosome, no male development occurs and the cortex of the genital ridge forms ovarian tissue.

10. The Y chromosome is male determining in humans, and it is a particular region of the Y chromosome that causes maleness, the sex-determining region (SRY). *SRY* encodes a product called the testis-determining factor (TDF), which causes the undifferentiated gonadal tissue to form testes. Individuals with the 47,XXY complement are males, whereas those with 45,XO are females. In *Drosophila,* it is the balance between the number of X chromosomes and the number of haploid sets of autosomes that determines sex. In contrast to

humans, XO *Drosophila* are males and the XXY complement is female.

11. In *primary* nondisjunction, half of the gametes contain two X chromosomes, whereas the complementary gametes contain no X chromosomes. In secondary nondisjunction, you get two normal gametes: one with two X chromosomes and one with no X. Fertilization, by a Y-bearing sperm cell, of those female gametes with two X chromosomes would produce the XXY Klinefelter syndrome. Fertilization of the "no-X" female gamete with a normal X-bearing sperm will produce Turner syndrome.

12. (a) female $X^{rw}Y$ $\times$ male $X^{+}X^{+}$

F_1: females: $X^{+}Y$ (normal)
males: $X^{rw}X^{+}$ (normal)

F_2: females: $X^{+}Y$ (normal)
$X^{rw}Y$ (reduced wing)

males: $X^{rw}X^{+}$ (normal)
$X^{+}X^{+}$ (normal)

(b) female $X^{rw}X^{rw}$ $\times$ male $X^{+}Y$

F_1: females: $X^{rw}X^{+}$ (normal)
males: $X^{rw}Y$ (reduced wing)

F_2: females: $X^{rw}X^{+}$ (normal)
$X^{rw}X^{rw}$ (reduced wing)

males: $X^{+}Y$ (normal)
$X^{rw}Y$ (reduced wing)

13. Males and females share a common placenta and, therefore, hormonal factors carried in blood. Hormones and other molecular species (transcription factors perhaps) triggered by the presence of a Y chromosome lead to a cascade of developmental events, which both suppress female organ development and enhance masculinization. Other mammals also exhibit a variety of similar effects depending on the sex of their uterine neighbors during development.

14. Because attached-X chromosomes have a mother-to-daughter inheritance and the father's X is transferred to the son, one would see daughters with the white eye phenotype and sons with the miniature wing phenotype. In addition, there would be YY male and attached-X/X females. The YY males are inviable, and only rare attached-X/X females survive.

Chapter 7 Sex Determination and Sex Chromosomes

15. If the male offspring had white eyes and the female offspring were phenotypically wild type, one might suspect that the attached-X had become unattached. All "expected" offspring would require that the detachment had occurred well before meiosis—early in germline formation. If it occurs <u>during</u> meiosis in some meiotic mother cells, we would see irregular numbers of the normal genotypes.

16. Because synapsis of chromosomes in meiotic tissue is often accompanied by crossing over, it would be detrimental to sex-determining mechanisms to have sex-determining loci on the Y chromosome transferred, through crossing over, to the X chromosome.

17. A *Barr body* is a differentially staining chromosome seen in some interphase nuclei of mammals with two X chromosomes. There will be one less Barr body than the number of X chromosomes. The Barr body is an X chromosome that is considered to be genetically inactive.

18. There is a simple formula for determining the number of Barr bodies in a given cell: $N - 1$, where N is the number of X chromosomes.

Klinefelter syndrome (XXY)	= 1
Turner syndrome (XO)	= 0
47,XYY	= 0
47,XXX	= 2
48,XXXX	= 3

19. The *Lyon hypothesis* states that the inactivation of the X chromosome occurs at random early in embryonic development. Such X chromosomes are in some way "marked," such that all clonally related cells have the same X chromosome inactivated.

20. Unless other markers, cytological or molecular, are available, one cannot test the Lyon hypothesis with homozygous X-linked genes. The test requires identification of allelic alternatives to see differences in X chromosome activity.

21. Females will display mosaic retinas with patches of defective color perception. Under these conditions, their color vision may be influenced.

22. Refer to the text and notice that the phenotypic mosaicism is dependent on the heterozygous condition of genes on the two X chromosomes. Dosage compensation and the formation of Barr bodies occur only when there are two or more X chromosomes. Males normally have only one X chromosome; therefore, such mosaicism cannot occur. Females normally have two X chromosomes. There are cases of male calico cats that are XXY.

23. Many organisms have evolved over millions of years with a balance of two doses of each gene product. Many genes required for normal cellular and organismic function in *both* males and females are located on the X chromosome. These gene products have nothing to do with sex determination or sex differentiation. Balance of their output is necessary for normal development; thus, dosage compensation evolved.

24. Like humans, *Drosophila* females contain two X chromosomes and males have only one X chromosome. Instead of X chromosome inactivation as seen in humans (mammals in general), male X-linked genes in *Drosophila* are transcribed at twice the rate of comparable genes on the X chromosome in *Drosophila* females.

25. In general, information about the primary sex ratio in humans is obtained from abortions and miscarriages. In addition, some studies (Barczyk, 2001) using "hamster oocyte—human sperm" have been successful in determining some of the causal factors involved in determining the primary sex ratio.

26. There are several possibilities that are discussed in the text. One could account for the significant departures from a 1:1 ratio of males to females by suggesting that at anaphase I of meiosis, the Y chromosome more often goes to the pole that produces the more viable sperm cells. One could also speculate that the Y-bearing sperm has a higher likelihood of surviving in the female reproductive tract, or that the egg surface is more receptive to Y-bearing sperm. At this time, the mechanism is unclear. As Pergament et al. (2002) explain:

"A number of environmental, physiological and genetic factors have been observed to impact on the primary sex ratio: sexual behaviour, variation in hormonal concentrations, natural disasters, environmental pollutants and timing of conception.

Nevertheless, no biological mechanism or interaction of factors has suitably explained this phenomenon, or that of the prenatal vulnerability of the male, the suspected higher sex ratio in spontaneous abortion and the male excesses in adult diseases related to the intrauterine environment."

27. Since there is a region of synapsis close to the SRY-containing section on the Y chromosome, crossing over in this region would generate XY translocations, which would lead to the condition described.

28. Because of the homology between the *red* and *green* genes, there exists the possibility for an irregular synapsis (see the following figure), which, following crossing over, would give a chromosome with only one (*green*) of the duplicated genes. When this X chromosome combines with the normal Y chromosome, the son's phenotype can be explained.

"Normal Synapsis"

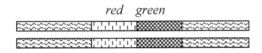

red   green

"Oblique Synapsis"

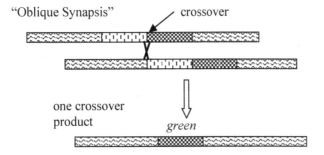

crossover

one crossover
product
green

29. Aromatase is responsible for the conversion of male hormones such as testosterone to female estrogens. Aromatase activity is high in developing ovaries and low in developing testes. Activity of the reptilian aromatase gene appears to be influenced by temperature and as such leads to a temperature-dependent mechanism of sexual differentiation in reptiles.

30. Since all haploids are male and half of the eggs are unfertilized, 50 percent of the offspring would be male at the start; adding the X_a/X_a types gives 25 percent more male; the remainder X_a/X_b would be female. Overall, 75 percent of the offspring would be male, and 25 percent would be female.

31. Since mention is made of "inbred" strains, it is likely that the diploid males are homozygous for a number of alleles, as is the case with *Bracon*.

32. The presence of the Y chromosome provides a factor (or factors) that leads to the initial specification of maleness and the formation of testes. Subsequent expression of secondary sex characteristics must be dependent on the interaction of the normal X-linked *Tfm* allele with testosterone. Without such interaction, differentiation takes the female path. To test the dominant nature of the *Tfm* allele, one could degenerate a XXY male that is heterozygous for the *Tfm* allele. Should the same testicular feminization phenotype occur, the dominant nature of the *Tfm* allele would be supported. If the *Tfm* phenotype was eliminated in the heterozygote, one would have support for the model that the normal *Tfm* allele is needed to interact with testosterone.

33. If one assumes that the somatic ovarian cell engaged in X chromosome inactivation, the ovarian somatic cell that Rainbow donated to create CC contained an activated *black* gene and an inactivated *orange* gene (from X-inactivation). This would mean that as CC developed, her cells did not change that inactivation pattern. Therefore, unlike Rainbow, CC developed without any cells that specified orange coat color. The result is CC's black and white tiger-tabby coat.

34. (a) The following figures depict only those chromosomes relevant to the *Mm* and *Dd* genotypes. With the *MmDd* genotype, both dyads separate intact to the secondary spermatocytes and are potentially capable of fertilizing the egg. (Only one configuration of the *MmDd* genotype is presented here.)

Primary Spermatocyte

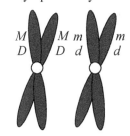

Secondary Spermatocytes

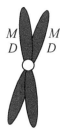
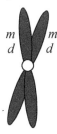

Following is the *Mmdd* genotype that leads to fragmentation of the *m*-bearing chromosome. Thus, only the *M*-bearing chromosome is available for fertilization.

Primary Spermatocyte

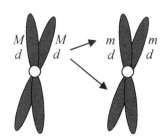

Secondary Spermatocytes

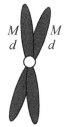
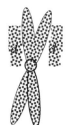

(b) There have been many attempts to control pest species by hampering the production or fertility of one sex. In this case, if a sex ratio distorter could be successfully integrated into a large enough pool of males, then female numbers may drop. Whether one could successfully manage a pest population with such a method remains to be tested.

35. In human males, one copy of the *SRY* gene provides for testis development; in chickens, two copies of *DMRT1* are required. The general architecture of sex determination in fowl is comparable to humans; however, it is somewhat reversed: females are the heterogametic sex, but the sex-determining genes function on the homogametic chromosomes of the male.

36. A number of experimental possibilities exist that can be explored with such gynandromorphs. For instance, do sex cells respond to signals carried in body fluids (nonautonomous) or are they cell specific (autonomous)? Reciprocal transplantation tests can be used to determine the influence of the anatomical environment for cellular differentiation. Since male/female gynandromorphs could be produced in the first place, it argues for an autonomous form of sex differentiation in contrast with that seen in mammals.

Chapter 8: Chromosome Mutations: Variation in Number and Arrangement

Concept Areas	Corresponding Problems
Variation in Chromosome Number	2, 3, 7, 8, 15, 16, 17, 18, 19, 32
Nondisjunction	1, 28, 29, 30
Human Variations	1, 4, 5, 6, 22, 27
Deletions	1, 3, 9, 12, 20
Duplications	1, 3, 9, 13
Inversions	1, 3, 10, 11, 21, 23
Translocations	14, 24, 25, 26, 31

Concepts and Processes Checklist

(Check topic when mastered – provide examples where appropriate – understand the context of each entry)

- **Variation in Chromosome Number**
  - terminology and origin
  - aneuploidy
  - euploidy
  - polyploidy
  - triploid
  - tetraploid
  - autopolyploidy
  - allopolyploidy
  - amphidiploidy
  - Klinefelter syndrome
  - Turner syndrome
  - nondisjunction
- **Monosomy and Trisomy**
  - haploinsufficient
  - $2n + 1$
  - Down syndrome
  - trisomy 21

- Down syndrome critical region
- DSCR
- **Origin of Extra 21st Chromosome**
  - nondisjunction at meiosis I
  - maternal age
  - genetic counseling
  - amniocentesis
  - chorionic villus sampling (CVS)
  - noninvasive prenatal genetic diagnosis
  - NIPGD
  - Down syndrome
  - human aneuploidy
  - Patau syndrome
  - 47,13+
  - Edwards syndrome
  - 47,18+
  - karyotype

- mouse model
- syntenic regions
- ortholog
- Hsa21
- Ts16
- Mmu 10, 16, 17
- **Polyploidy**
  - autopolyploidy
  - autotriploids
  - autotetraploids
  - colchicines
  - G1 cyclins
  - allopolyploidy
  - allotetraploid
  - amphidiploids
  - American cotton
  - *Gossypium*
  - *Brassica oleracea*
  - *Triticum*
  - *Secale*
  - *Triticale*
- **Endopolyploidy**
  - *Gerris*
- **Variation Occurs in Composition…**
  - deletion or deficiency
  - terminal
  - intercalary
  - compensation loop
  - cri du chat syndrome
  - segmental deletion
  - partial monosomy
- **A Duplication Is a Repeated Segment…**
  - duplication
  - gene redundancy
  - ribosomal RNA genes
  - rDNA
  - gene amplification
  - nucleolar organizer region (NOR)
  - *Bar* mutation in *Drosophila*
- **Gene Duplication in Evolution**
  - gene families
- **Copy Number Variations**
- **Inversions Rearrange the Linear…**
  - inversion
  - paracentric
  - pericentric
  - gametic consequences
  - inversion heterozygote
  - inversion loop
  - dicentric chromatid
  - acentric chromatid
  - evolutionary advantages
  - balancer chromosomes
- **Translocations Alter the Location…**
  - reciprocal translocation
  - alternate segregation
  - adjacent segregation
  - semisterility
- **Translocations in Humans**
  - familial Down syndrome
  - Robertsonian translocation

- ○ 14/21 translocation
- ○ D/G translocation
- ○ balanced translocation carrier
- ○ **Fragile Sites in Human…**
  - ○ fragile site
  - ○ Martin-Bell syndrome
- ○ fragile-X syndrome
- ○ trinucleotide repeat
- ○ genetic anticipation
- ○ *FHIT* gene
- ○ *WWOX* gene
- ○ tumor suppressor gene

F8.1 Illustration of the chromosomal configurations of euploid and aneuploid genomes of *Drosophila melanogaster.*

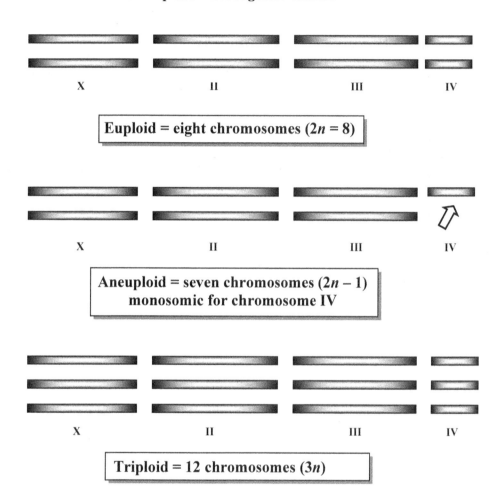

Drosophila melanogaster **female**

Answers to Now Solve This

3-1. A Turner syndrome female has the sex chromosome composition of XO. If the father had hemophilia, it is likely that the Turner syndrome individual inherited the X chromosome from the father and no sex chromosome from the mother. If nondisjunction occurred in the mother, either during meiosis I or meiosis II, an egg with no X chromosome can be the result. See the text for a diagram of primary and secondary nondisjunction.

3-2. The sterility of interspecific hybrids is often caused from a high proportion of univalents in meiosis I. As such, viable gametes are rare, and the likelihood of two such gametes "meeting" is remote. Even if partial homology of chromosomes allows some pairing, sterility is usually the rule. The horticulturist may attempt to reverse the sterility by treating the sterile hybrid with colchicine. Such a treatment, if successful, may double the chromosome number, and each chromosome would then have a homolog with which to pair during meiosis.

3-3. The rare double crossovers within the boundaries of a paracentric or pericentric inversion produce only minor departures from the standard chromosomal arrangement as long as the crossovers involve the same two chromatids. With two-strand double crossovers, the second crossover negates the first. However, three-strand and four-strand double crossovers have consequences that lead to anaphase bridges as well as a high degree of genetically unbalanced gametes.

Chapter 8 Chromosome Mutations: Variation in Number and Arrangement

Solutions to Problems and Discussion Questions

1. (a) Before the advent of polymorphic markers, maternal involvement in trisomy 21 was strongly suspected because of the striking influence of maternal age on incidence. **(b)** Karyotype analysis of spontaneously aborted fetuses has shown that a significant percentage of abortuses are trisomic and every chromosome can be involved. Other forms of aneuploidy (monosomy, nullisomy) are less represented. **(c)** A variety of studies, many tracing to early work with specialized (polytene) chromosomes in *Drosophila* and aneuploidy in other organisms, demonstrated that as chromosome structures or numbers are altered, phenotypic consequences are likely. **(d)** By examining the polytene chromosomes of *Drosophila*, Bridges and Muller determined that the Bar-eye phenotype was caused by a chromosomal duplication of the 16A region on the X chromosome. In addition, unequal crossing over that resulted in reduced or increased numbers of 16A regions reverted or enhanced the Bar-eye phenotype, respectively.

2. Your essay can draw from many examples discussed in the text as examples of deletions, duplications, inversions, translocations, and copy number variations.

3. With frequent exceptions, especially in plants, organisms typically inherit one chromosome complement (*haploid* = n = one representative of each chromosome) from each parent. Such organisms are *diploid*, or $2n$. When an organism contains complete multiples of the n complement ($3n$, $4n$, $5n$, etc.), it is said to be *euploid* in contrast with aneuploid in which complete haploid sets do not occur. An example of an aneuploid is *trisomic* where a chromosome is added to the $2n$ complement. In humans, trisomy 21 would be symbolized as $2n + 1$ or 47,+21.

Monosomy is an aneuploid condition in which one member of a chromosome pair is missing, thus producing the chromosomal formula of $2n - 1$. Haplo-IV is an example of monosomy in *Drosophila*. *Trisomy* is the chromosomal condition of $2n + 1$ in which an extra chromosome is present. Down syndrome is an example in humans (47,+21). See the text and notice that all the chromosomes are present in the diploid state except chromosome 21.

Patau syndrome is a chromosomal condition in which there is an extra D group chromosome. Such individuals are 47,+13 and have multiple congenital malformations. *Edwards syndrome* is a chromosomal condition in which there is an extra E group chromosome (47,+18). Individuals with Edwards syndrome have multiple congenital malformations and reduced life expectancy.

Polyploidy refers to instances in which there are more than two haploid sets of chromosomes in an individual cell. *Autopolyploidy* refers to cases of polyploidy in which the chromosomes in the individual originate from the same species. *Allopolyploidy* involves instances in which the chromosomes originate from the hybridization of two different species, usually closely related. *Autotetraploids* arise within a species, whereas *amphidiploids* arise from two taxa followed by chromosome doubling.

Paracentric inversions require breakpoints that do not flank the centromere, whereas *pericentric* inversions do.

4. haploid = 9, tetraploid = 36, trisomic = 19, monosomic = 17

5. Before the advent of polymorphic markers, maternal involvement in trisomy 21 was strongly suspected because of the striking influence of maternal age on incidence.

6. Karyotype analysis of spontaneously aborted fetuses has shown that a significant percentage of abortuses are trisomic and every chromosome can be involved. Other forms of aneuploidy (monosomy, nullisomy) are less represented.

7. Because an allotetraploid has a possibility of producing bivalents at meiosis I, it would be considered the most fertile of the three. Having an even number of chromosomes to match up at the metaphase I plate, autotetraploids would be considered to be more fertile than autotriploids.

8. American cultivated cotton has 26 pairs of chromosomes: 13 large and 13 small. Old-world cotton has 13 pairs of large chromosomes, and American wild cotton has 13 pairs of small chromosomes. It is likely that an interspecific hybridization occurred followed by chromosome doubling. These events probably produced a fertile amphidiploid (allotetraploid). Experiments have been conducted to reconstruct the origin of American cultivated cotton.

9. Basically, the synaptic configurations produced by chromosomes bearing a deletion or duplication (on one homolog) are very similar. There will be point-for-point pairing in all sections that are capable of pairing. The section that has no homolog will "loop out" as in the text.

10. Although there is the appearance that crossing over is suppressed in inversion "heterozygotes," the phenomenon extends from the fact that the crossover chromatids end up being abnormal in genetic content. As such, they fail to produce viable (or competitive) gametes or lead to zygotic or embryonic death. Notice in the text that the crossover chromatids end up genetically unbalanced.

11. Examine the text and notice that in a paracentric inversion, there are two genetically balanced chromatids (normal and inverted) and two, those resulting from a single crossover in the inversion loop, that are genetically unbalanced and abnormal (dicentric and acentric). The dicentric chromatid will often break, thereby producing highly abnormal fragments, whereas the acentric fragment is often lost in the meiotic process. In a pericentric inversion, all the chromatids have centromeres, but the two chromatids involved in the crossover are genetically unbalanced. The balanced chromatids are of normal or inverted sequence.

12. Modern globin genes resulted from a duplication event in an ancestral gene about 500 million years ago. Mutations occurred over time and a chromosomal aberration separated the duplicated genes, leaving the eventual α cluster on chromosome 16 and the eventual β cluster on chromosome 11.

13. In a work entitled *Evolution by Gene Duplication*, Ohno suggests that gene duplication has been essential in the origin of new genes. If gene products serve essential functions, mutation and therefore evolution would not be possible unless these gene products could be compensated for by products of duplicated, normal genes. The duplicated genes, or the original genes themselves, would be able to undergo mutational "experimentation" without necessarily threatening the survival of the organism.

14. It is likely that when certain combinations of genes are of selective advantage in a specific and stable environment, it would be beneficial to the organism to protect that gene combination from disruption through crossing over. By having the genes in an inversion, crossover chromatids are not recovered and therefore are not passed on to future generations. Translocations offer an opportunity for new gene combinations by associations of genes from nonhomologous chromosomes. Under certain conditions such new combinations may be of selective advantage. Meiotic conditions have evolved so that segregation of translocated chromosomes yields a relatively uniform set of gametes.

15. The primrose, *Primula kewensis*, with its 36 chromosomes, is likely to have formed from the hybridization and subsequent chromosome doubling of a cross between the two other species, each with 18 chromosomes. An example of this type of allotetraploidy (amphidiploidy) is seen in the text.

16. Given the basic chromosome set of nine unique chromosomes (a haploid complement), other forms with the "*n* multiples" are forms of autopolyploidy. In the illustration below, the *n* basic set is multiplied to various levels as is the autotetraploid in the example.

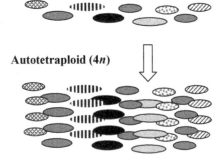

Basic set of nine unique chromosomes (*n*)

Autotetraploid (4*n*)

Individual organisms with 27 chromosomes (3*n*) are more likely to be sterile because there are trivalents at meiosis I, which cause a relatively high number of unbalanced gametes to be formed.

17. Set up the cross in the usual manner, realizing that recessive genes in the haplo-IV individual will be expressed.

Let b = bent bristles; b^+ = normal bristles.

(a)

$$\_/b \quad \times \quad b^+/b^+ \quad \Rightarrow$$

F$_1$:

$\_/b^+$ = normal bristles

b/b^+ = normal bristles

F$_2$:

$$\_/b^+ \quad \times \quad b/b+ \quad \Rightarrow$$

$\_/b^+$ = normal bristles

$\_/b$ = bent bristles

b^+/b^+ = normal bristles

b/b^+ = normal bristles

(b)

$$\_/b^+ \quad \times \quad b/b \quad \Rightarrow$$

F$_1$:

$\_/b$ = bent bristles

b/b^+ = normal bristles

F$_2$:

$$\_/b \quad \times \quad b/b^+ \quad \Rightarrow$$

$\_/b^+$ = normal bristles

$\_/b$ = bent bristles

b^+/b = normal bristles

b/b = bent bristles

18. The cross would be as follows:

$WWWW \times wwww$

(assuming that chromosomes pair as bivalents at meiosis)

F$_1$: $WWww$

F$_2$:   1 WW 4 Ww 1 ww

1 WW	fill in Punnett square
4 Ww	35 W phenotypes and 1 w phenotype
1 ww	

19. Given some of the information in the above problem, the expression would be as follows:

$(35/36 \ W:1/36 \ w)(35/36 \ A:1/36 \ a) \quad \Rightarrow$

    $(35/36)^2$ $W\_\_\_A\_\_\_$

    $35/(36)^2$ $W\_\_\_aaaa$

    $35/(36)^2$ $wwwwA\_\_\_$

    $1/(36)^2$ $wwwwaaaa$

20. Although a number of mechanisms for *bobbed* reversion have been documented, one based on meiotic recombination occurs through "unequal crossing over." When redundant chromosomal regions synapse, homologs can misalign. If crossing over occurs in the misaligned segments, one chromatid can gain chromosomal material at the expense of the other chromatid. As a chromosome gains rRNA genes, it harbors a selective advantage and produces flies that outcompete those with nonreverted *bobbed* mutations. Eventually, a stock that originally contained *bobbed Drosophila* contains what appear to be wild-type flies over time.

21. When a crossover occurs within a paracentric inversion, there are two genetically balanced chromatids (normal and inverted) and two, those resulting from a single crossover in the inversion loop, that are genetically unbalanced and abnormal (dicentric and acentric). The dicentric chromatid will often break, thereby producing highly unbalanced fragments, whereas the acentric fragment is often lost in the meiotic process. In a pericentric inversion, all the chromatids have centromeres, but the two chromatids involved in the crossover are genetically unbalanced. The balanced chromatids are of normal or inverted sequence.

22. (a) In all probability, crossing over in the inversion loop of an inversion (in the heterozygous state) had produced defective, unbalanced chromatids, thus leading to stillbirths and/ or malformed children. **(b)** It is probable that a significant proportion (perhaps 50 percent) of the children of the man will be similarly influenced by the inversion. **(c)** Since the karyotypic abnormality is observable, it may be possible to detect some of the abnormal chromosomes of the fetus by amniocentesis or CVS. However, depending on the type of inversion and the ability to detect minor changes in banding patterns, not all abnormal chromosomes may be detected.

23. Considering that there are at least three map units between each of the loci and that only four phenotypes are observed, it is likely that genes *a b c d* are included in an inversion, and crossovers that do occur among these genes are not recovered because of their genetically unbalanced nature. In a sense, the minimum distance between loci *d* and *e* can be estimated as 10 map units:

$$(48 + 52/1000)$$

However, this is actually the distance from the *e* locus to the breakpoint that includes the inversion.

The "map" is therefore as drawn below:

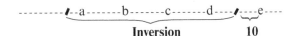

24. (a) Reciprocal translocation

(b)

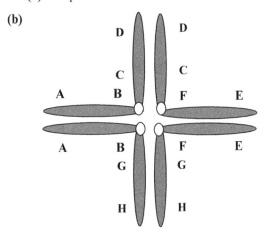

(c) Notice that all chromosomal segments are present, and there is no apparent loss of chromosomal material. However, if the breakpoints for the translocation occurred within genes, then an abnormal phenotype may be the result. In addition, a gene's function is sometimes influenced by its position (its neighbors, in other words). If such "position effects" occur, then a different phenotype may result.

25. It is likely that the translocation is the cause of the miscarriages. Segregation of the chromosomal elements will produce approximately half unbalanced gametes.

The chance of a normal child is approximately one in two; however, half of the normal children will be translocation carriers.

26. The symbolism t(14;21) indicates that a translocation (t) has occurred between chromosomes 14 and 21. Generally, a Down syndrome individual with a t(14;21) karyotype has 46 chromosomes.

27. (a) The father must have contributed the abnormal X-linked gene.

(b) Since the son is XXY and heterozygous for anhidrotic dysplasia, he must have received both the defective gene and the Y chromosome from his father. Thus, nondisjunction must have occurred during meiosis I.

(c) This son's mosaic phenotype is caused by X-chromosome inactivation, a form of dosage compensation in mammals.

28. Nondisjunction of the X chromosome could have occurred such that a daughter cell lost one copy of the X chromosome. The earlier the event occurred, the larger percentage of 45,X tissue would be observed. The distribution of the 45,X tissue would be dependent on the cell line within the developing embryo where the event occurred.

29. Notice that a chromosome in this question is defined as having two sisters joined at the centromere. This is the expected chromosome structure at the end of meiosis I.

(a) In light of this information, meiosis I must have produced the abnormal oocytes with more or less than 24 chromosomes, indicating multiple conditions of nondisjunction. More likely, the oocytes consisted of "22 1/2" chromosomes, those 22 normal dyads and a single monad.

(b) The result will be a monosomic and a normal zygote, assuming that the half chromosome (monad) migrates, intact, to one pole or the other.

(c) In all likelihood, premature division of the centromere (at meiosis I) probably causes the single (non-duplicated) chromosome at meiosis II.

(d) We generally consider nondisjunction occurring at meiosis I to consist of intact chromosomes, two sister chromatids, failing to separate appropriately.

These data indicate that some forms of aneuploidy result from premature division of the centromere at meiosis I as in the figure below.

**Synapsis of homologs
(bivalents, tetrads)**

⇩

$2n = 4$

G1, S, G2 ⇨

Meiosis I

"Equational" division at meiosis I leads to sister chromatid separation

30. It is likely that mitotic nondisjunction contributed to the mosaic condition. If one of the X chromosomes failed to be included in a daughter mitotic cleavage cell, then a substantial proportion of the child's cells would be XO. Expression of Turner syndrome characteristics would depend on the percentage and location of the XO cell population.

31. This female will produce meiotic products of the following types:

normal: $18 + 21$
translocated: $18/21$
translocated plus 21: $18/21 + 21$
deficient: 18 only

Note: The $18/21 + 18$ gamete is not formed because it would require separation of primarily homologous chromosomes at anaphase I.

Fertilization with a normal $18 + 21$ sperm cell will produce the following offspring:

normal: 46 chromosomes
translocation carrier: 45 chromosomes $18/21 + 18 + 21$
trisomy 21: 46 chromosomes $18/21 + 21 + 21$
monosomic: 45 chromosomes $18 + 18 + 21$, lethal

32. *Trisomic rescue* is a condition in which an original trisomic zygote occurs, but a particular chromosome is lost. In the diagram below, two chromosomes originally came from the father (solid) and one came from the mother (striped). The one from the mother was eliminated during mitosis, leaving the two chromosomes from the father.

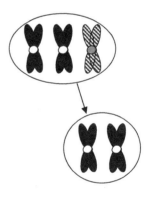

Monosomic rescue occurs when a chromosome is originally present in a zygote and, usually through mitotic nondisjunction, a duplicate of that chromosome occupies the cell.

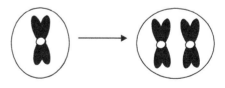

Gamete complementation occurs when a cell without either homolog of a given chromosome is fertilized by a gamete with two copies of that homolog. The resulting zygote contains a homologous chromosome pair from one parent.

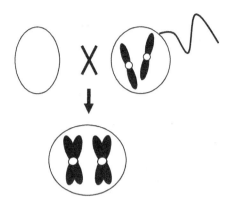

Isochromosome formation occurs when a chromosome contains two copies of one arm and has lost the homolog. Such a homolog loss can

originate in mitosis or meiosis. The isochromosome compensates for the nullisomic condition. Effectively, the chromosome is "uniparental" because most of the chromosomal material of a given homolog is from one parent.

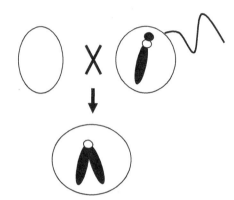

Chapter 9: Extranuclear Inheritance

Concept Areas	Corresponding Problems
Extranuclear Inheritance	2, 10, 17
Maternal Effect	1, 2, 7, 8, 14, 15, 16
Organelle Heredity	1, 3, 4, 5, 6, 11, 13, 18, 19
Infectious Heredity	9
Endosymbiotic Theory	12

Concepts and Processes Checklist

(Check topic when mastered – provide examples where appropriate – understand the context of each entry)

- **Organelle Heredity Involves DNA in Chloroplasts and Mitochondria**
  - transmitted from maternal parent
  - chloroplast
  - mitochondrion
  - heteroplasmy

- **Chloroplasts: Variegation in Four O'Clock Plants**
  - Correns, 1908
  - white, green, variegated leaves
  - *Mirabilis jalapa*
  - cytoplasmic transmission
  - chloroplast DNA

- **Chloroplast Mutations in *Chlamydomonas***
  - unicellular green alga
  - two mating types
  - mt^+, mt^-
  - streptomycin resistance (str^R)
  - Sager, 1954
  - uniparental inheritance

- **Mitochondrial Mutations: Early Studies in *Neurospora* and Yeast**
  - Mitchell and Mitchell, 1952
  - *Neurospora crassa*
  - pink bread mold
  - poly
  - *mi-1* (maternal inheritance)
  - cytochrome proteins
  - ATP synthesis
  - Ephrussi, 1956
  - petite
  - *Saccharomyces cerevisiae*
  - facultative anaerobe
  - fermentation
  - segregational petites
  - neutral petites
  - aerobic respiration
  - suppressive petites
  - dominant-negative mutation

Chapter 9 Extranuclear Inheritance

- **Knowledge of Mitochondrial and Chloroplast DNA Helps Explain Organelle Heredity**
  - organelle DNA
  - cytoplasmic inheritance
- **Organelle DNA and the Endosymbiotic Theory**
  - DNA similar to bacterial DNA
  - free-living protobacteria
  - engulfed by primitive eukaryotic cells
  - symbiotic relationship
  - endosymbiotic theory
  - miniscule mitochondrial genome
- **Molecular Organization and Gene Products of Chloroplast DNA**
  - autonomous genetic system
  - chloroplast DNA (cpDNA)
  - 100 to 225 kb in length
  - cpDNA much larger than mtDNa
  - introns in cpDNA
  - *Chlamydomonas*, 75 copies of cpDNA
  - ribosomal RNAs
  - transfer RNAs
  - ribosomal proteins
  - RNA polymerase
  - photosynthetic enzymes
  - ribulose-1-5-bisphosphate carboxylase
  - Rubisco

- **Molecular Organization and Gene Products of Mitochondrial DNA**
  - mtDNA smaller than cpDNA
  - 16 to 18 kb, but varies greatly
  - yeast mtDNA is 75 kb
  - introns mostly absent
  - two ribosomal RNAs
  - 22 transfer RNAs
  - 13 polypeptides (oxidative respiration)
  - multichain proteins
  - two density strands
  - ribosomes vary from $55S$ to $80S$
  - nuclear gene involvement
  - endosymbiotic theory
- **Mutations in Mitochondrial DNA Cause Human Disorders**
  - human mitochondria
  - 16,569 base pairs
  - vulnerable to mutations
  - no histone proteins
  - reactive oxygen species (ROS)
  - dispersion of mitochondria in zygote
  - heteroplasmy
  - maternal inheritance
  - myoclonic epilepsy and ragged red fiber disease (MERRF)
  - tRNA^{Lys} has A-to-G transition
  - Leber's hereditary optic neuropathy (LHON)
  - NADH dehydrogenase

108

- Kearns-Sayre syndrome (KSS)

- deletion mutations

- **Mitochondria, Human Health, and Aging**

  - mitochondrial dysfunction

  - future prevention of transmission

  - mitochondrial replacement

  - mitochondrial swapping

- **In Maternal Effect, the Maternal Genotype Has a Strong Influence during Early Development**

  - maternal effect

  - genotype of the mother

- *Lymnaea* **Coiling**

  - maternal effect

- sinistral

- dextral

- ovum donors

- genotype of the egg parent

- spindle cleavage division

- **Embryonic Development in *Drosophila***

  - Lewis

  - Nüsslein-Volhard

  - Wieschaus

  - 1995 Nobel Prize

  - *bicoid* (bcd^+)

  - anterior portion of fly

  - RNA deposited anteriorly

  - diluted posteriorly

Chapter 9 Extranuclear Inheritance

F9.1 Illustration of the common pattern seen in many cases of extranuclear inheritance. The condition of the female (egg) parent has a stronger influence on the phenotype of the offspring than the male (sperm/pollen) parent. Reciprocal crosses give different results in offspring.

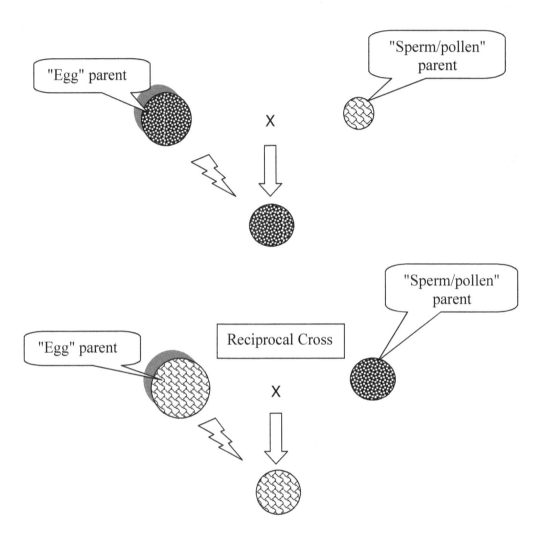

Chapter 9 Extranuclear Inheritance

Answers to Now Solve This

9-1. The mt^+ strain is the donor of the cpDNA since the inheritance of resistance or sensitivity is dependent on the status of the mt^+ gene. In this organism, chloroplasts obtain their characteristics from the mt^+ strain, whereas mitochondria obtain their characteristics from the mt^- strain.

9-2. See the text for a comparison of results involving various *petite* strains.

(a) neutral

(b) segregational (nuclear mutations)

(c) suppressive

9-3. In many cases, molecular components of mitochondria are recruited from the cytoplasm, having been synthesized from nuclear genes.

9-4. From an organismic standpoint, individuals with the most severe mitochondrial defects tend to be less reproductively successful. At the cellular level, mitochondria with mutations in protein-coding genes tend to be selected against. Such purifying selection tends to favor nonmutant mitochondria (Stewart, J., et al., PLOS, 2008).

Chapter 9 Extranuclear Inheritance

Solutions to Problems and Discussion Questions

1. (a) In general, organelle heredity is detected when the maternal parent has more influence than the paternal parent over the phenotype of the offspring. In addition, assuming other factors such as X-linked inheritance can be eliminated, different results from reciprocal crosses support inheritance by extranuclear elements.

(b) Whereas *segregational petites* exhibited Mendelian inheritance, both *neutral* and *suppressive petites* followed non-Mendelian patterns that were consistent with the involvement of an extranuclear agent.

(c) Electron micrographs show that DNA of mitochondria and chloroplasts looks like that seen in bacteria. In addition, the molecular components, notably ribosomal RNAs, are more like those in prokaryotes than eukaryotes.

(d) When eggs from a *Dd* (but sinistral because of its parent) snail are self-fertilized, all the offspring, even those that are *dd*, coil dextrally.

(e) A maternal effect is likely when the phenotype of the offspring is determined not by the mother's phenotype or its own genotype, but by the mother's genotype. The genotype of the sperm is not influential in determining the direction of shell coiling in offspring.

2. Your essay should be based on the fact that in organelle heredity, an organelle is responsible for the inheritance pattern, whereas in a maternal effect, organelles are not involved. In maternal effect, the effect persists for one generation only and is solely dependent on the genotype of the mother.

3. The *mt$^+$* strain (resistant for the nuclear and chloroplast genes) contributes the "cytoplasmic" component of streptomycin resistance, which would negate any contribution from the *mt$^-$* strain. Therefore, all the offspring will have the streptomycin resistance phenotype. In the reciprocal cross, with the *mt$^+$* strain being streptomycin sensitive, half of the offspring would be streptomycin resistant since there is an equal likelihood of obtaining the nuclear resistant gene from *mt$^-$* or the nonresistant gene from *mt$^+$*.

4. Because the ovule source furnishes the cytoplasm to the embryo and thus the chloroplasts, the offspring will have the same phenotype as the plant providing the ovule.

(a) green

(b) white

(c) white, variegated, or green (as illustrated below)

(d) green

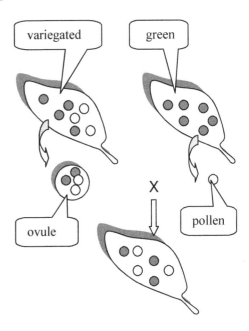

5. As with any description of dominance, one looks to the phenotype of the diploid heterozygote. In this problem, the heterozygote is of normal phenotype; therefore, the *segregational petite* gene is recessive.

6. Examine the text and notice that the inheritance patterns for the two, *segregational* and *neutral*, are quite different. The segregational mode is dependent on nuclear genes, whereas that of the *neutral* type is dependent on cytoplasmic influences, namely mitochondria. If the two are crossed as stated in the problem, then one would expect, in the diploid zygote, the *segregational* allele to be "covered" by normal alleles from the *neutral* strain. On the other hand, as the nuclear genes are again "exposed" in the haploid state of the ascospores, one would expect a 1:1 ratio of normals to petites. The petite phenoytpe is caused by the nuclear *segregational* gene.

7. The case with *Lymnaea* involves a maternal effect in which the *genotype* of the mother influences

112

the *phenotype* of the *immediate* offspring in a non-Mendelian manner. Notice that in the above statement, it is the maternal genotype that determines the phenotype of the offspring, regardless of its own genotype. Since both of the parents are *Dd*, the parent contributing the eggs must be *Dd*. Therefore, all of the offspring must have the phenotype of the mother's genotype, which is dextral.

8. In a maternal effect, the *genotype* of the mother influences the *phenotype* of her immediate offspring in a non-Mendelian manner. The fact that all of the offspring (F_1) showed a dextral coiling pattern indicates that one of the parents (maternal parent) contains the *D* allele. Taking these offspring and seeing that their progeny (call these F_2) occur in a 1:1 ratio indicate that half of the offspring (F_1) are *dd*. In order to have these results, one of the original parents must have been *Dd*, whereas the other must have been *dd*.

Parents: *Dd* × *dd*

Offspring (F_1):   1/2 *Dd*,   1/2 *dd*

(all dextral because of the maternal genotype)

Progeny (F_2):

All those from *Dd* parents will be dextral; all those from *dd* parents will be sinistral.

---

9. It appears as if some factor normally provided by the *gs*[+] allele is necessary for normal development and/or functioning of the female offspring's gonads. Without this product, the daughters are sterile, thus the term "grandchildless." Because the female provides so much vital material and information to the egg, including the cytoplasm necessary for germ-line determination, it is not surprising that such maternal-effect genes exist.

10. Since there is no evidence for segregation patterns typical of chromosomal genes and Mendelian traits, some form of extranuclear inheritance seems possible. If the *lethargic* gene is dominant, then a maternal effect may be involved. In that case, some of the F_2 progeny would be hyperactive because maternal effects are temporary, affecting only the immediate progeny. If the lethargic condition is caused by some infective agent, then perhaps injection experiments could be used. If caused by a mitochondrial defect, then the condition would persist in all offspring of lethargic mothers, through more than one generation.

11. Since an initial mutation does not involve all copies of mtDNA within the oocyte, the original state is heteroplasmic, but the mutated mtDNA is rare. If the new mutation confers no selective advantage to the host cell, the frequency of the mutant mtDNa is likely to diminish. However, if the mutation confers a selective advantage to the cell, it is likely to gain in frequency. Depending on a number of factors, including chance as well as the extent of the selective advantage, an mtDNA mutation may become prominent. However, in most cases, it will be competed out by normal mitochondria especially since the mutation influences a vital function (translation).

12. The endosymbiotic theory states that mitochondria and chloroplasts arose independently around 2 billion years ago from free-living protobacteria. These bacteria brought the capacity for aerobic respiration and photosynthesis to primitive eukaryotic cells. Because such organelles have prokaryotic origins, a deeper understanding of extranuclear DNA is possible. As we understand more of the molecular biology of prokaryotes, we automatically gain insight to the behavior of extranuclear DNA.

13. Mitochondrial defects often involve processes of oxidative phosphorylation and/or other essential mitochondrial functions that are dependent not only on the mitochondrial genome, but also on the nuclear genome. When a nuclear genome is transferred, it may contain mutant genes that negatively influence mitochondrial function that were compensated for in the original donor cells, but not in the recipient. In addition, enucleated eggs invariably contain both normal and defective mitochondria. When a nuclear genome is transferred to an enucleated egg, mitochondrial defects may arise from an uncompensated defective nuclear genome, the heteroplasmic condition of the egg, or a combination of the two. A disease occurs when the mitochondrial mutational load exceeds a tissue-specific threshold, which is generally low in highly metabolic tissues such as brain, heart, and muscle.

14. Developmental phenomena that occur early are more likely to be under maternal influence than those occurring late. Anterior/posterior and dorsal/ventral orientations are among the earliest to be established, and in organisms in which their study is experimentally and/or genetically approachable, they often show considerable maternal influence. Maternal-effect genes yield products that are not carried over for more than one generation, as is the case with organelle and infectious heredity. Crosses that illustrate the transient nature of a maternal effect could include the following:

Female *Aa* × male *aa* ----> all offspring of the A phenotype. Take a female A phenotype from the above cross and conduct the following mating (note that only half of the offspring from the above cross will be *aa*): *aa* × male *Aa*.

All offspring will be of the a phenotype because all of the offspring will reflect the *genotype* of the mother, not her *phenotype*. This cross illustrates that maternal effects last only one generation. In actual practice, the results of this cross may give a typical 1:1 ratio because the mother may be *Aa* or *aa*.

15. (a) The presence of *bcd⁻/bcd⁻* males can be explained by the maternal effect: mothers were *bcd⁺/bcd⁻*.

(b) The cross

    female *bcd⁺/bcd⁻* × male *bcd⁻/bcd⁻*

will produce an F_1 with normal embryogenesis because of the maternal effect. In the F_2, any cross having *bcd⁺/bcd⁻* mothers will have phenotypically normal embryos. Offspring from any cross involving homozygous *bcd⁻/bcd⁻* mothers will have problems with embryogenesis.

16. (a) Since mitochondrial defects are passed from mother to offspring, one would expect no defects being transferred through the grandfather. With the grandmother expressing the mitochondrial defect, one would expect adherence to a mother-to-offspring inheritance pattern throughout the pedigree.

(b) Each time the defect became homozygous, a mitochondrial disease would probably appear. In the heterozygous state, heteroplasmy would probably result, and a mild form of the disease might result. As defective mitochondria are produced, typical "mother-to-offspring" transmission might follow.

17. (a) Since these disorders involve pools of defective mitochondrial DNA in virtually all cells of the body and a certain percentage of healthy mitochondria is necessary for normal function, a difficulty arises in developing a cure. Somehow the defective mitochondria would need to be corrected for a cure to be achieved, and that appears to be technologically impossible at this time. An alternative, general approach seems reasonable. If one could suppress the replication of mutant mitochondria and favor the replication of normal mitochondria, perhaps a cure would be achieved. In addition to the application of certain drugs and/or restriction endonucleases to select against mutated mitochondria, some evidence suggests that resistance training may increase the level of normal mitochondria in muscle cells.

(b) Mitochondria can be successfully microinjected into mammalian oocytes, where they reproduce and behave as typical, ATP-producing organelles. Through this method, it may be possible to alter the heteroplasmic ratio by microinjection, thereby reducing the likelihood of a child being born with a mitochondrial disease (Smith, P., and Lightowlers, R. 2010. *Journal of Inherited Metabolic Disease*; Van Blerkom, J., et al. 1998. *Human Reproduction*).

18. (a) Note: to provide a meaningful pedigree, several individuals are added to the pedigree that are not listed in the table. Refer to Chapter 3 for information regarding symbols used.

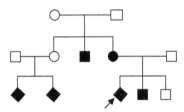

(b, c) If one looks solely at the above pedigree, one could argue that the pattern follows a typical Mendelian recessive. If that's the case, all individuals not showing the phenotype would be heterozygous. However, given that a mitochondrial DNA mutation was identified among affected family members, the pedigree is also consistent with organelle inheritance. Heteroplasmy explains variation in expression and transmission. Although this may seem like an erroneous conclusion at first, consider the range of mutant mitochondria presented in the table. The maternal grandmother has 56 percent mutant mtDNA and could pass a mixed population of mitochondria to her offspring, two of which are symptomatic with percentages of mutant mtDNA above 90 percent. The two maternal cousins (of unknown sex) inherited, by chance, pools of mitochondria with relatively high frequencies (90 percent and 91 percent) of mutant mtDNA and are therefore symptomatic. It appears as if the threshold for phenotypic expression is 85 percent and above.

(d) Transmission of a trait by organelle heredity occurs primarily through the mother, whereas single gene mutations (albinism) can be transmitted through either parent. In addition, because of heteroplasmy, phenotypic expression may vary and transmission patterns may complicate interpretations from pedigrees.

19. (a) The two likely sources of heteroplasmy are likely to be new mutations and/or cytoplasmic inheritance from the mother.

(b) The most likely genetic condition within a given mitochondrion would be some sort of mutator gene such as a faulty polymerase.

Chapter 10: DNA Structure and Analysis

Concept Areas	Corresponding Problems
Central Dogma	1, 2, 3, 7, 8, 9, 26
Transformation	4, 5
Differential Labeling of Macromolecules	6
Genetic Variation	9
Model Building	10, 13, 14, 15, 16, 26, 34
Nucleic Acid Structure	1, 10, 11, 12, 13, 14, 17, 18, 19, 26, 27, 28, 29
Genomic Complexity	1
Analytical Methods	6, 20, 21, 22, 23, 24, 30, 31, 32, 33, 34, 35, 36, 37
Hybridization	24, 31
Mutation	29, 30

Concepts and Processes Checklist

(Check topic when mastered – provide examples where appropriate – understand the context of each entry)

- **The Genetic Material Must Exhibit Four Characteristics**
  - replication
  - storage
  - expression of information
  - variation by mutation
  - partitioned by mitosis and meiosis
  - information flow
  - transcription
  - messenger RNA (mRNA)
  - transfer RNA (tRNA)
  - ribosomal RNA (rRNA)
  - translation
  - central dogma of molecular genetics
  - "DNA makes RNA, which makes proteins"

- **Until 1944, Observations Favored Protein as the Genetic Material**
  - Miescher, 1868
  - nuclein
  - Levene, 1910
  - nucleotides
  - tetranucleotide hypothesis
  - Chargaff, 1940s

- **Evidence Favoring DNA as the Genetic Material...**
  - Avery, MacLeod, McCarty, 1955
  - beginning of molecular genetics

- **Transformation: Early Studies**
  - Griffith
  - *Diplococcus pneumonia*
  - *Streptococcus pneumoniae*

- virulent
- avirulent
- polysaccharide capsule
- shiny-surfaced colonies (*S*)
- rough colonies (*R*)
- serotypes I, II
- II*R*, III*S*
- transformation

- **Transformation: The Avery, MacLeod, and McCarty Experiment**
  - "active factor"
  - deoxyribonuclease (DNase)
  - ribonuclease (RNase)
  - extremely rough (ER)
  - *Haemophilus influenza*
  - *Bacillus subtilis*
  - *Shigella paradysenteriae*
  - *Escherichia coli*

- **The Hershey-Chase Experiment**
  - bacteriophage T2
  - 1952
  - lytic cycle
  - ^{32}P, ^{35}S
  - radioactive labeling

- **Transfection Experiments**
  - protoplasts (spheroplasts)
  - transfection

- **Indirect and Direct Evidence Supports the Concept That DNA Is the Genetic Material in Eukaryotes**

- **Indirect Evidence: Distribution of DNA**
  - nuclear location
  - correlation to ploidy

- **Indirect Evidence: Mutagenesis**
  - ultraviolet (UV) light
  - action spectrum, 260 nm, 280 nm

- **Direct Evidence: Recombinant DNA Studies**
  - recombinant DNA technology
  - transgenic animals

- **RNA Serves as the Genetic Material in Some Viruses**
  - RNA core
  - tobacco mosaic virus
  - RNA replicase
  - retroviruses
  - reverse transcription
  - reverse transcriptase
  - HIV

- **Knowledge of Nucleic Acid Chemistry Is Essential to the Understanding of DNA Structure**

- **Nucleotides: Building Blocks of Nucleic Acids**
  - nucleotides
  - nitrogenous bas
  - pentose sugar
  - phosphate group
  - purine
  - pyrimidine
  - adenine
  - guanine
  - cytosine
  - thymine
  - uracil
  - ribose

- deoxyribose
- 2-deoxyribose
- nucleoside

- **Nucleoside Diphosphates and Triphosphates**
  - nucleoside monophosphate (NMP)
  - nucleoside diphosphate (NDP)
  - nucleoside triphosphate (NTP)
  - adenosine triphosphate (ATP)
  - guanosine triphosphate (GTP)

- **Polynucleotides**
  - phosphodiester bond
  - C-5′ end
  - C-3′ end
  - polynucleotide chain
  - variation
  - 1000 nucleotides = 4^{1000} combinations

- **The Structure of DNA Holds the Key to Understanding Its Function**
  - Chargaff
  - Wilkins
  - Franklin
  - Pauling
  - Crick
  - Watson
  - 1940 to 1953
  - journal *Nature*
  - base composition
  - X-ray diffraction

- **Base-Composition Studies**
  - Chargaff
  - adenine proportional to thymine

- guanine proportional to cytosine
- purines (A + G) = pyrimidines (C + T)
- percentage of (G + C)
- percentage of (A + T)

- **X-Ray Diffraction Analysis**
  - Pauling
  - Franklin
  - Wilkins
  - Astbury

- **The Watson-Crick Model**
  - 1953
  - two chains, right-handed double helix
  - antiparallel
  - bases stacked
  - nitrogenous bases paired
  - A = T, G = C
  - 34 Å per turn (3.4 nm)
  - major groove
  - minor groove
  - 20 Å diameter (2.0 nm)
  - 5′-to-3′ orientation
  - 3′-to-5′ orientation
  - Z-DNA
  - complementarity
  - hydrogen bond
  - electrostatic attraction
  - G,C three hydrogen bonds
  - A,T two hydrogen bonds
  - hydrophobic nitrogenous bases
  - horizontal stacking

- sugar-phosphate backbone
- "Molecular Structure of Nucleic Acids: A Structure for Deoxyribose Nucleic Acid," published in *Nature*

- **Alternative Forms of DNA Exist**
  - A-DNA
  - B-DNA
  - single X-ray analysis
  - C-DNA
  - P-DNA
  - D-DNA
  - E-DNA
  - Z-DNA
  - left-handed double helix

- **The Structure of RNA Is Chemically Similar to DNA, but Single Stranded**
  - most single stranded, but exceptions
  - ribosomal RNA (rRNA)
  - messenger RNA (mRNA)
  - transfer RNA (tRNA)
  - uracil replaces thymine in RNA
  - sedimentation behavior
  - Svedberg coefficient (*S*)
  - ribosomes
  - telomerase RNa
  - small nuclear RNA (snRNA)
  - antisense RNA
  - microRNA (miRNA)
  - short interfering RNA (siRNA)

- **Many Analytical Techniques Have Been Useful During the Investigation of DNA and RNA**

- **Absorption of Ultraviolet Light**
  - 254 to 260 nm

- **Denaturation and Renaturation of Nucleic Acids**
  - denature
  - hyperchromic shift
  - melting profile
  - melting temperature (T_m)
  - perfect complementarity

- **Molecular Hybridization**
  - DNA:RNA duplex
  - radioisotope tag
  - DNA blotting
  - DNA microarray analysis

- **Fluorescent *in situ* Hybridization (FISH)**
  - probe
  - complementarity
  - biotin
  - avidin, streptavidin
  - fluorescein

- **Reassociation Kinetics and Repetitive DNA**
  - rate of reassociation
  - reassociation kinetics
  - repetitive DNA sequences
  - unique DNA sequences

- **Electrophoresis of Nucleic Acids**
  - electrophoresis
  - resolution of molecules
  - electrical field
  - agarose gel

F10.1 Illustration of relationships among DNA, its functions, and related products.

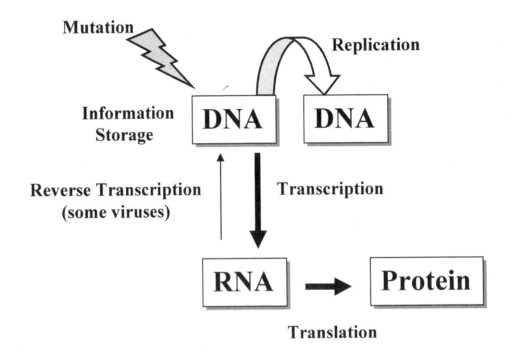

Chapter 10 DNA Structure and Analysis

Answers to Now Solve This

10-1. In theory, the general design would be appropriate in that some substance, if labeled, would show up in the progeny of transformed bacteria. However, since the amount of transforming DNA is extremely small compared with the genomic DNA of the recipient bacterium and its progeny, it would be technically difficult to assay for the labeled nucleic acid. In addition, it would be necessary to know that the small stretch of DNA that caused the genetic transformation was actually labeled.

10-2. Guanine = 17.5 percent; adenine and thymine both = 32.5 percent.

10-3. Assuming that the value of 1.13 is statistically different from 1.00, one can conclude that rubella is a single-stranded RNA virus.

Chapter 10 DNA Structure and Analysis
Solutions to Problems and Discussion Questions

1. (a) Major lines of evidence that DNA is the genetic material originally came from experiments using bacteria and bacteriophages. Transformation studies showed that DNA is the genetic material in bacteria, and differential labeling (proteins and nucleic acids) of bacteriophage T2 showed that DNA is the genetic material in some viruses.

(b) Both direct and indirect studies have shown that DNA is the genetic material in eukaryotes. Other than in mitochondria and chloroplasts, DNA is localized in the nucleus where its quantity varies with ploidy (n, $2n$) as one would predict for the genetic material. In addition, the action spectrum of UV light overlaps the absorption spectrum of DNA. Direct evidence comes from recombinant DNA studies in which transgenic organisms can be generated with transferred DNA.

(c, d) Given base composition studies showing proportional amounts of A and T, and G and C, and X-ray diffraction studies, Watson and Crick showed that hydrogen bonding between the bases provided attraction and stability for a DNA double helix. DNA melting supports this arrangement.

(e) Rapidly renaturing sequences were discovered by Britten and Kohne. They suggested and later showed that such sequences were repetitive.

2. Your essay should include a description of structural aspects including sugar and base content comparisons. In addition, you should mention complementation aspects, strandedness, flexibility, and conformation.

3. Prior to 1940, most of the interest in genetics centered on the transmission of similarity and variation from parents to offspring (transmission genetics). Whereas some experiments examined the possible nature of the hereditary material, abundant knowledge of the structural and enzymatic properties of proteins generated a bias that worked to favor proteins as the hereditary substance. In addition, proteins were composed of as many as 20 different subunits (amino acids), thereby providing ample structural and functional variation for the multiple tasks that must be accomplished by the genetic material. The tetranucleotide hypothesis (structure) provided insufficient variability to account for the diverse roles of the genetic material.

4. Griffith performed experiments with different strains of *Diplococcus pneumoniae* in which a heat-killed pathogen, when injected into a mouse with a live non-pathogenic strain, eventually led to the mouse's death. A summary of this experiment is provided in the text. Examination of the dead mouse revealed living pathogenic bacteria. Griffith suggested that the heat-killed virulent (pathogenic) bacteria transformed the avirulent (non-pathogenic) strain into a virulent strain. Avery and coworkers systematically searched for the transforming principle originating from the heat-killed pathogenic strain and determined it to be DNA. Taylor showed that transformed bacteria are capable of serving as donors of transforming DNA, indicating that the process of transformation involves a stable alteration in the genetic material (DNA).

5. Transformation is dependent on a macromolecule (DNA) that can be extracted and purified from bacteria. During such purification, however, other macromolecular species may contaminate the DNA. Specific degradative enzymes, proteases, RNase, and DNase were used to selectively eliminate components of the extract, and, if transformation is concomitantly eliminated, then the eliminated fraction is the transforming principle. DNase eliminates DNA and transformation; therefore, it must be the transforming principle.

6. Nucleic acids contain large amounts of phosphorus and no sulfur, whereas proteins contain sulfur and no phosphorus. Therefore, the radioisotopes ^{32}P and ^{35}S will selectively label nucleic acids and proteins, respectively. The Hershey–Chase experiment was based on the premise that the substance injected into the bacterium is the substance responsible for producing the progeny phage and, therefore, must be the hereditary material. The experiment demonstrated that most of the ^{32}P-labeled material (DNA) was injected, whereas the phage ghosts (protein coats) remained outside the bacterium. Therefore, the nucleic acid must be the genetic material.

7. Actually, phosphorus is found in approximately equal amounts in DNA and RNA. Therefore, labeling with ^{32}P would "tag" both RNA and DNA. However, the T2 phage, in its mature state, contains very little, if any, RNA; therefore, DNA would be interpreted as being the genetic material in T2 phage.

8. The early evidence would be considered indirect in that at no time was there an experiment, like transformation in bacteria, in which genetic information in one organism was transferred to another using DNA. Rather, by comparing DNA content in various cell types (sperm and somatic cells) and observing that the *action* and *absorption* spectra of ultraviolet light were correlated, DNA was considered to be the genetic material. This suggestion was supported by the fact that DNA was shown to be the genetic material in bacteria and some phages. Direct evidence for DNA being the genetic material comes from a variety of observations including gene transfer, which has been facilitated by recombinant DNA techniques.

9. Some viruses contain a genetic material composed of RNA. The tobacco mosaic virus is composed of an RNA core and a protein coat. "Crosses" can be made in which the protein coat and RNA of TMV are interchanged with another strain (Holmes ribgrass). The source of the RNA determines the type of lesion; thus, RNA is the genetic material in these viruses. Retroviruses contain RNA as the genetic material and use an enzyme known as *reverse transcriptase* to produce DNA that can be integrated into the host chromosome. See F10.1.

10. The structure of deoxyadenylic acid is given below and in the text. Linkages among the three components require the removal of water (H_2O).

11. The numbering of the carbons on the sugar is especially important (see following diagram). Examine the text for the numbers on the carbons and nitrogens of the bases:

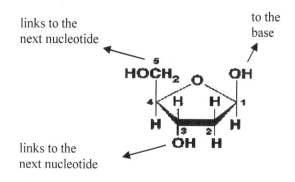

links to the
next nucleotide

to the
base

links to the
next nucleotide

12. Examine the structures of the bases in the text. The other bases would be named as follows:

Guanine:	2-amino-6-oxypurine
Cytosine:	2-oxy-4-aminopyrimidine
Thymine:	2, 4-dioxy-5-methylpyrimidine
Uracil:	2, 4-dioxypyrimidine

13. Examine the text for the format for this drawing. Note that the complementary strand must be drawn in the antiparallel orientation.

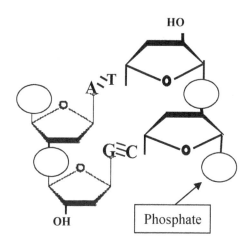

14. The following are characteristics of the Watson-Crick double-helix model for DNA:

The base composition is such that A = T, G = C, and (A + G) = (C + T). Bases are stacked 0.34 nm (3.4 Angstoms) apart and in a plectonic, antiparallel manner. There is one complete turn for each 3.4 nm that constitutes 10 bases per turn. Hydrogen bonds hold the two polynucleotide chains together, each being formed by phosphodiester linkages between the five-carbon sugars and the phosphates. There are two hydrogen bonds forming the A to T pair and three forming the G to C pair. The double helix exists as a twisted structure, approximately 20 Angstroms in diameter, with a topography of major and minor grooves. The hydrophobic bases are located in the center of the molecule; the hydrophilic phosphodiester backbone is on the outside.

15. In addition to creative "genius" and perseverance, model-building skills, and the conviction that the structure would turn out to be "simple" and have a natural beauty in its simplicity, Watson and Crick employed the X-ray diffraction information of Franklin and Wilkins and the base ratio information of Chargaff.

16. Because in double-stranded DNA, A = T and G = C (within limits of experimental error), the data presented would have indicated a lack of pairing of these bases in favor of a single-stranded structure or some other non-hydrogen-bonded structure.

Alternatively, from the data it would appear that A = C and T = G, which would negate the chance for typical hydrogen bonding since opposite charge relationships do not exist. Therefore, it is quite unlikely that a tight helical structure would form at all. In conclusion, Watson and Crick might have concluded that hydrogen bonding is not a significant factor in maintaining a double-stranded structure.

17. A covalent bond is a relatively strong bond that involves the sharing of electrons between two or more atoms. Hydrogen bonds, much weaker than covalent bonds, are formed as a result of

electrostatic attraction between a covalently bonded hydrogen atom and an atom with an unshared electron pair. The hydrogen atom assumes a partial positive charge, while the unshared electron pair—characteristic of covalently bonded oxygen and nitrogen atoms—assumes a partial negative charge. These opposite charges are responsible for the weak chemical attraction (Klug et al.).

Complementarity, responsible for the chemical attraction between adenine and thymine (uracil) and guanine and cytosine, is responsible for DNA and RNA assuming their double-stranded character. Complementarity is based on hydrogen bonding.

18. Three main differences between RNA and DNA are the following:

(1) uracil in RNA replaces thymine in DNA,
(2) ribose in RNA replaces deoxyribose in DNA, and
(3) RNA often occurs as both single- and partially double-stranded forms, whereas DNA most often occurs in a double-stranded form.

19. Although there are many types of RNA, the three main types described in this section are presented below:

ribosomal RNA: rRNA combines with proteins to form ribosomes that function to align mRNA and charged tRNA molecules during translation.

transfer RNA: tRNAs are involved in protein synthesis in that they represent a "link" between the codes in DNA (as reflected in mRNA) and the ordering of amino acids in proteins. Transfer RNAs are specific in that each species is attached to only one type of amino acid.

messenger RNA: The genetic code in DNA is transferred to the site of protein synthesis by a relatively short-lived molecule called messenger RNA. In eukaryotes, mRNA carries genetic information from the nucleus to the cytoplasm. It is the sequence of bases in mRNA that specifies the order of amino acids in proteins.

20. The nitrogenous bases of nucleic acids (nucleosides, nucleotides, and single- and double-stranded polynucleotides) absorb UV light maximally at wavelengths of 254 to 260 nm. Using this phenomenon, one can often determine the presence and concentration of nucleic acids in a mixture. Since proteins absorb UV light maximally at 280 nm, this is a relatively simple way of dealing with mixtures of biologically important molecules. UV absorption is greater in single-stranded molecules (hyperchromic shift) as compared with double-stranded structures; therefore, one can easily determine, by applying denaturing conditions, whether a nucleic acid is in the single- or double-stranded form. In addition, A-T rich DNA denatures more readily than G-C rich DNA; therefore, one can estimate base content by denaturation kinetics.

21. Various treatments, heat, and certain chemical environments cause separation of the hydrogen bonds that hold together the complementary strands of DNA. Under these conditions, double-stranded DNA is changed to single-stranded DNA.

22. *A hyperchromic effect* is the increased absorption of UV light as double-stranded DNA (or RNA for that matter) is converted to single-stranded DNA. As illustrated in the text, the change in absorption is quite significant, with a structure of higher G-C content *melting* at a higher temperature than an A-T rich nucleic acid. If one monitors the UV absorption with a spectrophotometer during the melting process, the hyperchromic shift can be observed. The T_m is the point on the profile (temperature) at which half (50 percent) of the sample is denatured.

23. Because G-C base pairs are formed with three hydrogen bonds, whereas A-T base pairs by two such bonds, it takes more energy (higher temperature) to separate G-C pairs.

24. The reassociation of separate complementary strands of a nucleic acid, either DNA or RNA, is based on hydrogen bonds forming between A-T (or U) and G-C.

25. In one of Watson and Crick's papers in *Nature*, they state,

> It has not escaped our notice that the specific pairing we have postulated immediately suggests a possible copying mechanism for the genetic material.

The model itself indicates that unwinding of the helix and separation of the double-stranded structure into two single strands immediately expose the specific hydrogen bonds through which new bases are brought into place.

26. (1) As shown, the extra phosphate is not normally expected.

(2) In the adenine ring, a nitrogen is at position 8 rather than position 9.

(3) The bond from the C-1' to the sugar should form with the N at position 9 (N-9) of the adenine.

(4) The dinucleotide is a "deoxy" form; therefore, each C-2' should not have a hydroxyl group. Notice the hydroxyl group at C-2' on the sugar of the adenylic acid.

(5) At the C-5 position on the thymine residue, there should be a methyl group.

(6) There are too many bonds between the N-3 and C-2 of thymine.

(7) There are too few bonds (should be a double bond) between the C-5 and C-6 of thymine.

27. (a) = right, (b) = left

28. Since cytosine pairs with guanine and uracil pairs with adenine, the result would be a base substitution of G:C to A:T after two rounds of replication.

29. Under this condition, the hydrolyzed 5-methyl cytosine becomes thymine.

30. Fluorescence *in situ* hybridization employs fluorescently labeled DNA that hybridizes to metaphase chromosomes and interphase nuclei. A FISH survey is considered interpretable if hybridization is consistent in 70 percent or more cells examined. Results are available in one to two days after the sample is tested. Because of the relatively high likelihood of aneuploidy for chromosomes 13, 18, 21, X, and Y, they are routine candidates for analysis.

31. One of the basic principles of gel electrophoresis is that shorter molecules migrate at a faster rate through a given gel than longer ones. Although a number of factors other than agarose concentration would be involved, depending on the length of the gel, it might be wise to use the 1.5 percent agarose recipe so that the short fragments will not reach the end of the gel, and enter the buffer, before the longer ones leave the wells.

32. (a) The X-ray diffraction studies would indicate a helical structure, for it is on the basis of such data that a helical pattern is suggested. The fact that it is irregular may indicate different diameters (base pairings), additional strands in the helix, kinking, or bending.

(b) The hyperchromic shift would indicate considerable hydrogen bonding, possibly caused by base pairing.

(c) Such data may suggest irregular base pairing in which purines bind purines (all the bases presented are purines), thus giving the atypical dimensions.

(d) Because of the presence of ribose, the molecule may show more flexibility, kinking, and/or folding.

Although there are several situations possible for this model, the phosphates are still likely to be far apart (on the outside) because of their strong like charges. Hydrogen bonding probably exists on the inside of the molecule, and there is probably considerable flexibility, kinking, and/or bending.

33. (a, b, c) Without knowing the exact bonding characteristics of hypoxanthine or xanthine, it may be difficult to predict the likelihood of each pairing type. It is likely that both are of the same class (purine or pyrimidine) because the names of the molecules indicate a similarity. In addition, the diameter of the structure is constant, which, under the model to follow, would be expected. In fact, hypoxanthine and xanthine are both purines.

Because there are equal amounts of A, T, and H, one could suggest that they are hydrogen bonded to one another; the same may be said for C, G, and X. Given the molar equivalence of erythrose and phosphate, an alternating sugar-phosphate-sugar backbone, as in "earth-type" DNA, would be acceptable. A model of a triple helix would be acceptable, since the diameter is constant. Given the chemical similarities to "earth-type" DNA, it is probable that the unique creature's DNA follows the same structural plan.

34. (1) Heat application would yield a hyperchromic shift if the DNA is double stranded. One could also get a rough estimation of the GC content from the kinetics of denaturation and the degree of sequence complexity from comparative renaturation studies.

(2) Determination of base content by hydrolysis and chromatography could be used for comparative purposes and could also provide evidence as to the strandedness of the DNA.

(3) Antibodies for Z-DNA could be used to determine the degree of left-handed structures, if present.

(4) Sequencing the DNA from both viruses would indicate sequence homology. In addition, through various electronic searches readily available on the Internet (Web site: http://blast.ncbi.nlm.nih.gov/Blast .cgi, for example), one could determine whether similar sequences exist in other viruses or in other organisms.

35. The way the question is stated suggests that DNA that is separated electrophoretically is of the same shape (long rod). In fact, DNA can exist in a variety of shapes, as seen in supercoiled plasmids, relaxed (nicked) plasmids, and linear molecules. Size comparisons with DNA must be such that linear molecules are compared with linear molecules and supercoiled with supercoiled, and so on. In comparing DNA migration with RNA, even though RNA molecules have the same charge to mass ratios, they also exist in a variety of shapes. Complementary intra-strand base pairing can make more compact structures compared with the more relaxed, open conformation. For electrophoretic size comparisons, RNA molecules must be denatured to eliminate secondary structural variables.

36. The mobility of DNA through a gel is dependent on a number of factors, including the concentration of the gel, strength of the current, ionic strength of the buffer, and the conformation of the DNA as stated in the problem. In general, superhelical/supercoiled DNA (form I) migrates the fastest, followed by linear DNA (form III). The slowest to migrate is usually the loose circle (form II).

37. In general, as the percentage of GC pairs increases, the T_m increases. This is to be expected because there are three hydrogen bonds that hold GC pairs together instead of two that hold AT pairs. Therefore, it takes more energy to break GC pairs than AT pairs.

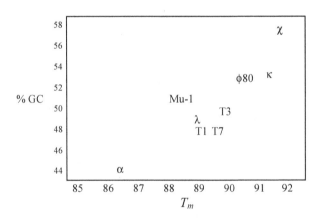

Chapter 11: DNA Replication and Recombination

Concept Areas	Corresponding Problems
Replication	1, 2, 3, 4, 5, 14, 16, 17, 18, 19, 25, 26, 27, 28, 29, 30, 31, 35
Nearest-Neighbor Analysis	10, 34
Enzymology	1, 6, 7, 8, 9, 11, 12, 13, 15, 21, 24
Conditional Mutations	20, 23, 32, 33
Gene Conversion	22

Concepts and Processes Checklist

(Check topic when mastered – provide examples where appropriate – understand the context of each entry)

- **DNA Is Reproduced by Semiconservative Replication**

    - Watson and Crick double helix

    - template function

    - complementarity

    - adenylic acid (A)

    - thymidylic acid (T)

    - guanidylic acid (G)

    - cytidylic acid (C)

    - semiconservative replication

    - conservative replication

    - dispersive replication

- **The Meselson-Stahl Experiment**

    - semiconservative replication

    - bacteria (*E. coli*)

    - $^{15}N_4Cl$ (ammonium chloride)

    - ^{14}N

    - sedimentation equilibrium centrifugation

- buoyant density gradient centrifucation

- "new" synthesis of DNA

- hybrid molecule

- intermediate density

- **Semiconservative Replication in Eukaryotes**

    - *Vicia faba*

    - Taylor, Woods, and Hughes, 1957

    - autoradiography

    - radioisotope

    - "grains"

    - colchicines

    - sister chromatid exchanges

- **Origins, Forks, and Units of Replication**

    - origin of replication

    - unidirectional or bidirectional

    - replication fork

    - replicon

- ○ *E. coli*
- ○ bacteriophages
- ○ 4.6 Mb
- ○ Cairns
- ○ bidirectional
- ○ *oriC*
- ○ *ter*

- ○ **DNA Synthesis in Bacteria Involves Five Polymerases, as Well as Other Enzymes**
  - ○ semiconservative and bidirectional

- ○ **DNA Polymerase I**
  - ○ Kornberg 1957
  - ○ *E. coli*
  - ○ cell-free system
  - ○ *in vitro* DNA synthesis
  - ○ all four deoxyribonucleoside triphosphates
  - ○ dNTPs
  - ○ template DNA
  - ○ 5'-carbon
  - ○ 3'-OH group
  - ○ chain elongation
  - ○ fidelity
  - ○ addition at 3'-OH end
  - ○ comparison of base compositions

- ○ **DNA Polymerase II, III, IV, and V**
  - ○ *polA1*
  - ○ DNA repair
  - ○ ultraviolet light (UV)
  - ○ radiation
  - ○ damage DNA
  - ○ DNA polymerase II

- ○ primer
- ○ excess of 100,000 daltons
- ○ 3' to 5' exonuclease activity
- ○ DNA polymerase III
- ○ 5' to 3' polymerization
- ○ *in vivo* replication
- ○ exonuclease activity
- ○ removal of primer
- ○ polymerase II, IV, and V
- ○ DNA repair
- ○ holoenzyme
- ○ core enzyme
- ○ sliding DNA clamp
- ○ sliding clamp loader
- ○ replisome

- ○ **Many Complex Issues Must Be Resolved during DNA Replication**
  - ○ antiparallel orientation
  - ○ two replication forks
  - ○ opposite direction
  - ○ localized unwinding
  - ○ RNA primer
  - ○ continuous synthesis
  - ○ discontinuous synthesis
  - ○ proofreading

- ○ **Unwinding the DNA Helix**
  - ○ *oriC*
  - ○ 245 nucleotide pairs
  - ○ repeating sequences (9mers and 13mers)
  - ○ DnaA
  - ○ DnaB

- DnaC
- helicase
- single-stranded binding proteins (SSBs)
- supercoiling
- DNA gyrase
- DNA topoisomerase
- double-stranded cuts
- replisome
- **Initiation of DNA Synthesis Using an RNA primer**
  - RNA primer 10–12 nucleotides
  - primase
  - provides free 3'-OH group
  - removal of RNA primer
- **Continuous and Discontinuous DNA Synthesis**
  - antiparallel
  - continuous DNA synthesis
  - leading strand
  - discontinuous DNA synthesis
  - lagging strand
  - Okazaki fragment
  - DNA ligase
  - *lig*
- **Concurrent Synthesis Occurs on the Leading and Lagging Strands**
  - DNA polymerase III
  - 1000 to 2000 nucleotides
  - looping
  - holoenzyme
  - core enzyme

- β-subunit clamp
- sliding clamp
- **Proofreading and Error Correction Occurs during DNA Replication**
  - noncomplementary nucleotide
  - proofreading
  - epsilon subunit
- **A Coherent Model Summarizes DNA Replication**
- **Replication Is Controlled by a Variety of Genes**
  - *polA1*
  - ligase-deficient
  - proofreading-deficient
  - conditional mutation
  - temperature-sensitive mutation
  - permissive
  - lethal knockouts
- **Eukaryotic DNA Replication Is Similar to Replication in Prokaryotes, but Is More Complex**
  - bidirectional
  - nucleosomes
  - linear chromosomes
- **Initiation at Multiple Replication Origins**
  - 2000 nucleotides per minute
  - 25 times slower than prokaryotes
  - autonomously replicating sequences (ARSs)
  - consensus sequence
  - 11 base pairs
  - prereplication complex (pre-RC)

- origin of replication complex (ORC)
- G1 phase of cell cycle
- kinases
- phosphorylation
- **Multiple Eukaryotic DNA Polymerases**
  - low processivity
  - polymerase switching
  - translesion synthesis (TLS)
- **Replication through Chromatin**
  - chromatin
  - histone proteins
  - nonhistone proteins
  - rapid reassociation
  - chromatin assembly factors (CAFs)
  - the ends of linear chromosomes are problematic during replication
  - telomeres
  - double-stranded breaks (DSBs)
- **Telomere Structure**
  - *Tetrahymena*
  - TTGGGG
  - G-rich
  - C-rich
  - TTAGGG
  - G-quartets
  - t-loops
- **Replication at the Telomere**
  - telomerase
  - gene-coding regions
  - guide and template
  - reverse transcription
- primase
- DNA polymerase
- DNA ligase
- TERC
- TERT
- **DNA Recombination, Like DNA Replication, Is Directed by Specific Enzymes**
  - genetic recombination
  - homologous molecules
  - homologous recombination
  - heteroduplex DNA molecules
  - branch migration
  - zipper-like action
  - Holliday structure
  - endonucleae
  - ligation
  - RecA protein
  - Rad51
  - Rad52
  - Rad55
  - Rad57
  - BRCA2
  - RecB, RecC, RecD
- **Gene Conversion, a Consequence of DNA Recombination**
  - gene conversion
  - *Neurospora*
  - no reciprocal product
  - correction of mismatch
  - 3:1 or 1:3

F11.1 Illustration of the mode of action of spleen phosphodiesterase.

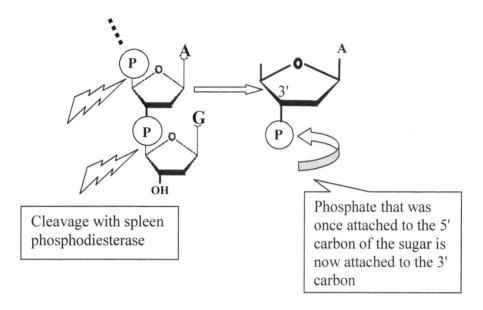

Cleavage with spleen phosphodiesterase

Phosphate that was once attached to the 5' carbon of the sugar is now attached to the 3' carbon

F11.2 Shorthand structures for 3' and 5' nucleotides.

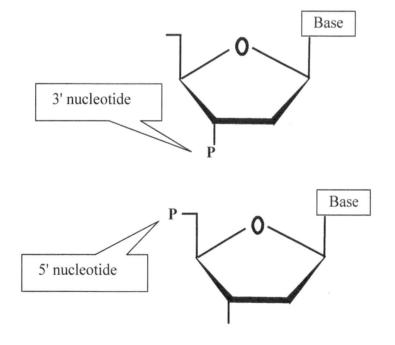

Base

3' nucleotide

Base

5' nucleotide

F11.3 Illustration of the influence of a conditional mutation on protein structure and function.

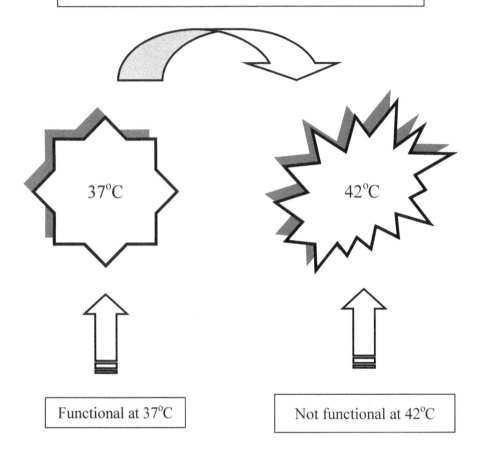

Changes in the environment of the protein may cause conformational changes in the protein to alter function of that protein.

37°C

42°C

Functional at 37°C

Not functional at 42°C

F11.4 Figure relating to problem #5 in the text depicts labeling pattern under conservative and dispersive replication patterns.

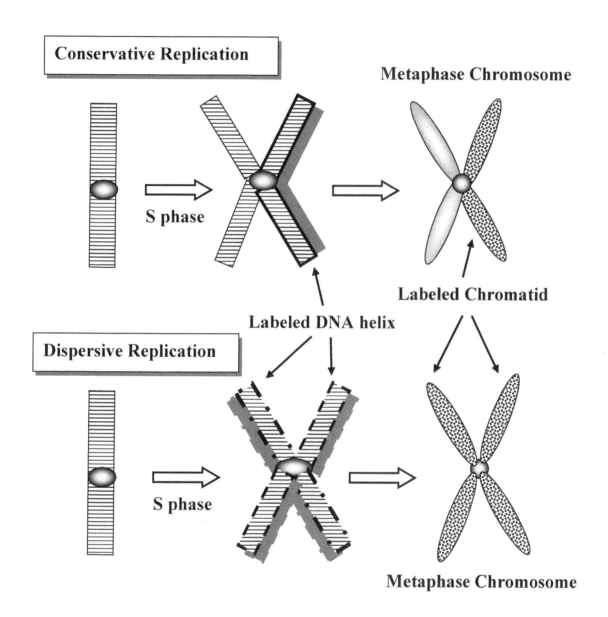

Conservative Replication

Metaphase Chromosome

S phase

Labeled Chromatid

Labeled DNA helix

Dispersive Replication

S phase

Metaphase Chromosome

Answers to Now Solve This

11-1. Under a conservative scheme, the first round of replication in ^{14}N medium produces one dense double helix and one light double helix in contrast with the intermediate density of the DNA in the semiconservative mode. Therefore, after one round of replication in the ^{14}N medium, the conservative scheme can be ruled out. After one round of replication in ^{14}N under a dispersive model, the DNA is of intermediate density, just as it is in the semiconservative model. However, in the next round of replication in ^{14}N medium, the density of the DNA is between the intermediate and light densities.

11-2. If the DNA contained parallel strands in the double helix and the polymerase would be able to accommodate such parallel strands, there would be continuous synthesis and no Okazaki fragments. Several other possibilities exist. If the DNA was replicated as single strands, the synthesis could begin at the free ends, and there would be no need for Okazaki fragments.

Chapter 11 DNA Replication and Recombination

Solutions to Problems and Discussion Questions

1. (a) Two classic experiments, one using *E. coli* and the other using *Vicia faba,* demonstrated, using density and radioisotope labeling, respectively, that replication is semiconservative in prokaryotes and eukaryotes. In both cases, daughter DNA molecules are each composed of one parental strand and one newly synthesized DNA strand.

(b) A mutant in DNA polymerase I (*polA1*) was nevertheless capable of synthesizing biologically active DNA, leading to the conclusion that at least one other enzyme is responsible for replicating DNA *in vivo.*

(c) *In vitro* studies by Kornberg and coworkers indicated that DNA strand elongation occurs by addition of nucleotides at the 3' end. During chain elongation, two of the outer phosphates of the precursor dNTP are cleaved, and the remaining phosphate attaches to the 3'-OH group of the deoxyribose. *In vivo* or *in vitro*, DNA polymerases, including polymerase III, are capable of only 5' to 3' synthesis.

(d) Two lines of evidence indicated that DNA synthesis is discontinuous. First, in newly formed DNA, relatively short nucleotide fragments are hydrogen bonded to the template strands. Second, these short nucleotide fragments accumulate in ligase-deficient mutants of *E. coli.*

(e) Because eukaryotic chromosomes are linear rather than circular, free ends exist. It was predicted that such free ends would create the problem of shortening because of the 5'–3' nature of DNA synthesis and the inability of DNA polymerases to initiate synthesis without a free 3'-OH. The finding of the telomerase enzyme and a number of terminal repeats at the ends of chromosomes provided supported the prediction of chromosome shortening and its solution.

2. Your essay should describe replication as the process of making daughter nucleic acids from existing ones. Synthesis refers to the precise series of steps, components, and reactions that allow such replication to occur.

3. The differences among the three models of DNA replication relate to the manner in which the new strands of DNA are oriented as daughter DNA molecules are produced.

Conservative: In the conservative scheme, the original double helix remains as a complete unit, and the new DNA double helix is produced as a single unit. The old DNA is completely conserved.

Semiconservative: In the semiconservative scheme, each daughter strand is composed of one old DNA strand and one new DNA strand. Separation of hydrogen bonds is required.

Dispersive: In the dispersive scheme, the original DNA strand is broken into pieces and the new DNA in the daughter strand is interspersed among the old pieces. Separation of the individual covalent, phosphodiester bonds is required for this mode of replication.

4. By labeling the pool of nitrogenous bases of the DNA of *E. coli* with the heavy isotope ^{15}N, it would be possible to "follow" the "old" DNA. This was accomplished by growing the cells for many generations in medium containing ^{15}N. Cells were transferred to ^{14}N medium so that "new" DNA could be detected. A comparison of the density of DNA samples at various times in the experiment (initial ^{15}N culture and subsequent cultures grown in the ^{14}N medium) showed that after one round of replication in the ^{14}N medium, the DNA was half as dense (intermediate) as the DNA from bacteria grown only in the ^{15}N medium. In a sample taken after two rounds of replication in the ^{14}N medium, half of the DNA was of the intermediate density and the other half was as dense as DNA containing only ^{14}N DNA.

5. Refer to the text for an illustration of the labeling of *Vicia* chromosomes under a Taylor, Woods, and Hughes experimental design. Notice that only those cells that pass through the S phase in the presence of the ^{3}H-thymidine are labeled and that each double helix (per chromatid) is "half labeled." See Figure F11.4 in this book for a graphic description of these conservative and dispersive replication patterns.

(a) Under a conservative scheme, all of the newly labeled DNA will go to one sister chromatid, and the other sister chromatid will remain unlabeled. In contrast to a semiconservative scheme, the first replicative round would produce one sister chromatid, which has labels on both strands of the double helix (see F11.4).

(b) Under a dispersive scheme, all of the newly labeled DNA will be interspersed with unlabeled DNA. Because these preparations (metaphase chromosomes) are highly coiled and condensed structures derived from the "spread-out" form at interphase (which includes the S phase), it is impossible to detect the areas where label is not found. Rather, both sister chromatids would appear as evenly labeled structures (see F11.4).

6. The *in vitro* replication requires a DNA template, a divalent cation (Mg^{2+}), and all four of the deoxyribonucleoside triphosphates: dATP, dCTP, dTTP, and dGTP. The lowercase "d" refers to the deoxyribose sugar.

7. Prior to the development of highly efficient methods of enzyme isolation, large cultures containing large numbers of bacterial cells were needed to yield even small quantities of enzymes.

8. Two general analytical approaches showed that the products of DNA polymerase I were probably copies of the template DNA. Because *base composition* can be similar without reflecting sequence similarity, the least stringent test was the comparison of base composition. By comparing *nearest-neighbor frequencies*, Kornberg determined that there is a very high likelihood that the product is of the same base sequence as the template.

9. The *in vitro* rate of DNA synthesis using DNA polymerase I is slow, being more effective at replicating single-stranded DNA than double-stranded DNA. In addition, it is capable of degrading as well as synthesizing DNA. Such degradation suggests that it functioned as a repair enzyme. In addition, DeLucia and Cairns discovered a strain of *E. coli* (*polA1*) that still replicates its DNA but is deficient in DNA polymerase I activity.

10. An exposed 3'-OH group is necessary for the attachment of the next nucleotide. The 3'-OH group is eventually removed in the form of water, and a covalent bond is formed to the 5'-phosphate of the added nucleotide.

11. The *polA1* mutation was instrumental in demonstrating that DNA polymerase I activity was not necessary for the *in vivo* replication of the *E. coli* chromosome. Such an observation opened the door for the discovery of other enzymes involved in DNA replication.

12. All three enzymes share several common properties. First, none can *initiate* DNA synthesis on a template, but all can *elongate* an existing DNA strand assuming there is a template strand as shown in the following figure. Polymerization of nucleotides occurs in the 5' to 3' direction, where each 5' phosphate is added to the 3' end of the growing polynucleotide.

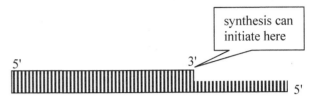

All three enzymes are large, complex proteins with a molecular weight in excess of 100,000 daltons, and each has 3' to 5' exonuclease activity. Refer to the text.

DNA polymerase I:
  5'–3' exonuclease activity
  present in large amounts
  relatively stable
  removal of RNA primer

DNA polymerase II:
  possibly involved in repair function

DNA polymerase III:
  essential for replication
  complex molecule

13. Refer to the text for a listing of the components of DNA polymerase III. The active form of the enzyme is called the holoenzyme. The region responsible for actual polymerization is called the "core" portion.

14. Given a stretch of double-stranded DNA, one could initiate synthesis at a given point and replicate strands either in one direction only (unidirectional) or in both directions (bidirectional) as shown below. Notice that in the text the synthesis of complementary strands occurs in a *continuous* $5' > 3'$ mode on the leading strand in the direction of the replication fork, and in a *discontinuous* $5' > 3'$ mode on the lagging strand opposite the direction of the replication fork. Such discontinuous replication forms Okazaki fragments.

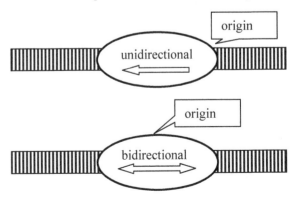

Chapter 11 DNA Replication and Recombination

15. *Helicase, dna*A, and *single-stranded* DNA *binding* proteins initially unwind, open, and stabilize DNA at the initiation point. DNA *gyrase*, a DNA topoisomerase, relieves supercoiling generated by helix unwinding. This process involves breaking both strands of the DNA helix.

16. (a) *Okazaki fragments* are relatively short (1000 to 2000 bases in prokaryotes) DNA fragments that are synthesized in a discontinuous fashion on the lagging strand during DNA replication. Such fragments appear to be necessary because template DNA is not available for $5' > 3'$ synthesis until some degree of continuous DNA synthesis occurs on the leading strand in the direction of the replication fork. The isolation of such fragments provides support for the scheme of replication shown in the text.

(b) *DNA ligase* is required to form phosphodiester linkages in gaps, which are generated when DNA polymerase I removes RNA primer and meets newly synthesized DNA ahead of it. Notice in the text that the discontinuous DNA strands are ligated together into a single continuous strand.

(c) *Primer RNA* is formed by RNA primase to serve as an initiation point for the production of DNA strands on a DNA template. None of the DNA polymerases are capable of initiating synthesis without a free 3' hydroxyl group. The primer RNA provides that group and thus can be used by DNA polymerase III.

17. The synthesis of DNA is thought to follow the pattern described in the text. The model involves opening and stabilizing the DNA helix, priming DNA synthesis with RNA primer, and moving replication forks in both directions, which includes elongation of RNA primers in continuous and discontinuous $5' > 3'$ modes and their removal by the exonucleolytic activity of DNA polymerase I. Okazaki fragments generated in the replicative process are joined together with DNA ligase. DNA gyrase relieves supercoils generated by DNA unwinding.

18. Eukaryotic DNA is replicated in a manner that is similar to that of *E. coli*. Synthesis is bidirectional, continuous on one strand and discontinuous on the other, and the requirements of synthesis (four deoxyribonucleoside triphosphates, divalent cation, template, and primer) are the same. Okazaki fragments of eukaryotes are about one-tenth the size of those in bacteria.

Because there is a much greater amount of DNA to be replicated and DNA replication is slower, there are multiple initiation sites for replication in eukaryotes (and increased DNA polymerase per cell) in contrast to the single replication origin in prokaryotes. Replication occurs at different sites during different intervals of the S phase. The proposed functions of four DNA polymerases are described in the text.

19. (a) In *E. coli*, 100 kb are added to each growing chain per minute. Therefore, the chain should be about 4,000,000 bp.

(b) Given $(4 \times 10^6 \text{ bp}) \times 0.34 \text{ nm/bp} =$

$$1.36 \times 10^6 \text{ nm or } 1.3 \text{ mm}$$

20. (a) no repair from DNA polymerase I and/or DNA polymerase III **(b)** no DNA ligase activity **(c)** no primase activity **(d)** only DNA polymerase I activity **(e)** no DNA gyrase activity.

21. DNA gyrase is a member of a group of enzymes called DNA topoisomerases that "undo" the twists and knots of supercoiling generated by the unwinding of DNA during replication. They generally bind to the ATP-binding site of DNA gyrase and block the energy of hydrolysis needed for gyrase function. By inhibiting DNA gyrase, DNA replication is stopped, which, in bacteria, reduces the intensity of an infection. Since cancer cells are actively replicating their DNA during cellular proliferation (discussed in Chapter 19), their replication is slowed by inhibitors of DNA gyrase. Because of structural differences between prokaryotic and eukaryotic DNA gyrases, different drugs are required for bacterial and cancer treatments.

22. *Gene conversion* is likely to be a consequence of genetic recombination in which nonreciprocal recombination yields products in which it appears that one allele is "converted" to another. Gene conversion is now considered a result of heteroduplex formation, which is accompanied by mismatched bases. When these mismatches are corrected, the "conversion" occurs.

23. (a) Because DNA polymerase III is essential for DNA chain elongation, it is necessary for replication of the *E. coli* chromosome. Thus, strains that are mutant for this enzyme must contain conditional mutations, and growth can be achieved at the permissive condition.

(b) The 3'–5' exonuclease activity is involved in proofreading. Thus, proofreading would be hampered in such mutant strains and a higher than expected mutation rate would occur.

24. Telomerase activity is present in germ-line tissue to maintain telomere length from one generation to the next. In other words, telomeres cannot shorten indefinitely without eventually eroding genetic information.

25. Since synthesis is bidirectional, one can multiply the rate of synthesis by two to come up with a figure of 18,000 bases replicated per five minutes (30 bases/second × 300 seconds). Dividing 1.6×10^8 by 1.8×10^4 gives 0.88×10^4, or about 8,800 replication sites.

26. If replication is conservative, the first autoradiographs (see metaphase I in the text) would have label distributed only on one side (chromatid) of the metaphase chromosome, as shown below.

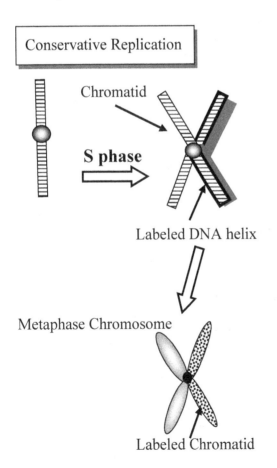

Conservative Replication

Chromatid

S phase

Labeled DNA helix

Metaphase Chromosome

Labeled Chromatid

27. (a) DNA polymerase would catalyze a bond between the 5' end of the last nucleotide added and the 3' end of the incoming nucleotide. In this reaction, the energy would be provided by the cleavage of the gamma and beta phosphates of the last nucleotide added to the chain rather than of the incoming nucleotide.

(b) If DNA polymerase removed a base, it would not be able to add any more bases to the chain because the penultimate base would have a monophosphate rather than a triphosphate, and there would be no source of energy for the polymerization reaction.

28. It is possible that the alien organism contains DNA that has parallel strands or only one DNA strand. In either case, the telomere problem would occur at one end of the chromosome. Since prokaryotic DNA is generally circular, therefore having no free ends, the alien organism is most likely a eukaryote.

29. (a) 5'ACCUAAGU **(b)** U

30. One could use a DNA strand that is stripped of its nucleosomes to determine whether Okazaki fragments are dependent on nucleosome periodicity. Since such an experiment would be *in vitro*, it may not represent a natural setting.

31. First, ^{3}H-thymidine would be incorporated into newly synthesized DNA. Second, under denaturing centrifugation conditions, the short Okazaki fragments are free to form a distinct peak of lower molecular weight DNA in a centrifugation profile. Third, as time passes, the Okazaki fragments that are synthesized on the lagging strand are joined by DNA ligase so that larger strands are created that form their own higher molecular weight peak.

32. Notice in strain *A* that DNA synthesis is reduced at both 30°C and 42°C, indicating that strain *A* is temperature sensitive. In addition, strain *A* is sensitive to novobiocin. Therefore, strain *A* is *gyr^{ts}*. Strain *B* is resistant to novobiocin but temperature sensitive and is therefore *gyr^{ts, r}*. Strain *C* is sensitive to novobiocin but not temperature sensitive and is therefore *wild type*. Strain *D* is resistant to novobiocin and not temperature sensitive and is therefore *gyr^r*.

33. (a) DNA, since one of the nitrogenous bases is T; also, notice the lack of an OH group at the

2' carbon. **(b)** 3' **(c)** Since spleen diesterase cuts between the 5' carbon and the phosphate, the original 5' phosphate is transferred to the 3' carbon of the 5' neighbor. Therefore, deoxyadenosine would obtain the phosphate at its 3' position.

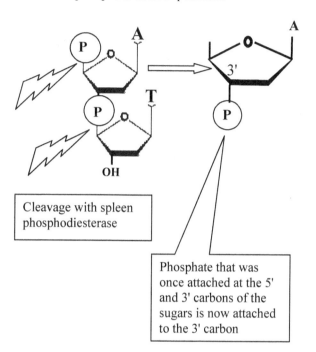

Cleavage with spleen phosphodiesterase

Phosphate that was once attached at the 5' and 3' carbons of the sugars is now attached to the 3' carbon

One can determine which model occurs in nature by comparing the pattern in which the labeled phosphate is shifted following spleen phosphodiesterase digestion. Focus your attention on the antiparallel model and notice that the frequency of which "C" (for example) is the 5' neighbor of "G" is not necessarily the same as the frequency of which "G" is the 5' neighbor of "C." However, in the parallel model (b), the frequency of which "C" is the 5' neighbor of "G" is the same as the frequency of which "G" is the 5' neighbor of "C." By examining such "digestion frequencies," it can be determined that DNA exists in the opposite polarity.

35. Because the semiconservative scheme predicts that *half* of the DNA in each daughter double helix is labeled, it would be difficult to envision a scheme in which three strands are replicated in such a semiconservative manner. It would seem that either the conservative or dispersive scheme would fit more appropriately. To examine the nature of replication, one could devise an experiment similar to that of Meselson and Stahl or Taylor, Woods, and Hughes.

34.

Initial Labeled Base	Labeled Base after Spleen Phosphodiesterase Digestion	
	ANTIPARALLEL	PARALLEL
G	A,T	C,T
C	G,A,G	G,A
T	C,T,G	C,T,A,G
A	T,C,A,T	T,C,A,G

Chapter 12: DNA Organization in Chromosomes

<u>Concept Areas</u>	<u>Corresponding Problems</u>
Viral and Bacterial Chromosomes	1, 2, 12, 13, 14, 19, 25
Specialized Chromosomes	1, 3, 4, 6
Organization of DNA in Chromatin	1, 2, 8, 9, 10, 11, 12, 15, 20, 21, 22, 23, 29
Organization of the Eukaryotic Genome	1, 5, 7, 11, 16, 17, 18, 24, 26, 27, 28

Concepts and Processes Checklist

(Check topic when mastered – provide examples where appropriate – understand the context of each entry)

- **Viral and Bacterial Chromosomes…**
    - DNA or RNA
    - ϕX174
    - lambda (λ)
    - packaging
    - nucleoid
    - DNA-binding proteins
    - HU and H-NS

- **Supercoiling Facilitates Compaction…**
    - supercoiled DNA
    - supercoil
    - linking number
    - energetically relaxed
    - energetically strained
    - left-handed supercoils
    - right-handed helix
    - closed circular molecules
    - topoisomers
    - topoisomerase

- **Specialized Chromosomes Reveal…**
    - polytene chromosomes
    - lampbrush chromosomes
    - chromomere
    - *Drosophila*
    - *Chironomus*
    - 5000 bands
    - lampbrush loops

- **DNA Is Organized into Chromatin…**
    - chromatin
    - interphase stage of cell cycle
    - histone
    - nonhistone protein
    - lysine
    - arginine
    - histone types (five)
    - nucleosome
    - nucleosome core particle
    - linker DNA

Chapter 12 DNA Organization in Chromosomes

- H1
- solenoid
- looped domains
- coiled chromatin fibers
- packing ratio
- chromatin remodeling
- histone tails
- acetylation
- methylation
- phosphorylation
- 5-methyl cytosine
- CpG island
- epigenetics
- heterochromatin, euchromatin
- position effect

- **Chromosome Banding Differentiates…**
  - chromosome-banding techniques
  - C-banding
  - G-bands
  - Giemsa staining

- **Eukaryotic Genomes Demonstrate…**
  - repetititive DNA
  - multiple-copy genes
  - tandem repeats
  - satellite DNA

- *in situ* hybridization
- centromere
- CEN region
- kinetochore
- alphoid family
- CENP-A
- CEN-P
- middle (moderately) repetitive DNA
- variable number tandem repeat
- VNTR
- minisatellite
- DNA fingerprinting
- microsatellite
- short tandem repeat
- STR
- SINEs, LINEs
- transposable sequences
- short interspersed element
- *Alu* family
- long interspersed element
- L1 family
- retrotransposon
- rRNA, 5.8*S*, 18*S*, 28*S*

- **The Vast Majority of a Eukaryotic…**
  - pseudogene

Chapter 12 DNA Organization in Chromosomes

Answers to Now Solve This

12-1. By having a circular chromosome, no free ends present the problem of linear chromosomes, namely, complete replication of terminal sequences.

12-2. Since eukaryotic chromosomes are "multirepliconic" in that there are multiple replication forks along their lengths, one would expect to see multiple clusters of radioactivity if labeled for a short period of time.

12-3. Volume of the nucleus = 4/3 πr^3

$= 4/3 \times 3.14 \times (5 \times 10^3 \text{ nm})^3$

$= 5.23 \times 10^{11} \text{ nm}^3$

Volume of the chromosome = $\pi r^2 \times \text{length}$

$= 3.14 \times 5.5 \text{ nm} \times 5.5 \text{ nm} \times (2 \times 10^9 \text{ nm})$

$= 1.9 \times 10^{11} \text{ nm}^3$

Therefore, the percentage of the volume of the nucleus occupied by the chromatin is

$= (1.9 \times 10^{11} \text{ nm}^3 / 5.23 \times 10^{11} \text{ nm}^3) \times 100$

$= \text{about } 36.3\%$

Chapter 12 DNA Organization in Chromosomes

Solutions to Problems and Discussion Questions

1. (a) Higher-level circular chromosomal structures have been revealed through both chemical and observational (microscopic) analyses.

(b) Using radioactively labeled RNA precursors followed by autoradiography, researchers discovered a high rate of RNA incorporation, indicating intense transcription.

(c) Early evidence came from endonuclease digestion that yielded DNA fragments of about 200 base pairs in length. Electron microscopic, X-ray, and neutron-scattering observations revealed the structure of nucleosomes and their relationship to DNA.

(d) Base sequences and organizational motifs of satellite DNA are common to many regions within and flanking centromeric DNA. In humans, most satellite DNA is of the alphoid family found mainly in centromeric regions that total up to 3 million base pairs. In addition, *in situ* hybridization of satellite DNA clusters in heterochromatic regions flanking centromeres. Rapid renaturation of DNA also indicates the presence of repetitive sequences.

2. Your essay should include a description of overall chromosomal configuration (linear, circular, etc.) as well as association with chromosomal proteins.

3. Bacteriophage λ has a linear, double-stranded DNA while in the phage coat and, upon infection, closes to form a circular chromosome. It contains about 50 kb. T2 phage also has a linear, double-stranded DNA chromosome; it is less than 200 kb. *E. coli* has a circular, double-stranded DNA chromosome of about 4.2×10^3 kb. Both intact phages are about 1/150 the size of *E. coli*. Since phages are obligate parasites of bacteria, they are dependent on their hosts for the manufacture of materials for their replication. Bacteria contain all genetic information for metabolism, replication, and *de novo* synthesis of numerous life-supporting materials. Phages, on the other hand, contain relatively few genes, namely, those needed to adsorb, inject, and produce progeny using primarily bacterial materials.

4. Polytene chromosomes are formed from numerous DNA replications, pairing of homologs, and absence of strand separation or cytoplasmic division. Each chromosome contains about 1000–5000 DNA strands in parallel register. They appear in specific tissues, such as salivary glands, of many dipterans such as *Drosophila*. They appear as comparatively long, wide fibers with sharp light and dark sections (bands) along their length. Such bands (chromomeres) are useful in chromosome identification, etc.

5. Most puffs represent active genes as evidenced by staining and uptake of labeled RNA precursors as assayed by autoradiography.

6. Lampbrush chromosomes are typically present in vertebrate oocytes and are so named because of their similar appearance to brushes used to clean kerosene lamp chimneys in the nineteenth century. They are also found in spermatocytes of some insects. They are found as diplotene stage structures and are active uncoiled versions of condensed meiotic chromosomes. Lampbrush chromosomes are typically viewed using light and electron microscopy.

7. Although greater DNA content per cell is associated with eukaryotes, one cannot universally equate genomic size with an increase in organismic complexity. There are numerous examples in which DNA content per cell varies considerably among closely related species. Because of the diverse cell types of multicellular eukaryotes, a variety of gene products are required, which may be related to the increase in DNA content per cell.

However, seeing the question in another way, it is likely that a much higher *percentage* of the genome of a prokaryote is actually involved in phenotype production than in a eukaryote.

Eukaryotes have evolved the capacity to obtain and maintain what appear to be large amounts of "extra," perhaps "junk," DNA. This concept will be examined in subsequent chapters of the text. Prokaryotes, on the other hand, with their relatively short life cycles, are extremely efficient in their accumulation and use of their genome.

Given the larger amount of DNA per cell and the requirement that the DNA be partitioned in an orderly fashion to daughter cells during cell division, certain mechanisms and structures (mitosis, nucleosomes, centromeres, etc.) have evolved for packaging and distributing the DNA. In addition, the genome is divided into separate entities (chromosomes) to perhaps facilitate the partitioning process in mitosis and meiosis.

8. Digestion of chromatin with endonucleases, such as micrococcal nuclease, gives DNA fragments of approximately 200 base pairs or multiples of such segments. X-ray diffraction data indicate a regular spacing of DNA in chromatin. Regularly spaced beadlike structures (nucleosomes) were identified by electron microscopy.

9. Nucleosomes are octomeric structures of two molecules of each histone (H2A, H2B, H3, and H4) except H1. Between the nucleosomes and complexed with linker DNA is histone H1. A 146-base-pair sequence of DNA wraps around the nucleosome.

10. As chromosome condensation occurs, a 300-Å fiber is formed. It appears to be composed of five or six nucleosomes coiled together. Such a structure is called a solenoid. These fibers form a series of loops that further condense into the chromatin fiber, which are then coiled into chromosome arms making up each chromatid.

11. *Heterochromatin* is chromosomal material that stains deeply and remains condensed when other parts of chromosomes, such as euchromatin, are otherwise pale and decondensed. Heterochromatic regions replicate late in S phase and are relatively inactive in a genetic sense because there are few genes present, or if they are present, they are repressed. Telomeres and the areas adjacent to centromeres are composed of heterochromatin.

12. (a) Since there are 200 base pairs per nucleosome (as defined in this problem) and 10^9 base pairs, there would be 5×10^6 nucleosomes. **(b)** Since there are 5×10^6 nucleosomes and nine histones (including H1) per nucleosome, there must be $9(5 \times 10^6)$ histone molecules: 4.5×10^7. **(c)** Since there are 10^9 base pairs present and each base pair is 3.4 Å, the overall length of the DNA is 3.4×10^9 Å. Dividing this value by the packing ratio (50) gives 6.8×10^7 Å.

13. The first step of this solution is to convert all of the given values to cubic Å, remembering that 1 μm = 10,000 Å. Using the formula πr^2 for the area of a circle and $4/3\ \pi r^3$ for the volume of a sphere, the following calculations apply:

Volume of DNA: 3.14×10 Å $\times 10$ Å $\times$
$$(50 \times 10^4 \text{ Å}) = 1.57 \times 10^8 \text{ Å}^3$$

Volume of capsid: 4/3 (3.14 $\times$ 400 Å $\times$
$$400 \text{ Å} \times 400 \text{ Å}) = 2.67 \times 10^8 \text{ Å}^3$$

Because the capsid head has a greater volume than the volume of DNA, the DNA will fit into the capsid.

14. One base pair occupies 0.34 nm; therefore, the equation would be as follows:

52 μm/(0.34 nm/bp) $\times$ 1000 nm/μm =
$$152{,}941 \text{ base pairs}$$

15. When the w^+ locus is rearranged such that it is now positioned next to heterochromatin, activity becomes intermittent, leading to a variegated eye in a w^+/w heterozygote or w^+/Y male. Heterochromatin is characterized as gene-poor and relatively inaccessible to DNA-binding factors needed for transcription. Specific regions of heterochromatin recruit histone deacetylases that modify histones and essentially silence such regions. As with X chromosome inactivation in mammals, heterochromatic regions can spread until they reach specific sequences that signal a block to additional silencing. Such spreading can be continuous or discontinuous. When the w^+ gene is juxtaposed to heterochromatin, apparently the normal regulatory signals are altered, and sporadic silencing that leads to variegation is the result. Once the w^+ gene is silenced, the w^+ gene in descendent cells is also silenced, leading to patches of white tissue.

16. Long interspersed elements (LINEs) are repetitive transposable DNA sequences in humans. The most prominent family, designated **L1**, is about 6.4 kb each and is represented about 100,000 times. LINEs are often referred to as retrotransposons because their mechanism of transposition resembles that used by retroviruses.

17. Except for identical twins, each individual possesses a virtually unique set of numerous VNTRs. Such variety provides a dependable, consistent, and unique DNA fingerprint for forensic applications.

18. First, the methylation patterns displayed by a particular disease must be stable and not change dramatically over time. Second, because DNA methylation patterns differ among individuals, specific patterns must be disease specific and not individual specific. Third, because disease-related changes in DNA methylation patterns often involve hundreds of genes, appropriate interpretation of pattern specifics requires expertise presently beyond our capabilities; however, some progress is being made (Tost, 2010).

19. In many cases, viruses specifically methylate the genetic apparatus associated with the immune response, thus dampening that response and enhancing viral infectivity.

20. Cancer cells undergo a variety of changes in histone acetylation compared to normal cells. Overacetylation (hyperacetylation) is often associated with increased gene activity. By introducing HDAC inhibitors, the attempt is to generally decrease gene activity. Although the mode of action of HDAC inhibitors is obscure, they are thought to act by promoting cell-cycle arrest by reducing the output of a relatively small number of genes.

21. Data by Sun et al. support the general observation that heterochromatic genes are less active than euchromatic genes, and, more specifically, the possibility that heterochromatin may contain genes that are repressed. Heterochromatin is located in eukaryotic chromosomes as differentially staining compared with euchromatin. It is relatively inactive genetically because of either a lack of genes or the presence of repressed genes. Heterochromatin replicates later in S phase than euchromatic segments. Centromeric and telomeric regions of chromosomes are typically heterochromatic.

22. The intimate relationships among histones, nucleosomes, and DNA in chromatin clearly account for structural remodeling of chromosomes as the cell cycle proceeds from interphase to metaphase. That nucleosomes are associated with chromatin during periods of gene activity begs the question as to the possible roles they play in influencing not only chromosome structure but also gene function. The finding that natural chemical modification of nucleosomal components increases gene activity, as indicated in the question, suggests that changes in the binding of nucleosomes to DNA (in this case due to methylation) enable genes to be more accessible to factors that promote gene function. In addition, the finding that heterochromatin,

containing fewer genes and more repressed genes, is undermethylated further supports the suggestion that histone modification is functionally related to changes in gene activity.

23. DNA replicates in a *semiconservative* fashion, with each daughter DNA double helix containing one new and one original single strand. Nucleosomes follow a *dispersive* pattern, with each daughter chromatid containing a mixture of new and original nucleosomes. One could test the distribution of nucleosomes by conducting an autoradiographic experiment similar to Taylor-Woods-Hughes, but instead of labeling the DNA with ^{3}H-thymidine, one would label some or all the histones H2A, H2B, H3, and H4 in nucleosomes.

24. Assuming a random distribution, dividing 3×10^9 base pairs, by 10^6 gives approximately 3000 base pairs, or 3 kbp between *Alu* sequences.

25. Bacteriophage λ is composed of a double-stranded, linear DNA molecule of about 48,000 base pairs. It is capable of forming a closed, double-stranded circular molecule because of a 12-base-pair, single-stranded, complementary "overhanging" sequence at the 5' end of each single strand.

26. The distribution of microsatellites varies in a taxon-related manner. Microsatellites are more common within genes of yeast and fungi and quite infrequent in genes of mammals. There appears to be a general decrease in within-gene microsatellites in more recently evolved organisms.

27. The general frequency and pattern of various trinucleotide repeat motifs are similar in all taxonomic groups. Within-gene trinucleotide repeats are the most frequent repeat motif in all taxonomic groups followed by hexanucleotide repeats. One explanation might be that various microsatellite types (mono, di, tri, etc.) are generated at different rates in different genomic regions (within and between genes). A second possibility is that selection acts differentially depending on the type and location of a repeat. The correlation between the high frequency of tri- and hexanucleotide repeats within genes and a triplet code specifying particular amino acids within genes may not be coincidental.

28. The basic issue here is to determine whether all the loci that are not from the mother can come from the father. That is, does the father's genotype provide the child's loci that are not provided by the mother? For example, at the *D9S302* locus, the mother contributed the child's 31 locus and the alleged father could have contributed the child's 32 locus. Since other men also have the 32 locus, one cannot say that the alleged father is the father; rather, one could say that the alleged father cannot be excluded as the source of the sperm that produced the child. Notice that in every case, the child includes at least one locus from the father and one from the mother, which is expected if the alleged father is indeed the real father. Without information as to the frequency of each marker in the general population, it is difficult to draw definitive conclusions.

29. Since both genes mentioned in the problem are located near the end of chromosome 16, it is possible that erosion of the end of the chromosome is related to each disease. Examination of the gene by *in situ* hybridization and molecular cloning indicates that thalassemia involves a terminal deletion in distal portion of 16p. To learn more about such conditions, visit http://www.ncbi.nlm.nih.gov/ and follow the OMIM link.

Chapter 13: The Genetic Code and Transcription

Concept Areas	Corresponding Problems
Genetic Code	2, 26, 28, 29
Deciphering the Code	1, 6, 7, 11
Characteristics of the Code	1, 3, 4, 5, 8, 9, 14, 16, 28, 29, 30
Information Flow	1, 2, 10, 12, 17, 18, 19, 20, 27, 32
RNA Structure and Function	1, 13, 15, 21, 23
RNA Processing	1, 22, 24, 25, 31, 33

Concepts and Processes Checklist

(Check topic when mastered – provide examples where appropriate – understand the context of each entry)

- **The Genetic Code Uses Ribonucleotide Bases . . .**
  - triplet code
  - codon
  - unambiguous
  - degenerate
  - initiation
  - termination
  - commaless
  - nonoverlapping
  - universal
  - collinear

- **Early Studies Established . . .**
  - mRNA (messenger RNA)
  - triplet nature
  - 20 amino acids
  - *rII* locus in T4
  - proflavin
  - contiguous sequence

- frameshift mutation
- *E. coli* K12
- plus, minus
- nonoverlapping code
- transfer RNA adaptor
- commaless code
- +++, – – –
- nonsense codon

- **Studies by Nirenberg . . .**
  - polynucleotide phosphorylase
  - cell-free system
  - RNA templates
  - ribonucleoside diphosphates
  - opposite direction
  - no DNA template
  - homopolymer codes
  - RNA homopolymers
  - RNA heteropolymers
  - triplet binding assay

- anticodon
- repeating copolymers
- termination codons

- **The Coding Dictionary Reveals . . .**
  - degeneracy
  - wobble hypothesis
  - ordered genetic code
  - chemically similar amino acids
  - initiation
  - termination
  - suppression
  - *N*-formylmethionine
  - fmet
  - initiator codon
  - termination codons
  - nonsense mutation

- **The Genetic Code . . .Confirmed**
  - MS2
  - colinearity
  - exceptions to universal code

- **Different Initiation Points . . .**
  - overlapping genes
  - ORF
  - open reading frame
  - overlapping ORFs
  - ϕX174

- **Transcription Synthesizes RNA . . .**
  - transcription
  - RNA migration
  - information flow

- **Studies with Bacteria and Phages . . .**

- **RNA Polymerase Directs . . .**
  - RNA polymerase
  - n(NTP)
  - NMPs
  - PP$_i$
  - holoenzyme
  - sigma (σ) factor
  - transcription components
  - template binding
  - initiation
  - chain elongation

- **Promoters, Template Binding . . .**
  - template binding
  - transcription start site
  - consensus sequences
  - Pribnow box
  - *cis*-acting elements
  - *trans*-acting elements
  - initiation
  - elongation
  - termination
  - hairpin secondary structure
  - termination factor
  - rho (ρ)
  - polycistronic mRNA
  - monocistronic RNA

- **Transcription in Eukaryotes . . .**
  - pre-mRNA
  - heterogeneous nuclear RNA
  - hnRNA

- transcription factors
- initiation of transcription
- RNA polymerase II
- RNAP II
- core-promoter
- proximal-promoter elements
- enhancers
- silencers
- Goldberg-Hogness box
- TATA box
- RNA polymerase I
- RNA polymerase II
- RNA polymerase III
- −30 upstream
- −10 upstream
- general transcription factors (GTFs)
- TFIIA, TFIIB, TFIID
- pre-initiation complex
- clamp
- initial transcript
- mature mRNA
- posttranscriptional modification
- 7-methylguanosine (7-mG) cap
- 5'-5' bonding
- poly-A sequence (3')
- AAUAAA
- **The Coding Regions . . .Interrupted**
  - intervening sequences
  - split genes

- introns
- exons
- heteroduplex
- *β*-globin gene
- ovalbumin gene
- *pro-α-2(1) collagen* gene
- *Tetrahymena*
- ribozyme
- self-excision
- group I introns
- spliceosome
- small nuclear RNAs (snRNAs)
- small nuclear ribonucleoproteins
- snRNPs or snurps
- U1, U2, . . ., U6
- acceptor sequence
- branch point
- transesterification reaction
- alternative splicing
- isoform
- **RNA Editing May Modify . . .**
  - RNA editing
  - substitution editing
  - insertion/deletion editing
  - gRNA (guide RNA)
  - ADAR enzymes
- **Transcription Has Been Visualized . . .**
  - polyribosomes

F13.1 Illustration of the processes, transcription and translation, involved in protein synthesis. Such relationships are often called the Central Dogma.

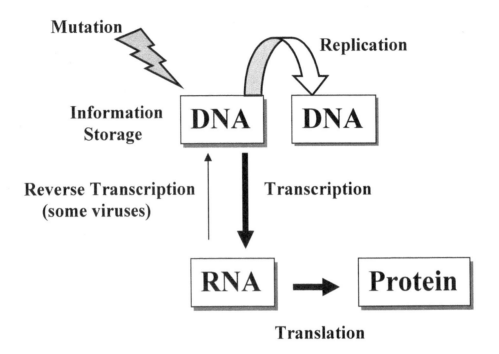

F13.2 Illustration of transcription in prokaryotes coupled with translation. Transcription involves production of RNA from a DNA template.

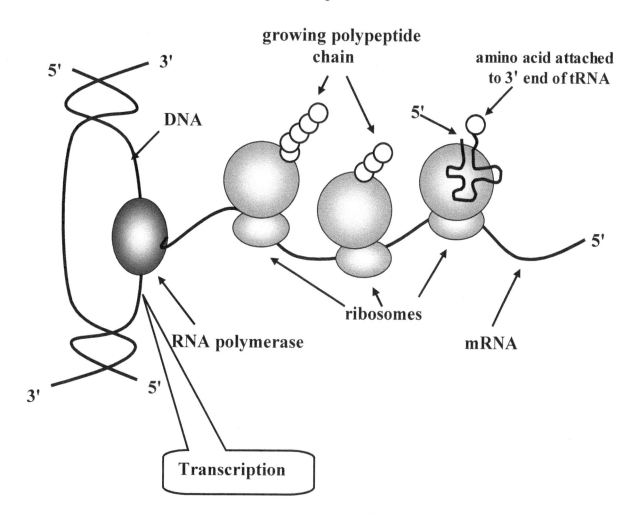

Chapter 13 *The Genetic Code and Transcription*

Chapter 13 The Genetic Code and Transcription

Answers to Now Solve This

13-1. (a.) The way to determine the fraction of each triplet that will occur with a random incorporation system is to determine the likelihood that each base will occur in each position of the codon (first, second, third) and then multiply the individual probabilities (fractions) for a final probability (fraction).

$$GGG \ = \ 3/4 \times 3/4 \times 3/4 \ = \ 27/64$$

$$GGC \ = \ 3/4 \times 3/4 \times 1/4 \ = \ 9/64$$
$$GCG \ = \ 3/4 \times 1/4 \times 3/4 \ = \ 9/64$$
$$CGG \ = \ 1/4 \times 3/4 \times 3/4 \ = \ 9/64$$

$$CCG \ = \ 1/4 \times 1/4 \times 3/4 \ = \ 3/64$$
$$CGC \ = \ 1/4 \times 3/4 \times 1/4 \ = \ 3/64$$
$$GCC \ = \ 3/4 \times 1/4 \times 1/4 \ = \ 3/64$$

$$CCC \ = \ 1/4 \times 1/4 \times 1/4 \ = \ 1/64$$

(b) Glycine:

GGG and one G_2C (adds up to 36/64)

Alanine:

one G_2C and one C_2G (adds up to 12/64)

Arginine:

one G_2C and one C_2G (adds up to 12/64)

Proline:

one C_2G and CCC (adds up to 4/64)

(c) With the wobble hypothesis, variation can occur in the third position of each codon.

Glycine:	GGG, GGC
Alanine:	CGG, GCC, CGC, GCG
Arginine:	GCG, GCC, CGC, CGG
Proline:	CCC, CCG

13-2. Assume that you have introduced a copolymer (ACACACAC . . .) to a cell-free protein-synthesizing system. There are two possibilities for establishing the reading frames: ACA, if one starts at the first base, and CAC, if one starts at the second base. These would code for two different amino acids (ACA = threonine; CAC = histidine) and would produce repeating polypeptides that would alternate *thr-his-thr-his* . . . or *his-thr-his-thr* . . . .

Because of a triplet code, a trinucleotide sequence will, once initiated, remain in the same reading frame and produce the same code all along the sequence regardless of the initiation site.

Given the sequence CUACUACUACUA, notice the different reading frames producing three sequences each containing the same amino acid.

Codons:	CUA	CUA	CUA	CUA . . .
Amino acids:	leu	leu	leu	leu . . .
	UAC	UAC	UAC	UAC . . .
	tyr	tyr	tyr	tyr . . .
	ACU	ACU	ACU	ACU . . .
	thr	thr	thr	thr . . .

152

If a tetranucleotide is used, such as ACGUACGUACGU . . .

Codons:	ACG	UAC	GUA	CGU	ACG
Amino acids:	thr	tyr	val	arg	thr
	CGU	ACG	UAC	GUA	CGU
	arg	thr	tyr	val	arg
	GUA	CGU	ACG	UAC	GUA
	val	arg	thr	tyr	val
	UAC	GUA	CGU	ACG	UAC
	tyr	val	arg	thr	tyr

Notice that the sequences are the same except that the starting amino acid changes.

13-3. Apply complementary bases, substituting U for T:

(a)

    Sequence 1: 3'-GAAAAAACGGUA-5'
    Sequence 2: 3'-UGUAGUUAUUGA-5'
    Sequence 3: 3'-AUGUUCCCAAGA-5'

(b)

    Sequence 1: met-ala-lys-lys
    Sequence 2: ser-tyr-(termination)
    Sequence 3: arg-thr-leu-val

(c) Apply complementary bases:

    3'-GAAAAAACGGTA-5'

Chapter 13 The Genetic Code and Transcription

Solutions to Problems and Discussion Questions

1. (a) The triplet nature of the code was suggested because, given 20 amino acids, minimal use of the four DNA bases would require three bases per amino acid, thus providing 64 possible code words. The nonoverlapping nature of the code was suggested because of the limitations that an overlapping code would place on peptide sequences. In addition, with an overlapping code, single nucleotide substitutions would often alter two adjacent amino acids, which was not observed in mutant proteins that had been examined at the time. The triplet, nonoverlapping nature of the code along with other characteristics were demonstrated primarily by studies on frameshift mutations in the *rII* locus of phage T4.

(b) An initial understanding about the composition (unordered) of codons came from homopolymer and heteropolymer RNAs introduced into an *in vitro* system. Assays of the relative amino acid composition of resulting polypeptides indicated the composition of the bases in codons, but not their actual sequence.

(c) The specific sequences of the triplet codes were determined by the triplet binding assay and repeating copolymers of known sequence. When added to a cell-free system, a direct analysis of codon assignments was possible.

(d) Since the complete sequence of the RNA phage MS2 was known, scientists matched that sequence with protein products of MS2, which supported the code as derived from previous studies.

(e) Work with *E. coli* infected with phage showed that the synthesis of proteins was under the direction of newly synthesized RNA. Others were able to show that newly synthesized RNA formed during a phage infection of bacteria would hybridize only with phage DNA, thus demonstrating the dependence of RNA on the template nature of DNA.

(f) The most direct evidence for the presence of noncoding sequences in RNA and therefore the presence of split genes comes from hybridization experiments. When mature mRNAs are hybridized to DNA containing the genes specifying that mRNA, heteroduplexes form, indicating that sequences in the DNA are not always represented in mRNA products. In addition, studies that compare the sequences of DNAs to their corresponding RNAs and proteins show that DNA often contains sequences that are not represented in RNA and protein products.

2. Your essay should include a description of the nature and structure of the genetic code, the enzymes and logistics of transcription, and the chemical nature of polymerization.

3. The reason that $(+ + +)$ or $(- - -)$ restored the reading frame is that the code is triplet. The translation system is "out of phase" until the third "+" or "−" is encountered.

(a) If the code contained six nucleotides (a sextuplet code), then the translation system is "out of phase" until the sixth "+" or "−" is encountered. In this case, the out-of-phase region would probably be longer and likely cause more amino acid alterations.

(b) Given a sextuplet code, restoration of the reading frames would occur only with the addition or loss of six nucleotides. Lay out a sequence such as

CATDOGPIGOWLCATDOGPIGOWLCAT...

and test this explanation.

4. The UUACUUACUUAC tetranucleotide sequence will produce the following triplets depending on the initiation point: UUA = leu, UAC = tyr, ACU = thr, CUU = leu. Notice that because of the degenerate code, two codons correspond to the amino acid leucine.

The UAUCUAUCUAUC tetranucleotide sequence will produce the following triplets depending on the initiation point: UAU = tyr, AUC = ileu, UCU = ser, CUA = leu. Notice that in this case, degeneracy is not revealed and all the codons produce unique amino acids.

5. From the repeating polymer ACACA . . . one can say that threonine is either CAC or ACA. From the polymer CAACAA . . . with ACACA . . . , ACA is the only codon in common. Therefore, threonine would have the codon ACA.

6. As in the previous problem, the procedure is to find those sequences that are the same for the first two bases, but that vary in the third base. Given that AGG = arg, then information from the AG copolymer indicates that AGA also codes for arg, and GAG must therefore code for glu.

Coupling this information with that of the AAG copolymer, GAA must also code for glu, and AAG must code for lys.

7. The basis of the technique is that if a trinucleotide contains bases (a codon) that are complementary to the anticodon of a charged tRNA, a relatively large complex is formed that contains the ribosome, the tRNA, and the trinucleotide. This complex is trapped in the filter, whereas the components by themselves are not trapped. If the amino acid on a charged, trapped tRNA is radioactive, then the filter becomes radioactive.

8. List the substitutions; then from the code table, apply the codons to the original amino acids. Select codons that provide single base changes.

Original		Substitutions
Original		**Substitutions**
threonine	----->	alanine
<u>AC</u>(U, C, A, or G)		<u>GC</u>(U, C, A, or G)
glycine	----->	serine
<u>GG</u>(U or C)		<u>AG</u>(U or C)
isoleucine	----->	valine
<u>AU</u>(U, C, or A)		<u>GU</u>(U, C, or A)

9. Apply the most conservative pathway of change.

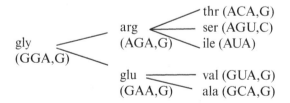

10. Polynucleotide phosphorylase generally functions in the degradation of RNA; however, in an *in vitro* environment, with high concentrations of the ribonucleoside diphosphates, the direction of the reaction can be forced toward polymerization. *In vivo*, the concentration of ribonucleoside diphosphates is low and the degradative process is favored.

11. Because poly U is complementary to poly A, double-stranded structures will be formed. In order for an RNA to serve as a messenger RNA, it must

be single stranded, thereby exposing the bases for interaction with ribosomal subunits and tRNAs.

12. Applying the coding dictionary, the following sequences are "decoded":

Sequence 1: met-pro-asp-tyr-ser-(term)

Sequence 2: met-pro-asp-(term)

The 12th base (a uracil) is deleted from Sequence 1, thereby causing a frameshift mutation, which introduced a terminating triplet UAA.

13. (a)

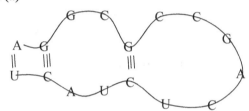

(b) TCCGCGGCTGAGATGA (use complementary bases, substituting T for U)

(c) GCU

(d) Assuming that the AGG . . . is the 5' end of the mRNA, then the sequence would be

arg-arg-arg-leu-tyr

14. Given the sequence GGA, by changing each of the bases to the remaining three bases and then checking the code table, one can determine whether amino acid substitutions will occur.

G G A	gly		G G U	gly
U G A	**term**		G G C	gly
C G A	**arg**		G G A	gly
A G A	**arg**		G G G	gly
G U A	**val**		U G U	**cys**
G C A	**ala**		C G U	**arg**
G A A	**glu**		A G U	**ser**
G G U	gly		G U U	**val**
G G C	gly		G C U	**ala**
G G A	gly		G A U	**asp**

15. (a) Starting from the 5' end and locating the AUG triplets, one finds two initiation sites leading to the following two sequences:

met-his-thr-tyr-glu-thr-leu-gly

met-arg-pro-leu-asp (or glu)

(b) In the shorter of the two reading sequences (the one using the internal AUG triplet), a UGA triplet was introduced at the second codon. Although not in the reading frames of the longer polypeptide (using the first AUG codon), the UGA triplet eliminates the product starting at the second initiation codon.

16. By examining the coding dictionary, one will notice that the number of codons for each particular amino acid (synonyms) is directly related to the frequency of amino acid incorporation stated in the problem.

17. The central dogma of molecular genetics and, to some extent, all of biology states that DNA produces, through transcription, RNA, which is "decoded" (during translation) to produce proteins. See F13.2 for a graphic description.

18. Several observations indicated that a "messenger" molecule exists. First, DNA, the genetic material, is located in the nucleus of a eukaryotic cell, whereas protein synthesis occurs in the cytoplasm. DNA, therefore, does not directly participate in protein synthesis. Second, RNA, which is chemically similar to DNA, is synthesized in the nucleus of eukaryotic cells. Much of the RNA migrates to the cytoplasm, the site of protein synthesis. Third, there is generally a direct correlation between the amounts of RNA and protein in a cell. More direct support was derived from experiments showing that an RNA other than that found in ribosomes was involved in protein synthesis, and shortly after phage infection, an RNA species is produced that is complementary to phage DNA.

19. RNA polymerase from *E. coli* is a complex, large (almost 500,000 daltons) molecule composed of subunits ($\alpha, \beta, \beta', \sigma$) in the proportion $\alpha2, \beta, \beta', \sigma$ for the holoenzyme. The β subunit provides catalytic function, whereas the sigma (σ) subunit is involved in recognition of specific promoters. The core enzyme is the protein without the sigma.

20. Ribonucleoside triphosphates and a DNA template in the presence of RNA polymerase and a divalent cation (Mg^{2+}) produce a ribonucleoside monophosphate polymer, DNA, and pyrophospate (diphosphate). Equimolar amounts of precursor ribonucleoside triphosphates, product ribonucleoside monophosphates, and

pyrophosphates (disphosphates) are formed. In *E. coli*, transcription and translation can occur simultaneously. Ribosomes add to the 5' end nascent mRNA and progress to the 3' end during translation. Although transcription/translation can be "visualized" in the *E. coli* (F13.2), the predominant components "visualized" are the strings of ribosomes (polysomes).

21. Whereas some folding (from complementary base pairing) may occur with mRNA molecules, they generally exist as single-stranded structures, which are quite labile. Eukaryotic mRNAs are generally processed such that the 5' end is "capped" and the 3' end has a considerable string of adenine bases. It is thought that these features protect the mRNAs from degradation. Such stability of eukaryotic mRNAs probably evolved with the differentiation of nuclear and cytoplasmic functions. Because prokaryotic cells exist in a more unstable environment (nutritionally and physically, for example) than many cells of multicellular organisms, rapid genetic response to environmental change is likely to be adaptive. To accomplish such rapid responses, a labile gene product (mRNA) is advantageous. A pancreatic cell, which is developmentally stable and exists in a relatively stable environment, could produce more insulin on stable mRNAs for a given transcriptional rate.

22. The immediate product of transcription of an RNA destined to become a mRNA often involves modification of the 5' end to which a 7-methylguanosine cap is added. In addition, a stretch of as many as 250 adenylic acid residues is often added to the 3' end after removal of a AAUAAA sequence. The vast majority of eukaryotic pre-mRNAs also contain intervening sequences that are removed, often in a variety of combinations, during the maturation process. In some organisms, RNA editing occurs in one of two ways: substitution editing whereby nucleotides are altered and insertion/deletion editing that changes the total number of bases.

Processing location	Example
5' end	Addition of 7-mG
3' end	Poly-A addition
internal	Removal of internal sequences
	RNA editing
	-substitution
	-insertion/deletion

23. It is likely that 3'-polyadenylation influences the overall configuration of RNA transcripts that then either by itself or in conjunction with proteins or other RNAs impacts the longevity of the transcript. Especially in eukaryotes, 3'-polyadenylation may also influence the transport of RNAs to and from cellular organelles. In addition, 3'-polyadenylation may facilitate or inhibit the association of RNAs to other cellular components, such as proteins, lipids, or nucleic acids.

24. RNA editing falls into two general categories. Substitution editing occurs when individual nucleotide bases are altered. It is very common in mitochondrial and chloroplast RNAs as well as some nuclear-derived eukatyotic RNAs. Apolipoprotein B occurs in a long and short form even though a single gene encodes both forms. The initial transcript is edited, which generates a stop codon that terminates the polypeptide at about half its length. The other category is insertion/deletion editing. The parasite that causes African sleeping sickness uses insertion/deletion editing of its mitochondrial RNAs in forming the initiation codon that then places the remaining sequence in proper reading frame.

25. Notice that C and U are both pyrimidines and A and I are both purines. Therefore, each conversion is not chemically radical. Both cases involve deamination, the removal of an NH_2 group.

26. (a) Notice that the first two bases in the triplet code are common to more codons than the last base. If there were fewer amino acids used in earlier times, perhaps the first two bases were primarily involved.

(b) Interestingly, all the amino acids mentioned as primitive use guanine as the first base in each codon. We might therefore suppose that the GNN configuration was the starting point of the present-day code. Within the GNN format, the second base is used to distinguish among the amino acids mentioned as primitive.

(c) It is interesting to note that what are considered as the most primitive amino acids are GNN coded, whereas the later-arriving amino acids are U(U,A,G) (U,C) coded. It would seem that some phenomenon could explain the differences in codon structure between primitive and late-arriving amino acids. It is likely that the addition of new amino acids to the codon field was a slow and mutation-prone process. Did the addition of late-arriving amino acids displace earlier codon assignments or were some of the late-arriving amino acids able to make use of codons that originally did not code for an amino acid? If this is the case, fewer and more restricted codon assignments would be available for late-arriving amino acids. Notice that each of the late-arriving amino acids has the same starting nucleotide as the present-day stop codons. Is it possible that what were once stop codons were used for late-arriving amino acids because this would be less disruptive to protein synthesis than displacing assignments at the time of their introduction? Much is left to be discovered regarding the structure of the genetic code.

27. In eukaryotes, protein synthesis occurs primarily in the cytoplasm, far from the location of DNA and the encoded information. In addition, whereas some of the basic amino acids would be able to associate directly with DNA, the acidic amino acids would be unable to do so. Thus, some sort of "adaptor" system was needed for DNA to direct amino acid assembly.

28. First, compute the frequency (percentages would be easiest to compare) for each of the random codons.

For 4/5C: 1/5A:

$CCC = 4/5 \times 4/5 \times 4/5 = 64/125$ (51.2%)

$C_2A = 3(4/5 \times 4/5 \times 1/5) = 48/125$ (38.4%)

$CA_2 = 3(4/5 \times 1/5 \times 1/5) = 12/125$ (9.6%)

$AAA = 1/5 \times 1/5 \times 1/5 = 1/125$ (0.8%)

For 4/5A: 1/5C:

$AAA = 4/5 \times 4/5 \times 4/5 = 64/125$ (51.2%)

$A_2C = 3(4/5 \times 4/5 \times 1/5) = 48/125$ (38.4%)

$AC_2 = 3(4/5 \times 1/5 \times 1/5) = 12/125$ (9.6%)

$CCC = 1/5 \times 1/5 \times 1/5 = 1/125$ (0.8%)

Proline:	C_3 and one of the C_2A triplets
Histidine:	one of the C_2A triplets
Threonine:	one C_2A triplet and one A_2C triplet
Glutamine:	one of the A_2C triplets
Asparagine:	one of the A_2C triplets
Lysine:	A_3

29.

(a) #1: nonsense mutation
#2: missense mutation
#3: frameshift mutation

(b) #1: mutation in third position to A or G
#2: change U to C in third triplet
#3: removal of a G in the UGG triplet (trp)

(c) termination

(d) All of the amino acids can be assigned specific triplets, including the third base of each triplet. Compare the sequences for the wild type and mutant #2. After removal of a G in the UUG triplet of tryptophan, the frameshift mutation shifts the first base of the following triplet to the third (often ambiguous) base of the previous triplet. The only tricky solution is with serine, which has six triplet possibilities, but it can still be resolved.

AUG UGG UAU CGU GGU AGU CCA ACA

(e) The mutation may be in a promoter or enhancer, although many posttranscriptional alterations are possible. Depending on the gene and the organism, the mutation may be in an intron/exon splice site, etc.

30. (a, b) Use the code table to determine the number of triplets that code each amino acid; then construct a graph and plot such as this one:

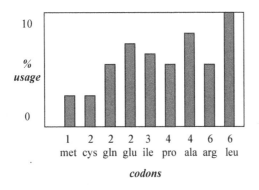

(c) There appears to be a weak correlation between the relative frequency of amino acid usage and the number of triplets for each.

(d) To continue to investigate this issue, one might examine additional amino acids in a similar manner. In addition, different phylogenetic groups use code synonyms differently. It may be possible to find situations in which the relationships are more extreme. One might also examine more proteins

to determine whether such a weak correlation is stronger with different proteins.

31.

(a)

gucccaaccaugcccaccgaucuuccgccugcuucugaagAUGC
GGGCCCAG

(b)

5' gtc cca acc **atg** ccc acc gat ctt ccg cct gct tct gaa
gAT GCG GGC CCA G

(c)

5' gtcccaaccatgcccaccgatcttccgcctgcttctgaag
ATG CGG GCC CAG

The two initiator codons are not in phase.

(d)

5' gtc cca acc **atg** ccc acc gat ctt ccg cct gct tct gaa
gAT GCG GGC CCA G

            met pro thr asp leu pro pro ala
ser glu asp ala gly pro

5' gtcccaaccatgcccaccgatcttccgcctgcttctgaag
ATG CGG GCC CAG

met arg ala gln

The amino acid sequences in the region of overlap are not the same.

(e) One might argue for the conservation of DNA by having the same region code for a multiple of products, and that might be the case in viruses and prokaryotes in which genomic efficiency is more of an issue. However, eukaryotes appear to be much less likely to evolve strategies that conserve DNA sequences *per se*. However, if functionally and/or structurally related products can be conveniently regulated by such an arrangement, then perhaps an evolutionary advantage exists. The most obvious disadvantage is that if a mutation occurs in the common region, then two gene products are altered instead of one.

32. The advantage would be that if sequence homologies can be identified for a variety of HIV isolates, then perhaps a single or a few vaccines could be developed for the multitude of subtypes that infect various parts of the world. In other words, the wider the match of a vaccine to circulating infectives is, the more likely the efficacy. On the other hand, the more finely aligned a vaccine is to the target, the more likely it is that new or previously undiscovered variants will escape vaccination attempts.

33. (a, b) Alternative splicing occurs when pre-mRNAs are spliced in more than one way to yield various combinations of exons in the final mRNA product. Upon translation of a group of alternatively spliced mRNAs, a series of related proteins, called isoforms, are produced. It is likely that alternative splicing evolved to provide a variety of functionally related proteins in a particular tissue from one original source. In other words, varieties of similar proteins can be produced by alternative splicing rather than by independent evolution.

Chapter 14: Translation and Proteins

Concept Areas	Corresponding Problems
Translation/Colinearity	8, 25, 26, 27
RNAs	1, 2, 3, 4, 5, 7, 8, 9, 10, 38
Punctuation/Code	1, 5, 7, 24
Information Flow	1, 20
One-Gene:One-Enzyme	1, 17
Pathways	1, 11, 12, 13, 14, 15, 16, 32, 33, 34
Proteins	1, 6, 18, 19, 21, 22, 23, 28, 29, 30, 39
Exon Shuffling	31
Antibiotic Resistance	35, 36
Antisense Therapy	37

Concepts and Processes Checklist

(Check topic when mastered – provide examples where appropriate – understand the context of each entry)

- **Translation of mRNA Depends…**

  - ribosomes
  - transfer RNA (tRNA)
  - triplet codons
  - anticodon
  - ribosomal proteins
  - monosome
  - 70S, 80S
  - 50S, 30S
  - 60S, 40S
  - 23S, 5S
  - 31 ribosomal proteins
  - 28S, 5.8S, 5S
  - 46 ribosomal proteins
  - 16S
  - 21 ribosomal proteins
  - 18S

- 33 ribosomal proteins
- rDNA
- tandem repeats
- spacer DNA
- chromosomal locations
- cognate amino acid
- posttranscriptional modification
- cloverleaf model of tRNA
- anticodon loop
- …pCpCpA-3'
- charging (aminoacylation)
- aminoacyl tRNA synthetase
- wobble
- 20 synthetases
- aminoacyladenylic acid
- isoaccepting tRNAs

Chapter 14 Translation and Proteins

- **Translation of mRNA…**
  - initiation
  - initiation factors (IFs)
  - *N*-formylmethionine (f-met)
  - Shine-Dalgarno sequence
  - initiation complex
  - P (peptidyl) site
  - A (aminoacyl) site
  - elongation
  - peptidyl transferase
  - ribozyme
  - E (exit) site
  - mRNA-tRNA-aa_2-aa_1
  - termination
  - stop codon
  - termination codon
  - nonsense codon
  - GTP-dependent release factor
  - polyribosomes
  - polysomes
- **High-Resolution Studies…**
  - X-ray diffraction
  - *Thermus thermophilus*
  - wobble hypothesis
  - cryo-EM
- **Translation Is More Complex…**
  - Kozak sequence
- **The Initial Insight That Proteins…**
  - alkaptonuria
  - consanguineous
- phenylketonuria (PKU)
- phenylalanine hydroxylase
- **Studies of *Neurospora*…**
  - one-gene:one-enzyme hypothesis
  - *Neurospora*
  - biosynthetic pathway
- **Studies of Human Hemoglobin…**
  - one-gene:one-protein hypothesis
  - one-gene:one polypeptide chain hypothesis
  - sickle-cell anemia
  - sickle-cell trait
  - HbA, HbS
  - starch gel electrophoresis
  - fingerprinting technique
  - molecular disease
  - α, β chains
  - HbA_2
  - delta (δ) chains
  - Gower 1
  - zeta (ζ) chains
  - epsilon (ϵ) chains
  - HbF, fetal hemoglobin
  - gamma (γ) chains
- **The Nucleotide Sequence of a Gene…**
  - colinearity
  - *trpA* gene
  - one-gene-one-enzyme
  - one-gene-one-polypeptide chain

161

Chapter 14 Translation and Proteins

- **Variation in Protein Structure...**
    - polypeptides
    - proteins
    - 20 amino acids
    - carboxyl group
    - amino group
    - radical (R) group
    - central (C) atom
    - nonpolar (hydrophobic)
    - polar (hydrophilic)
    - positively charged
    - negatively charged
    - peptide bond
    - primary structure
    - secondary structure
    - α helix
    - β-pleated sheet
    - fibroin
    - tertiary structure
    - basic amino acids
    - acidic amino acids
    - quaternary structure
    - oligomeric
    - protomer
    - subunit

- **Posttranslational Modification...**
    - N-terminal removal
    - modification of amino acids
    - carbohydrate side chains
    - trimming
    - signal sequences removed

- protein targeting
- metal complexes
- protein folding
- chaperones
- heat-shock proteins
- upiquitins
- polyubiquitin-protein complex
- proteasome
- scrapie
- bovine spongiform encephalopathy
- mad cow disease
- Creutzfeldt-Jakob disease
- prion
- sickle-cell anemia
- Huntington disease
- Alzheimer disease
- Parkinson disease

- **Proteins Function in Many...**
    - hemoglobin
    - myoglobin
    - collagen
    - keratin
    - actin
    - myosin
    - tubulin
    - immunoglobulins
    - transport proteins
    - hormones
    - receptors

Chapter 14 Translation and Proteins

- ○ histones
- ○ transcription factors
- ○ enzymes
- ○ biochemistry
- ○ biological catalysis
- ○ energy of activation
- ○ active site
- ○ catabolism
- ○ anabolism

- ○ **Proteins Are Made Up of One…**
  - ○ protein domains
  - ○ catalytic domains
  - ○ DNA-binding domains
  - ○ exon shuffling
  - ○ LDLs
  - ○ *EGF*
  - ○ intron-early
  - ○ intron-late

F14.1 Polarity constraints associated with simultaneous transcription and translation in prokaryotes. The RNA polymerase is moving downward (arrow) in this sketch.

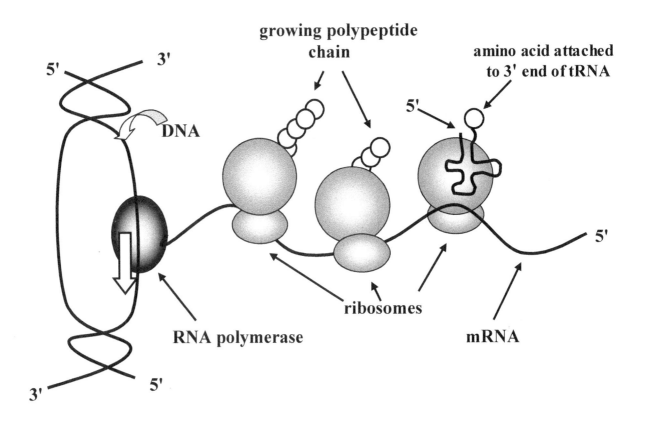

Chapter 14 Translation and Proteins

Answers to Now Solve This

14-1. One can conclude that the amino acid is not involved in recognition of the codon.

14-2. The best way to approach these types of problems, especially when the data are organized in the form given, is to realize that the substance (supplement) that "repairs" a strain, as indicated by a (+), is *after* the metabolic block for that strain. In addition, and most important, the substance that "repairs" the highest number of strains is either *the end product* or is *closest to the end product*.

Looking at the table, notice that the supplement tryptophan "repairs" all the strains. Therefore, it must be at the end of the pathway or at least after all the metabolic blocks (defined by each mutation). Indole "repairs" the next highest number of strains (3); therefore, it must be second from the end. Indole glycerol phosphate "repairs" two of the four strains, so it is third from the end. Anthranilic acid "repairs" the least number of strains, so it must be early (first) in the pathway.

Minimal medium is void of supplements, and mutant strains involving this pathway would not be expected to grow (or be "repaired"). The pathway, therefore, would be as follows:

AA----->IGP----->I----->TRY

To assign the various mutations to the pathway, keep in mind that if a supplement "repairs" a given mutant, the supplement must be after the metabolic block. Applying this rationale to the above pathway, the metabolic blocks are created at the following locations:

```
        trp 8     trp 2      trp 3  trp 1
precursor--\->AA--\->IGP--\->I--\->TRY
```

14-3. With the codes for valine being GUU, GUC, GUA, and GUG, single base changes from glutamic acid's GAA and GAG can cause the glu>>>val switch. The normal glutamic acid is a negatively charged amino acid, whereas valine carries no net charge and lysine is positively charged. Given these significant charge changes, one would predict some, if not considerable, influence on protein structure and function. Such changes could stem from internal changes in folding or interactions with other molecules in the RBC, especially other hemoglobin molecules.

165

Chapter 14 Translation and Proteins

Solutions to Problems and Discussion Questions

1. (a) The base sequences in tRNA suggested a cloverleaf secondary structure due to within-strand complementary base pairing. Such a model was later supported by X-ray crystallography and denaturation studies. **(b)** When UAA, UGA, or UAG triplets occur at internal sites in genes, premature translation termination occurs and verifies the chain-terminating function of these triplets. **(c)** Examination of nutritional mutations in *Neurospora* showed that upsets in metabolic pathways could result from mutant genes that segregated and assorted in typical fashion. In some cases, sufficient information was available to show that defective enzymes caused the metabolic upset. Thus, mutant genes must be responsible for the production of defective enzymes. **(d)** Since enzymes are proteins, it is reasonable to conclude that genes make proteins. In addition, early work on hemoglobin showed that one gene was responsible for making one of the polypeptide chains in hemoglobin. **(e)** A variety of experiments, ranging from sequencing of DNA and respective proteins to transformation and transfection experiments with known DNAs, directly confirm the genetic code. **(f)** Mutations that alter the amino acid sequence of a protein often alter its structure and surface chemistry. Since phenotypes (functions) are altered by mutations, structural changes in proteins are usually accompanied by alterations in function. The classic example that demonstrates the structure/function relationship of proteins is the comparison between normal (HbA) and mutant (HbS) hemoglobin. An amino acid substitution alters the structure of HbS and also alters its function.

2. When involved in protein synthesis, a functional ribosome will contain the following components: mRNA, charged tRNA, large and small ribosomal subunits, elongation and perhaps initiation factors, peptidyl transferase, GTP, Mg^{2+}, nascent proteins, and possibly GTP-dependent release factors. Together, these components order and form peptide bonds between adjacent amino acids, thereby assembling proteins.

3. Transfer RNAs are "adaptor" molecules in that they provide a way for amino acids to interact with sequences of bases in nucleic acids. Amino acids are specifically and individually attached to the 3' end of tRNAs, which possess a three-base sequence

(the anticodon) that can base-pair with three bases of mRNA (codons). Messenger RNA, on the other hand, contains a copy of the triplet codes, which are stored in DNA. The sequences of bases in mRNA interact, three at a time, with the anticodons of tRNAs.

Enzymes involved in transcription include the following: RNA polymerase (*E. coli*) and RNA polymerase I, II, III (eukaryotes). Those involved in translation include the following: aminoacyl tRNA synthetases, peptidyl transferase, and GTP-dependent release factors.

4. It was reasoned that there would not be sufficient affinity between amino acids and nucleic acids to account for protein synthesis. For example, acidic amino acids would not be attracted to nucleic acids. With an adaptor molecule, specific hydrogen bonding could occur between nucleic acids, and specific covalent bonding could occur between an amino acid and a nucleic acid tRNA.

5. The sequence of base triplets in mRNA constitutes the sequence of codons. A three-base portion of the tRNA constitutes the anticodon.

6. Since there are three nucleotides that code for each amino acid, there would be 423 code letters (nucleotides), 426 including a termination codon. This assumes that other features, such as the poly-A tail, the 5' cap, and noncoding leader sequences, are omitted.

7. Dividing 20 by 0.34 gives the number of nucleotides (about 59) occupied by a ribosome. Dividing 59 by 3 gives the approximate number of triplet codes, approximately 20.

8. The steps involved in tRNA charging are outlined in the text. An amino acid in the presence of ATP, Mg^{2+}, and a specific aminoacyl synthetase produces an amino acid–AMP enzyme complex (+ PP$_i$). This complex interacts with a specific tRNA to produce the aminoacyl tRNA.

9. The four sites in tRNA that provide for specific recognition are the following: attachment of the specific amino acid, interaction with the aminoacyl tRNA synthetase, interaction with the ribosome, and interaction with the codon (anticodon).

10. Isoaccepting tRNAs are those tRNAs that recognize and accept only one type of amino acid. In some way, each of the 20 different aminoacyl tRNA synthetases must be able to recognize either the base composition and/or tertiary structure of each of the isoaccepting tRNA species. Otherwise, the fidelity of translation would be severely compromised. The most direct solution to the problem would be to have each synthetase recognize each anticodon. Another reasonable consideration might involve the variable loop, which, in conjunction with the anticodon, might enable such specificity. In reality, there are several characteristics of each tRNA that are involved: one or more of the anticodon bases, portions of the acceptor arm, and a particular base that lies near the CCA terminus.

11. Phenylalanine is an amino acid that, like other amino acids, is required for protein synthesis. Whereas too much phenylalanine and its derivatives cause PKU in phenylketonurics, too little will restrict protein synthesis.

12. Both phenylalanine and tyrosine can be obtained from the diet. Most natural proteins contain these amino acids.

13. Tyrosine is a precursor to melanin, which is a skin pigment. Individuals with PKU fail to convert phenylalanine to tyrosine, and even though tyrosine is obtained from the diet, at the population level, individuals with PKU have a tendency for less skin pigmentation.

14. When an expectant mother returns to consumption of phenylalanine in her diet, she subjects her baby to higher than normal levels of phenylalanine throughout its development. Since increased phenylalanine is toxic, many (approximately 90 percent) newborns are severely and irreversibly retarded at birth. Expectant mothers (who are genetically phenylketonurics) should return to a low phenylalanine intake during pregnancy.

15. (a) In this cross, two gene pairs are operating because the F_2 ratio is a modification of a 9:3:3:1 ratio, which is typical of a dihybrid cross. If one assumes that homozygosity for either or both of the two loci gives white, then let strain A be *aaBB* and strain B be *AAbb*. The F_1 is *AaBb* and pigmented (purple). The typical F_2 ratio would be as follows:

9/16	A_B_	purple
3/16	aaB_	white
3/16	A_bb	white
1/16	aabb	white

If a pathway exists that has the following structure, then the genetic and biochemical data are explained.

(b) For this condition, with the pink phenotype present, leave the symbols the same; however, change the Y compound such that when accumulated, a pink phenotype is produced:

9/16	A_B_	purple
3/16	aaB_	white
3/16	A_bb	**pink**
1/16	aabb	white

16. In general, the rationale for working with a branched chain pathway is similar to that stated in the previous problem. Since thiamine "repairs" each of the mutant strains, it must, as stated in the problem, be the final synthetic product.

Remembering the "one-gene:one-enzyme" statement, each metabolic block should occur only in one place, so even though pyrimidine and thiazole supplements each "repair" only one strain, they will not occupy the same step; rather, a branched pathway is suggested. Consider that pyrimidine and thiazole are products of distinct pathways and that both are needed to produce the end product, thiamine, as indicated below:

17. The fact that enzymes are a subclass of the general term *protein*, a *one-gene:one-protein* statement might seem to be more appropriate. However, some proteins are made up of subunits, each different type of subunit (polypeptide chain) being under the control of a different gene. Under this circumstance, the *one-gene:one-polypeptide* statement might be more reasonable.

It turns out that many functions of cells and organisms are controlled by stretches of DNA that either produce no protein product (operator and promoter regions, for example) or have more than one function, as in the case of overlapping genes and differential mRNA splicing. A simple statement regarding the relationship of a stretch of DNA to its physical product is difficult to justify.

18. The electrophoretic mobility of a protein is based on a variety of factors, primarily the net charge of the protein and, to some extent, the conformation in the electrophoretic environment. Both are based on the type and sequence (primary structure) of the component amino acids of a protein. The interactions (hydrogen bonds) of the components of the peptide bonds, hydrophobic, hydrophilic, and covalent interactions (as well as others) are all dependent on the original sequence of amino acids and take part in determining the final conformation of a protein. A change in the electrophoretic mobility of a protein would therefore indicate that the amino acid sequence had been changed.

19. The following types of normal hemoglobin are presented in the text:

Hemoglobin	Polypeptide chains
HbA	$2\alpha2\beta$ (alpha, beta)
HbA$_2$	$2\alpha2\delta$ (alpha, delta)
HbF	$2\alpha2\gamma$ (alpha, gamma)
Gower 1	$2\zeta2\varepsilon$ (zeta, epsilon)

The *alpha* and *beta* chains contain 141 and 146 amino acids, respectively. The *zeta* chain is similar to the alpha chain, whereas the other chains are like the beta chain. Each chain represents a primary structure of amino acids connected by covalent peptide bonds. Secondary structures are determined by hydrogen bonding between components of the peptide bonds. Alpha helices and beta-pleated sheets result. Tertiary structures are formed from interactions between the amino acid side chains, whereas the quaternary level results from the associations of chains shown above.

20. Sickle-cell anemia is coined as a *molecular* disease because it is well understood at the molecular level; there is a base change in DNA, which leads to an amino acid change in the β chain of hemoglobin.

It is a *genetic* disease in that it is inherited from one generation to the next. It is not contagious, as might be the case of a disease caused by a microorganism. Diseases caused by microorganisms may not necessarily follow family blood lines, whereas genetic diseases do.

21. In the late 1940s, Pauling demonstrated a difference in the electrophoretic mobility of HbA and HbS (sickle-cell hemoglobin) and concluded that the difference had a chemical basis. Ingram determined that the chemical change occurs in the primary structure of the globin portion of the molecule using the fingerprinting technique. He found a change in the sixth amino acid in the β chain.

22. It is possible for an amino acid to change without changing the electrophoretic mobility of a protein under standard conditions. If the amino acid is substituted with an amino acid of like charge and similar structure, there is a chance that factors that influence electrophoretic mobility (primarily net charge) will not be altered. Other techniques such as chromatography of digested peptides may detect subtle amino acid differences.

23. One would expect individuals with HbC to suffer some altered hemoglobin function and, perhaps, be resistant to malaria as well. In fact, HbC homozygotes suffer mild hemolytic anemia (a benign hemoglobinopathy). The HbC gene is distributed particularly in malarial-infested areas, suggesting that some resistance to malaria is conferred. Recent studies indicate that HbC may be protective against severe forms of malaria, but not to more uncomplicated forms.

24. All of the substitutions involve one base change.

Chapter 14 Translation and Proteins

25. "Fine-mapping," meaning precise mapping of mutations *within* a gene, is possible in some phage systems because many recombinants can often be generated relatively easily. Having the precise intragenic location of mutations as well as the ability to isolate the products, especially mutant products, allows scientists to compare the locations of lesions within genes. Mutations occurring near the 5' end of a gene will produce proteins with defects near the N-terminus. In this problem, the lesions cause chain termination; therefore, the nearer the mutations are to the 5' end of the mRNA, the shorter will be the polypeptide product and thus the demonstration of the colinear relationship of genes and proteins.

26. *Colinearity* refers to the sequential arrangement of subunits, amino acids, and nitrogenous bases in proteins and DNA, respectively. Sequencing of genes and products in MS2 phages and studies on mutations in the A subunit of the *tryptophan synthetase* gene indicate a colinear relationship.

27. Yanofsky's work on the *trpA* locus in bacteria involved the mapping of mutations and the finding that a relationship exists between the position of the mutation in a gene and the amino acid change in a protein. Work with the MS2 by Fiers showed, by sequencing of the coat protein (129 amino acids) and the gene (387 nucleotides), a linear relationship as predicted by the code word dictionary. Because Fiers showed a direct relationship between codons, amino acids and punctuation (initiation and termination), one would consider it direct evidence for colinearity.

28. As stated in the text, the four levels of protein structure are the following:

Primary: the linear arrangement or sequence of amino acids. This sequence determines the higher level structures.

Secondary: α-helix and β-pleated sheet structures generated by hydrogen bonds between components of the peptide bond.

Tertiary: folding that occurs as a result of interactions between the amino acid side chains. These interactions include, but are not limited to, the following: covalent disulfide bonds between cysteine residues, interactions of hydrophilic side chains with water, and interactions of hydrophobic side chains with each other.

Quaternary: the association of two (dimer) or more polypeptide chains. Called *oligomeric,* such a protein is made up of more than one protein chain.

29. There are probably as many different types of proteins as there are different types of structures and functions in living systems. The text lists the following:

Oxygen transport: hemoglobin, myoglobin
Structural: collagen, keratin, histones
Contractile: actin, myosin
Immune system: immunoglobins
Cross-membrane transport: a variety of proteins in and around membranes, such as receptor proteins
Regulatory: hormones, perhaps histones
Catalytic: enzymes

30. Enzymes function to regulate catabolic and anabolic activities of cells. They influence (lower) the *energy of activation,* thus allowing chemical reactions to occur under conditions that are compatible with living systems. Enzymes possess active sites and/or other domains that are sensitive to the environment. The active site is considered to be a crevice, or pit, that binds reactants, thus enhancing their interaction. The other domains mentioned above may influence the conformation and therefore function of the active site.

31. An exon often encodes a functional domain within a protein, rather than some random part of the protein. The exon shuffling proposal hypothesizes that such an arrangement facilitates the mixing of domains. Evidence supporting exon shuffling comes from discoveries of DNA sequences related to functional domains of proteins that appear to have been recruited during evolution. In addition, the partial architectures of genes with respect to exons appear to be conserved but also modified as if altered by shuffling. The "intron-early" theory suggests that introns appeared early in evolution but were selected against. This model is supported by DNA sequence data whereby similar gene architecture is shared by distantly related species. The "intron-late" theory suggests that introns arose late in evolution with the origin of eukaryotes. The fact that introns are almost totally absent in prokaryotes and infrequent in yeast supports this view.

32. Even though three gene pairs are involved, notice that because of the pattern of mutations, each cross may be treated as monohybrid **(a)** or dihybrid **(b, c)**.

(a) F$_1$:   *AABbCC* = speckled

   F$_2$: 3   *AAB_CC* = speckled
      1   *AAbbCC* = yellow

(b) F$_1$:   *AABbCc* = speckled

   F$_2$: 9   *AAB_C_* = speckled
      3   *AAB_cc* = green
      3   *AAbbC_* = yellow⎤
      1   *AAbbcc* = yellow⎦ 4

(c) F$_1$:   *AaBBCc* = speckled

   F$_2$: 9   *A_BBC_* = speckled
      3   *A_BBcc* = green
      3   *aaBBC_* = colorless⎤
      1   *aaBBcc* = colorless⎦ 4

33. Because cross **(a)** is essentially a monohybrid cross, there would be no difference in the results if crossing over occurred (or did not occur) between the *A* and *B* loci.

34. A cross of the following nature would satisfy the data:

   AABBCC × *aabbcc*

Offspring in the F$_2$:

   27   *A_B_C_* = purple
   9   *A_B_cc* = pink
   9   *A_bbC_* = rose
   9   *aaB_C_* = orange
   3   *A_bbcc* = pink
   3   *aaB_cc* = pink
   3   *aabbC_* = rose
   1   *aabbcc* = pink

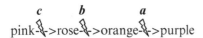

      c   *b*   *a*
   pink-↯->rose-↯->orange-↯->purple

The above hypothesis could be tested by conducting a backcross as given below:

   AaBbCc × *aabbcc*

The cross should give a

4(pink):2(rose):1(orange):1(purple) ratio

35.

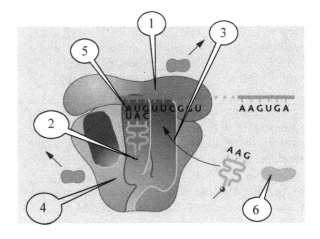

36.

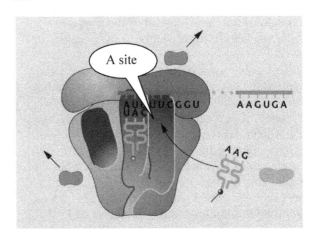

37. (a) Since protein synthesis is dependent on the passage of mRNA from DNA to ribosomes, any circumstance that compromises the flow will cause a reduction in protein synthesis. The more specific the binding of the antisense oligonucleotide to the target mRNA, the more specific the influence on protein synthesis. The ideal situation would be one in which a particular species of antisense oligonucleotide impacted on one and only one mRNA and therefore protein population.

(b) Clearly, a length of around 15 to 16 nucleotides is most effective in causing RNA degradation.

(c) A number of factors, including length of the oligonucleotide, are probably involved *in vivo*. It is likely that stability of the oligonucleotide is dependent on its base composition and length. The oligonucleotide must be small enough to diffuse effectively throughout the cell in order to "locate" the targeted mRNA, and it must not assume a folded conformation, which blocks opportunities for base pairing. Since the oligonucleotide is so much smaller than the target mRNA, it is also likely that the actual location of binding to the target is important in mRNA degradation. One of the main problems of antisense therapy is the introduction of the oligonucleotide into the interior of target cells.

38. (a) Considering the pedigree, it would appear that the gene is inherited as a dominant because to be recessive, all three individuals from outside the blood line would have to be heterozygous, an unlikely event. In addition, one would expect that a mutation in a tRNA synthetase would have considerable negative impact on glycine-bearing protein synthesis.

(b) On the other hand, because affected individuals in the pedigree are heterozygous, sufficient glycyl tRNA synthetase activity must be present to provide vital functions.

(c) Mutational and physiological perturbations, especially when occurring early in development, often cause neuropathologies. This is because of the highly sensitive nature of nerve cell development, and perhaps because axons are typically quite long, reduction of synthesis of glycine-bearing proteins inhibits required widespread distribution of such proteins within axons.

39. (a) To interact with the aqueous environment of a cell, polar amino acids would most likely populate the protein surface.

(b) A sequence of two positively charged amino acids and one negatively charged amino acid, in that sequence, would most likely be most effective.

(c) D-amino acids are not natural and may be more able to be specifically designed for a given function with a narrower range of side effects.

(d) Rational drug design marries knowledge of specific physiological functions of cellular structures with the possibility of designing an agent that targets that, and only that, function.

Chapter 15: Gene Mutation, DNA Repair, and Transposition

Concept Areas	Corresponding Problems
Mutations in General	2
Random and Adaptive Mutations	1, 3, 5, 6
Classes of Mutations	1, 3, 4, 7, 8
Detection of Mutations	17, 23
Induced Mutations	1, 10, 11, 12, 19, 25, 26
Molecular Basis of Mutation	9, 16, 19, 28, 32
Case Studies, Human Impact	15, 18, 20, 24, 29, 33
Transposition	21, 22, 30, 31
Repair of DNA	1, 13, 14, 27
UV Radiation and Skin Cancer	25, 26, 27, 29

Concepts and Processes Checklist

(Check topic when mastered – provide examples where appropriate – understand the context of each entry)

- **Gene Mutations Are Classified…**
  - alteration in DNA sequence
  - coding or noncoding regions
  - somatic cells or germ cells
  - point mutation
  - base mutation
  - missense mutation
  - nonsense mutation
  - silent mutation
  - frameshift mutation
  - transition
  - transversion
  - loss-of-function
  - gain-of-function
  - null mutation
  - visible mutation
  - nutritional mutation
  - biochemical mutation
  - behavioral mutation
  - regulatory mutation
  - lethal mutation
  - conditional mutation
  - temperature-sensitive mutation
  - neutral mutation
  - autosomal mutations
  - X-linked mutations
  - Y-linked mutations
  - homogametic
  - hemizygous
  - spontaneous mutations
  - induced mutations
  - mutation rate
  - mutation hot spots
  - human mutation rates

- SNPs
- fluctuation test
- Luria-Delbrück
- adaptive mutations
- random mutations
- **Spontaneous Mutations Arise...**
  - tautomers
  - replication slippage
  - depurination
  - apurinic site
  - deamination
  - oxidative damage
  - reactive oxidants
  - superoxides
  - hydroxyl radicals
  - hydrogen peroxide
  - transposable elements
- **Induced Mutations Arise...**
  - mutagens
  - base analogs
  - 5-bromouracil
  - 2-amino purine
  - bromodeoxyuridine
  - alkylating agents
  - ultraviolet radiation
  - electromagnetic spectrum
  - pyrimidine dimmers
  - ionizing radiation
  - X rays
  - gamma rays
  - cosmic rays
- ionizing radiation
- free radicals
- radon gas
- radioactive pharmaceuticals
- **Single-Gene Mutations Cause...**
  - polygenic
  - monogenic
  - single-base pair mutations
  - β-thalassemia
  - β-globin
  - *HBB* gene
  - expandable DNA repeats
  - trinucleotide repeat sequences
  - fragile-X syndrome
  - myotonic dystrophy
  - Huntington disease
  - glutamine tracks
- **Organisms Use DNA Repair...**
  - DNA repair
  - DNA polymerase III
  - proofreading
  - mismatch repair
  - DNA methylation
  - adenine methylase
  - endonuclease
  - exonuclease
  - postreplication repair
  - SOS repair
  - homologous recombination repair
  - photoreactivation repair
  - UV damage

- excision repair
- base excision repair
- DNA glycosylase
- apyrimidinic site
- apurinic site
- AP endonuclease
- nucleotide excision repair
- xeroderma pigmentosum (XP)
- unscheduled DNA synthesis
- somatic cell hybridization
- heterokaryon
- complementation
- double-strand break repair
- homologous recombination

- **The Ames Test Is Used to Assess…**
  - *Salmonella typhimurium*
  - carcinogens

- **Geneticists Use Mutations…**
  - model organisms
  - *E. coli*
  - *Saccharomyces cerevisiae*
  - *Drosophila melanogaster*
  - *Caenorhabditis elegans*
  - *Arabidopsis thaliana*
  - *Mus musculus*
  - conditional mutation
  - screening for mutations
  - selecting for mutations
  - genetic screen

- **Transposable Elements Move…**
  - transposable elements
  - transposons
  - insertion sequences (IS)
  - transposase
  - inverted terminal repeats (ITRs)
  - Tn elements
  - *Ac-Ds* system in maize
  - *dissociation (Ds)*
  - *activator (Ac)*
  - autonomous movement
  - mobile controlling element
  - *Copia* and *P* elements
  - *Drosophila*
  - 30 families
  - direct terminal repeat
  - hybrid dysgenesis
  - germ-line transformations
  - human transposable elements
  - transposable elements, LINEs, SINEs
  - LINE insertions–human genes
  - *Alu* element
  - transposable elements and evolution
  - 1/50–100 human births
  - 0.2 percent of human mutations
  - recombinase

F15.1 Graphic representation of the relationship between mutation and Darwinian evolutionary theory. Mutation provides the original source of variation on which natural selection operates.

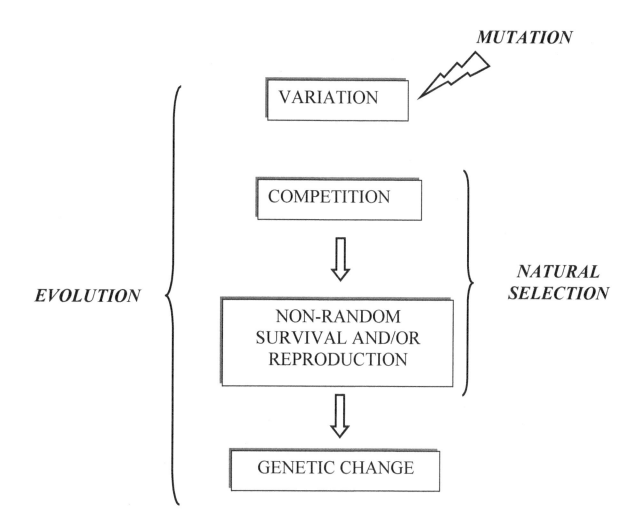

F15.2 Illustration of the difference between somatic and germ-line mutations. Somatic mutations are not passed to the next generation, whereas those in the germ line may be passed to offspring.

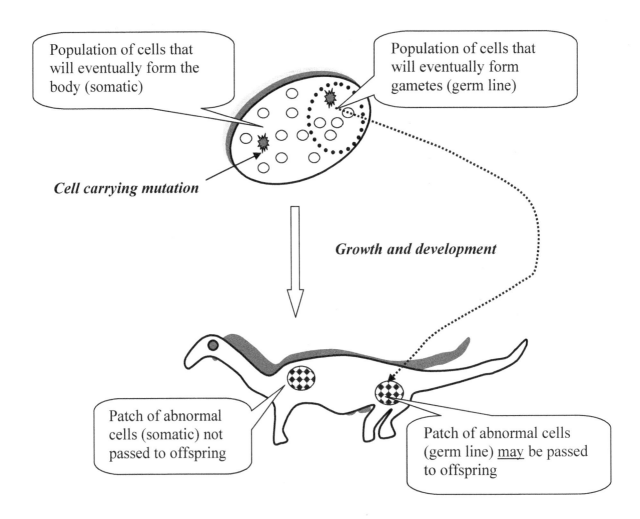

Answers to Now Solve This

15-1. The phenotypic influence of any base change is dependent on a number of factors, including its location in coding or noncoding regions, its potential in dominance or recessiveness, and its interaction with other base sequences in the genome. If a base change is located in a noncoding region, there may be no influence on the phenotype; however, some noncoding regions, in a traditional sense, may influence other genes and/or gene products. If a mutation occurring in a coding region acts as a full recessive, there should be no influence on the phenotype. If mutant gene acts as a dominant, then there would be an influence on the phenotype. Some genes interact with other genes in a variety of ways that would be difficult to predict without additional information.

15-2. There are several ways in which an unexpected mutant gene may enter a pedigree. If a gene is incompletely penetrant, it may be present in a population and only express itself under certain conditions. It is unlikely that the gene for hemophilia behaved in this manner. If a gene's expression is suppressed by another mutation in an individual, it is possible that offspring may inherit a given gene and not inherit its suppressor. Such offspring would have hemophilia. Since all genetic variations must arise at some point, it is possible that the mutation in the Queen Victoria family was new, arising in the father. Lastly, it is possible that the mother was heterozygous and, by chance, no other individuals in her family were unlucky enough to receive the mutant gene.

15-3. Any agent that inhibits DNA replication, either directly or indirectly, through mutation and/or DNA crosslinking will suppress the cell cycle and may be useful in cancer therapy. Since guanine alkylation often leads to mismatched bases, they can frequently be repaired by a variety of mismatched repair mechanisms. However, DNA crosslinking can be repaired by recombinational mechanisms; thus, for such agents to be successful in cancer therapy, suppressors of DNA repair systems are often used in conjunction with certain cancer drugs. See Wang, Z., et al. 2001. *J Natl. Cancer Inst.* 93(19):1434–6.

15-4. Ethylmethane sulfonate (EMS) alkylates the keto groups at the sixth position of guanine and at the fourth position of thymine. In each case, base-pairing affinities are altered and transition mutations result. Altered bases are not readily repaired, and once the transition to normal bases occurs through replication, such mutations avoid repair altogether.

Chapter 15 Gene Mutation, DNA Repair, and Transposition
Solutions to Problems and Discussion Questions

1. (a) When no known agents are involved and a mutation occurs and there is no indication of a mutation in the "family line," that mutation is considered to have arisen spontaneously.

(b) Numerous studies, beginning with those of Muller (1927) and Stadler (1928), showed that the occurrence of mutations could be associated with X rays. Since that time, various chemicals and radiation have been tested by a number of screening strategies. When the frequency of mutation in a test organism increases when exposed to a given agent, that agent is classified as a mutagen.

(c) In addition to postreplication, SOS, photoreactivation, and excision repair, various proofreading functions have been discovered in polymerases. Each has provided evidence that many mutations, once generated, may trigger repair.

2. Your essay should include a brief description of the genomic differences between diploid and haploid organisms and, with the exception of phenomena such as cell death, disease, and cancer, mutational circumstances are attributable to both groups of organisms.

3. Mutations that occur as a result of natural biological and/or chemical processes are considered spontaneous. They are relatively rare in comparison to induced mutations, which are more directed to the physical or chemical properties of DNA.

4. When conducting genetic screens, one assumes that all the cells of an organism are genetically identical. Therefore, the organism responds to the screen enabling detection of the mutation. Since a somatic mutation first appears in a single cell, it is highly unlikely that the organism will be sufficiently altered to respond to a screen because none of the other cells in that organism will have the same mutation. That's not to say that somatic mutations can't influence the organism. Cancer cells generally originate from a single altered cell and can have a profound influence on the fate of an organism.

5. It is true that *most* mutations are thought to be deleterious to an organism. A gene is a product of perhaps a billion or so years of evolution, and it is only natural to suspect that random changes will probably yield negative results. However, *all* mutations may not be deleterious. Those few, rare variations that are beneficial will provide a basis for possible differential propagation of the variation. Such changes in gene frequency represent the basis of the evolutionary process. See F15.1.

6. As stated in the previous question, a functional sequence of nucleotides, a gene, is likely to be the product of perhaps a billion or so years of evolution. Each gene and its product function in an environment that has also evolved, or coevolve. A coordinated output of each gene product is required for life. Deviations from the norm, caused by mutation, are likely to be disruptive because of the complex and interactive environment in which each gene product must function. However, on occasion a beneficial variation occurs.

7. A diploid organism possesses at least two copies of each gene (except for "hemizygous" genes), and in most cases, the amount of product from one gene of each pair is sufficient for production of a normal phenotype. Recall that the condition of "recessive" is defined by the phenotype of the heterozygote. If output from one normal (nonmutant) gene in a heterozygote gives the same phenotype as in the normal homozygote, where there are two normal genes, the normal allele is considered "dominant."

Genotypes	Phenotype, if mutant is	
	recessive	dominant
wild/wild	wild	wild
wild/mutant	wild	mutant
mutant/mutant	mutant	mutant

8. A *conditional* mutation is one that produces a wild-type phenotype under one environmental condition and a mutant phenotype under a different condition. A conditional *lethal* is a gene that under one environmental condition leads to premature death of the organism.

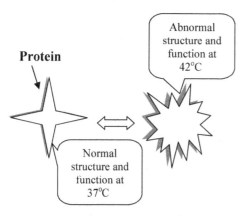

9. Watson and Crick recognized that various tautomeric forms, caused by single proton shifts, could exist for the nitrogenous bases of DNA. Such shifts could result in mutations by allowing hydrogen bonding of normally noncomplementary bases. As stated in the text, important tautomers involve keto-enol pairs for thymine and guanine, and amino-imino pairs for cytosine and adenine.

10. All three of the agents are mutagenic because they cause base substitutions. Deaminating agents oxidatively deaminate bases such that cytosine is converted to uracil and adenine is converted to hypoxanthine. Uracil pairs with adenine, and hypoxanthine pairs with cytosine. Alkylating agents donate an alkyl group to the amino or keto groups of nucleotides, thus altering base-pairing affinities. Note that 6-ethyl guanine acts like adenine, thus pairing with thymine. Base analogs such as 5-bromouracil and 2-amino purine are incorporated as thymine and adenine, respectively, yet they base pair with guanine and cytosine, respectively.

11. Frameshift mutations are likely to change more than one amino acid in a protein product because as the reading frame is shifted, new codons are generated. In addition, there is the possibility that a nonsense triplet could be introduced, thus causing premature chain termination. If a single pyrimidine or purine has been substituted, then only one amino acid is influenced.

12. X rays are of higher energy and shorter wavelength than UV light. They have greater penetrating ability and can create more disruption of DNA.

13. The delay or arrest of cell division provides an opportunity for normal DNA repair mechanisms to operate. Apoptosis is an organismic survival mechanism that eliminates a cell and its descendents that may eventually harm the organism.

14. *Photoreactivation* can lead to repair of UV-induced damage. An enzyme, photoreactivation enzyme, will absorb a photon of light to cleave thymine dimers. *Excision repair* involves the products of several genes, DNA polymerase I and DNA ligase, to clip out the UV-induced dimer, fill in, and join the phosphodiester backbone in the resulting gap. The excision repair process can be activated by damage that distorts the DNA helix.

Recombinational repair is a system that responds to DNA that has escaped other repair mechanisms at the time of replication. If a gap is created on one of the newly synthesized strands, a "rescue operation or SOS response" allows the gap to be filled. Many different gene products are involved in this repair process, for example, *recA* and *lexA*. In SOS repair, the proofreading by DNA polymerase III is suppressed; therefore, this is called an "error-prone system."

15. Because mammography involves the use of X rays and X rays are known to be mutagenic, it has been suggested that frequent mammograms may do harm. This subject is presently under considerable debate. At the 2002 World Health Organization conference in Barcelona, Spain, the conclusion was that "mammograms can prevent breast cancer deaths in one in 500 women ages 50 to 69."

16. There are numerous regions upstream from coding regions in a gene that are sensitive to mutation. Many mutations upset the regions that signal transcription factor and/or polymerase, thereby influencing transcription. Mutations within introns may affect intron splicing or other factors that determine mRNA stability or translation.

17. In the *Ames assay,* the compound to be tested is incubated with a mammalian liver extract to simulate an *in vivo* environment. This solution is then placed on culture plates with an indicator microorganism, *Salmonella typhimurium*, which is defective in its normal repair processes. The frequency of mutations in the tester strains is an indication of the mutagenicity of the compound.

18. *Xeroderma pigmentosum* is a form of human skin cancer caused by perhaps several rare autosomal genes, which interfere with the repair of damaged DNA. Studies with heterokaryons provided evidence for complementation, indicating that there may be as many as seven different genes involved. The photoreactivation repair enzyme appears to be involved. Since cancer is caused by mutations in several types of genes, interfering with DNA repair can enhance the occurrence of these types of mutations.

19. Transposable elements occur in a variety of sizes in bacteria, and each contains a gene for transposition as well as inverted terminal repeats. They may contain genes for antibiotic resistance in bacteria and as such create a considerable health risk to humans. Several classes of transposable elements have been discovered in maize, most notable being dissociation (*Ds*) and activator (*Ac*). There are more than 30 families of transposable elements in *Drosophila*, each present about 20 to 50 times in the genome. The human genome contains a number of transposable elements, which vary in size from one kilobase to more than six kilobases in length. Together, they may make up almost half of the human genome. Each transposable element is composed of terminal repeats and each can move within or between genomes.

20. It is possible that through the reduction of certain environmental agents that cause mutations, mutation rates might be reduced. On the other hand, certain industrial and medical activities actually concentrate mutagens (radioactive agents and hazardous chemicals). Unless human populations are protected from such agents, mutation rates might actually increase. If one asks about the accumulation of mutations (not rates) in human populations as a result of improved living conditions and medical care, then it is likely that as the environment becomes less harsh (through improvements), more mutations will be tolerated as selection pressure decreases. In addition, as individuals live longer and have children at a later age, some studies indicate that older males accumulate more gametic mutations.

21. In some cases, chromosome breakage occurs that has significant influence on gene function. In other cases, deletions may occur that also influence gene function.

22. Transposons cause changes in DNA in a variety of ways, including massive chromosomal alterations. In most cases, changes in DNA are harmful to organisms; in rare cases, an evolutionary advantage occurs because the new genetic variation confers a selective advantage.

23. Given that the cells were treated and then allowed to complete one round of replication, the final computation of the mutation rate should be divided by two (two cells are plated for each cell treated). The general expression for the mutation rate is the number of mutant cells divided by the total number of cells. In this case, the equation would be as follows:

$$\frac{18 \times 10^1}{6 \times 10^7}$$

$$\text{or} \qquad 3 \times 10^{-6}$$

Now dividing by two (as stated above) gives

$$1.5 \times 10^{-6}$$

24. Unscheduled DNA synthesis represents DNA repair. One can determine complementation groupings by placing each heterokaryon giving a "−" into one group and those giving a "+" into a separate group. For instance, *XP1* and *XP2* are placed into the same group because they do not complement each other. However, *XP1* and *XP5* do complement ("+"); therefore, they are in different groups. Completing such pairings allows one to determine the following groupings:

XP1	*XP4*	*XP5*
XP2		*XP6*
XP3		*XP7*

The groupings (complementation groups) indicate that there are at least three "genes" that form products necessary for unscheduled DNA synthesis. All of the cell lines that are in the same complementation group are defective in the same product.

25. Your study should include examination of the following short-term aspects: immediate assessment of radiation amounts distributed in a matrix of the bomb sites as well as a control area not receiving bomb-induced radiation and radiation exposure as measured by radiation sickness and evidence of radiation poisoning from tissue samples, abortion rates, birthing rates, and chromosomal studies.

Long-term assessment should include sex-ratio distortion (males being more influenced by X-linked recessive lethals than females), chromosomal studies, birth and spontaneous abortion rates, cancer frequency and type, and genetic disorders. In each case, data should be compared with a suitable control site to see if changes are bomb related. In addition, to attempt to determine cause-effect, it is often helpful to show a dose response. Thus, by comparing the location of individuals at the time of exposure with the matrix of radiation amounts, one may be able to determine whether those most exposed to radiation suffer the most physiologically and genetically. If a positive correlation is observed, then statistically significant conclusions may be possible.

26. Approximately 78 percent of the radiation exposure to humans comes from natural sources. Although diagnostic X rays do contribute about 10 percent of the exposure, other forms of human-made forms of radiation contribute only a relatively small amount. That's not to say that human-made radiation exposure is not a factor in causing mutations; rather, it is not a major factor.

27. Any condition that causes mutations in genes or DNA repair systems is likely to increase the rate of cancer. Specifically, mismatch repair defects are common in hereditary nonpolypopsis colon cancer, leukemias, lymphomas, and tumors of the ovary, prostate, and endometrium. The link between mutant mismatch repair systems and cancer is seen in mice engineered to have defects in mismatch repair genes. Such mice are cancer prone.

28. Since Betazoids have a four-letter genetic code and the gene is 3332 nucleotides long, the protein involved must be 833 amino acids in length.

(mr-1) Codon 829 specifies an amino that is very close to the end (carboxyl) of the gene. Whereas a nonsense mutation would terminate translation prematurely, the protein would be shortened by only five amino acids. Thus, the protein's ability to fold and perform its cellular function must not be seriously altered. Because of the direction of translation (5' to 3' on the mRNA), the carboxyl-terminal amino acids in

a protein are the last to be included in folding priorities and are sometimes less significant in determining protein function.

(mr-2) Since the phenotype is mild, this amino acid change does not completely inactivate the protein, but it does change its activity to some extent. Perhaps the substitution causes the protein to fold in a slightly aberrant manner, allowing it to have some residual function but preventing it from functioning entirely normally. Additionally, even if the protein folds similar to the wild-type protein, charge or structural differences in the protein's active site may be only mildly influenced.

(mr-3) This deletion contains a total of 68 nucleotides, which account for 17 amino acids. Since Betazoids' codons contain four nucleotides, the mRNA reading frames are maintained subsequent to the deletion. Protein function significantly depends on the relative positions of secondary levels of structure: α-helices and β-sheets. If the deleted section is a "benign" linker between more significant protein domains, then perhaps the protein can tolerate the loss of some amino acids in a part of the protein without completely losing its function.

(mr-4) Amino acid specified by codon 192 must be critical to the function of the protein. Altering this amino acid must disrupt a critical region of the protein, thus causing it to lose most or all of its activity. If the protein is an enzyme, this amino acid could be located in its active site and be critical for the ability of the enzyme to bind and/or influence its substrate. One might expect that the amino acid alteration is rather radical, such as that seen in the generation of sickle-cell anemia. HbS is caused by the substitution of a valine (no net charge) for glutamic acid (negatively charged).

(mr-5) A deletion of 11 base pairs, a number that is not divisible by four, will shift the reading frames subsequent to its location. Even though this deletion is smaller than the deletion discussed above (83–150) and is located in the same region, it causes a reading frame shift, and some or all of the amino acids that are added downstream from the mutation may be different from those in the normal protein. The reason that all will not likely change is the result of the synonyms in the code. There is also the possibility that a nonsense triplet may be introduced in the "out-of-phase" region, thus causing premature

chain termination. Because this mutation occurs early in the gene, most of the protein will be affected. This may well explain the severe insensitive phenotype.

29. Individuals with xeroderma pigmentosum (XP) are much more likely to contract skin cancer in youth than non-XP individuals. By age 20, approximately 80 percent of the XP population has skin cancer compared with approximately 4 percent in the non-XP group. XP individuals lack one or more genes involved in DNA repair.

30. It is probable that the IS occupied or interrupted normal function of a controlling region related to the *galactose* genes, which are in an operon with one controlling upstream element.

31. First, although less likely, one might suggest that transposons, for one reason or another, are more likely to insert in noncoding regions of the genome. One might also suggest that they are more stable in such regions. Second, and more likely, it is possible that transposons insert rather randomly and that selection eliminates those that have interrupted coding regions of the genome. Since such regions are more likely to influence the phenotype, selection is more likely to influence such regions.

32. (a) Nonsense mutation in coding regions: shortened product somewhat less than 375 amino acids depending on where the chain termination occurred. **(b)** Insertion in Exon 1, causing frameshift: a variety of amino acid substitutions and possible chain termination downstream. **(c)** Insertion in Exon 7, causing frameshift; a variety of amino acid substitutions and possible chain termination downstream involving less of the protein than the insertion in Exon 1. **(d)** Missense mutation: an amino acid substitution. **(e)** Deletion in Exon 2, causing frameshift: depending on the size of the deletion, a few too many amino acids may be missing. The frameshift would cause additional amino acid changes and possible termination. **(f)** Deletion in Exon 2, in frame: amino acids missing from Exon 2 without additional changes in the protein. **(g)** Large deletion covering Exons 2 and 3: significant loss of amino acids toward the N-terminal side of the protein.

33. (a) (1) When a region of DNA contains repeated segments, it is possible that the alignment of these segments may be offset as pictured in the following. Should there be a crossover between the elements within a segment, shortening and lengthening of the segments can occur. (Note: both of the figures that follow were obtained from http://biol.lf1.cuni.cz/ucebnice/en/repetitive_dna.htm)

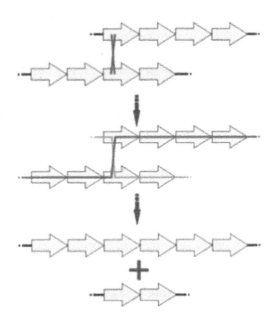

(2) When a loop forms because of within-strand base pairing of complementary repeats within a repetitive segment, it provides an opportunity for the polymerase to add repeats by continuing to replicate beyond the loop, as shown below.

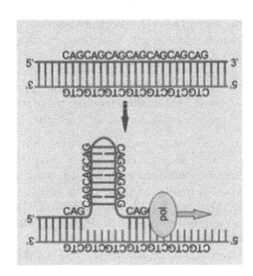

(b) A variety of regulatory signals occur both upstream and downstream from the coding regions of genes. Repeats often upset such regulatory signals. Although introns are normally removed from RNAs during maturation, repeats with introns may upset the splicing process or may actually influence regulatory sequences that are contained in introns.

(c) The coding region of a gene specifies a sequence of amino acids in a protein. Having a stretch of repetitive amino acids, even if short, may have a profound influence on protein function. Trinucleotide repeat expansion probably occurs to the same degree within and outside exons, but there is stronger selection against protein sequence changes. Changes in upstream and downstream sequences would also be significantly influenced by repeat expansion and be selected against.

Chapter 16: Regulation of Gene Expression in Prokaryotes

Concept Areas	Corresponding Problems
Overview	1, 2
Lactose Metabolism in E. coli: Inducible	1, 2, 4, 5, 6, 7, 8, 9, 10, 15, 27
Arabinose Operon	16
Positive and Negative Control	3, 18, 19, 21
Model Systems	4, 11, 14, 19, 20, 22, 23, 24, 26
Tryptophan Operon	1, 2, 17, 25
Attenuation	12, 13, 17

Concepts and Processes Checklist

(Check topic when mastered – provide examples where appropriate – understand the context of each entry)

- **Prokaryotes Regulate Gene...**

  - response to the environment

  - adaptive enzymes

  - constitutive enzyme

  - inducible

  - inducer

  - repressible

  - negative control

  - positive control

- **Lactose Metabolism in *E. coli***

  - lactose metabolism

  - galactose

  - glucose

  - *cis*-acting

  - *trans*-acting

  - *lac* operon

  - structural gene

  - β-galactosidase

  - permease

- transacetylase

- *lacZ, lacY*

- *lacA*

- gratuitous inducer

- isopropylthiogalactoside (IPTG)

- constitutive mutation

- repressor gene

- operator region

- operon model

- allosteric

- I^-, I^+, I^s, O^c

- merozygote

- equilibrium dialysis

- IPTG-binding protein

- **Catabolite-Activating Protein (CAP)**

  - catabolite repression

  - promoter retion

  - 5' upstream

- cyclic adenosine monophosphate (cAMP)
- adenyl cyclase
- ATP
- CAP-cAMP complex
- cooperative binding
- **Crystal Structure Analysis…**
  - confirmation of operon model
  - repression loop
  - multiple operators
- **The Tryptophan (*trp*) Operon…**
  - normally inactive repressor
  - tryptophan
  - corepressor
  - evidence for *trp* operon
  - leader sequence
  - evolving concept of the gene
- **Alterations to RNA Secondary Structure…**
  - attenuation

- hairpin
- terminator
- antiterminator
- antiterminator hairpin
- regulation of transcription
- riboswitches
- terminator structure
- secondary structures
- metabolite-sensing RNA sequence
- aptamer
- expression platform
- 5'-UTR
- terminator conformation
- antiterminator conformation
- **The *ara* Operon Is Controlled…**
  - arabinose (*ara*) operon
  - two regulatory regions
  - CAP-binding site

F16.1 Illustration of general processes of *negative* and *positive* control. If *negative* control is operating, the regulatory protein inhibits transcription. With *positive* control, transcription is stimulated.

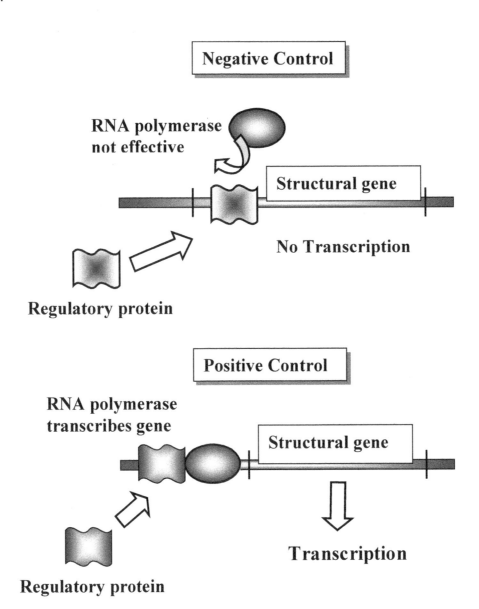

F16.2 Illustration of the nature of the product of the *I* gene. It can act "at a distance" because it is a protein that can diffuse through the cytoplasm and thus act in *trans*. There is no protein product of the operator gene; therefore, it can only act in *cis*.

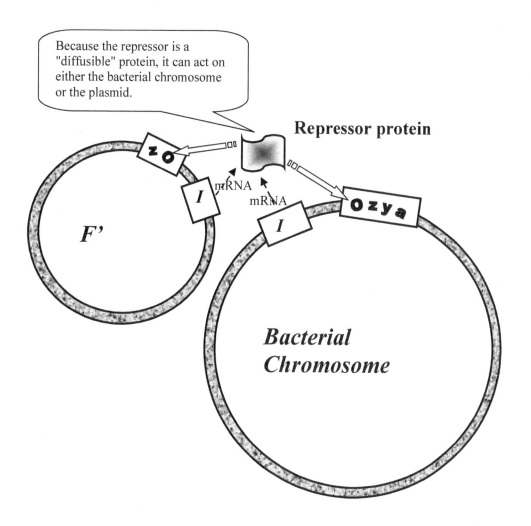

Chapter 16 Regulation of Gene Expression in Prokaryotes

<u>**Answers to Now Solve This**</u>

16-1. (a) Due to the deletion of a base early in the *lac Z* gene, there will be "frameshift" of all the reading frames downstream from the deletion, thereby altering many amino acids. It is likely that either premature chain termination of translation will occur (from the introduction of a nonsense triplet in a reading frame) or the normal chain termination will be ignored. Regardless, a mutant condition for the *Z* gene will be likely. If such a cell is placed on a lactose medium, it will be incapable of growth because β-galactosidase is not available. **(b)** If the deletion occurs early in the *A* gene, one might expect impaired function of the *A* gene product, but it will not influence the use of lactose as a carbon source.

16-2. In order to understand this question, it is necessary that you understand the negative regulation of the *lactose* operon by the *lac* repressor as well as the positive control exerted by the CAP protein. Remember, if lactose is present, it inactivates the *lac* repressor. If glucose is present, it inhibits adenyl cyclase, thereby reducing, through a lowering of cAMP levels, the positive action of CAP on the *lac* operon. **(a)** With no lactose and no glucose, the operon is off because the *lac* repressor is bound to the operator; although CAP is bound to its binding site, it will not override the action of the repressor. **(b)** With lactose added to the medium, the *lac* repressor is inactivated and the operon is transcribing the structural genes. With no glucose, the CAP is bound to its binding site, thus enhancing transcription. **(c)** With no lactose present in the medium, the *lac* repressor is bound to the operator region; since glucose inhibits adenyl cyclase, the CAP protein will not interact with its binding site. The operon is therefore "off." **(d)** With lactose present, the *lac* repressor is inactivated; however, since glucose is also present, CAP will not interact with its binding site. Under this condition, transcription is severely diminished and the operon can be considered to be "off."

Chapter 16 Regulation of Gene Expression in Prokaryotes

Solutions to Problems and Discussion Questions

1. (a) From 1900 on, scientists have known that when certain additives are supplied to growth media, organisms respond with the production of certain enzymes. Such enzymes were referred to as adaptive in contrast to constitutive enzymes that are produced regardless of particular medium additives. **(b)** Beginning with studies by Monod in 1946, it was determined that when lactose is added to a medium *E. coli* respond with the production of enzymes involved in lactose metabolism. When lactose was removed, such enzymes decreased in concentration. **(c)** Although a repressor molecule was originally suggested by Jacob and Monod from *cis*-acting O^c mutations, its isolation was achieved by others. Using a mutant of *E. coli* that produces relatively large amounts of the repressor, Gilbert and his colleagues were able to show that a repressor binds specifically to DNA containing the operator portion of the *lac* operon. **(d)** Radioactive IPTG, a sulfur-containing analog of lactose, was shown to bind to the *lac* repressor. Extracts of I^- constitutive cells, having no *lac* repressor activity, did not bind IPTG. The IPTG-binding substance was shown to be a protein using labeled (radioactive sulfur) amino acids. **(e)** Contrary to the *lac* system in which a material in the medium (lactose) causes the synthesis of *lac*-utilizing structural proteins, addition of tryptophan to the medium represses the transcription of proteins for the synthesis of tryptophan.

2. Your essay should include a description of the evolutionary advantages of the efficient response to environmental resources and challenges (antibiotics, for example) when such resources are present. Having related functions in operons provides for coordinated responses.

3. Refer to F16.1 to see that under *negative* control, the regulatory molecule interferes with transcription, whereas in *positive* control, the regulatory molecule stimulates transcription. Negative control is seen in the *lactose* and *tryptophan* systems, as well as a portion of the *arabinose* regulation. Catabolite repression and a portion of the *arabinose* regulatory systems are examples of positive control. Negative control requires a molecule to be removed from the DNA for transcription to occur. Positive control requires a molecule to be added to the DNA for transcription to occur.

4. In an *inducible system*, the repressor that normally interacts with the operator to inhibit transcription is inactivated by an *inducer*, thus permitting transcription. In a *repressible system*, a normally inactive repressor is *activated* by a corepressor, thus enabling it (the activated repressor) to bind to the operator to inhibit transcription. Because the interaction of the protein (repressor) has a negative influence on transcription, the systems described here are forms of *negative control* (see F16.1).

5. Refer to the text and to F16.1 and F16.2 to get a good understanding of the lactose system before starting.

$I^+O^+Z^+$ = **Inducible** because a repressor protein can interact with the operator to turn off transcription.

$I^-O^+Z^+$ = **Constitutive** because the repressor gene is mutant; therefore, no repressor protein is available.

$I^-O^cZ^+$ = **Constitutive** because the repressor protein is mutant, and the operator cannot bind the RNA polymerase.

$I^-O^cZ^+/F'O^+$ = **Constitutive** because there is no functional repressor. (See F16.2.)

$I^+O^cZ^+/F'O^+$ = **Constitutive** because there is a constitutive operator (O^c) next to a normal Z gene. Remembering that this operator functions in *cis* and is not influenced by the repressor protein, constitutive synthesis of β-galactosidase will occur.

$I^sO^+Z^+$ = **Repressed** because the product of the I^s gene is *insensitive* to the inducer lactose and thus cannot be inactivated. The repressor will continually interact with the operator and shut off transcription regardless of the presence or absence of lactose.

$I^sO^+Z^+/F'I^+$ = **Repressed** because, as in the previous case, the product of the I^s gene is insensitive to the inducer lactose and thus cannot be inactivated. The repressor will continually interact with the operator and shut off transcription regardless of the presence or absence of lactose. The fact that there is a normal I^+ gene is of no consequence because once a repressor from I^s binds to an operator, the presence of normal repressor molecules will make no difference.

6. Refer to the text and to F16.2 to get a good understanding of the lactose system before starting.

$I^+O^+Z^+$ = Because of the function of the active repressor from the I^+ gene, and no lactose to influence its function, there will be **no enzyme made**.

$I^+O^cZ^+$ = There will be a **functional enzyme made** because the constitutive operator is in *cis* with a Z gene. The lactose in the medium will have no influence because of the constitutive operator. The repressor cannot bind to the mutant operator.

$I^-O^+Z^-$ = There will be a **nonfunctional enzyme made** because with I^- the system is constitutive, but the Z gene is mutant. The absence of lactose in the medium will have no influence because of the nonfunctional repressor. The mutant repressor cannot bind to the operator.

$I^-O^+Z^-$ = There will be a **nonfunctional enzyme made** because with I^- the system is constitutive, but the Z gene is mutant. The lactose in the medium will have no influence because of the nonfunctional repressor. The mutant repressor cannot bind to the operator.

$I^-O^+Z^+/F'I^+$ = There will be **no enzyme made** because in the absence of lactose, the repressor product of the I^+ gene will bind to the operator and inhibit transcription.

$I^+O^cZ^+/F'O^+$ = Because there is a constitutive operator in *cis* with a normal Z gene, there will be **functional enzyme made**. The lactose in the medium will have no influence because of the mutant operator.

$I^-O^+Z^-/F'I^+O^+Z^+$ = Because there is lactose in the medium, the repressor protein will not bind to the operator and transcription will occur. The presence of a normal Z gene allows **functional and nonfunctional enzymes to be made**. The repressor protein is diffusible, working in *trans*.

$I^-O^+Z^-/F'I^+O^+Z^+$ = Because there is no lactose in the medium, the repressor protein (from I^+) will repress the operators and there will be **no enzyme made**.

$I^sO^+Z^+/F'O^+$ = With the product of I^s, there is binding of the repressor to the operator and therefore **no enzyme made**. The lack of lactose in the medium is of no consequence because the mutant repressor is insensitive to lactose.

$I^+O^cZ^+/F'O^+Z^+$ = The arrangement of the constitutive operator (O^c) with the Z gene will cause a **functional enzyme to be made**.

7. The mutations described are consistent with the structure of the *lac* repressor. The N-terminal portion of the repressor is involved in DNA binding; the C-terminal portion is more involved in association with lactose and its analogs.

8. A single *E. coli* cell contains very few molecules of the *lac* repressor. However, the *lac* I^q mutation causes a 10× increase in repressor protein production, thus facilitating its isolation. With the use of dialysis against a radioactive gratuitous inducer (IPTG), Gilbert and Müller-Hill were able to identify the repressor protein in certain extracts of *lac* I^q cells. The material that bound the labeled IPTG was purified and shown to be heat labile and to have other characteristics of protein. Extracts of *lac* I^- cells did not bind the labeled IPTG.

9. First, mutations could be isolated, suggesting that these mutations functioned in *trans*. At that time, gene products were assumed to be proteins, and the *trans* aspect strengthened the thought that a protein was involved. The IPTG-binding protein was labeled with sulfur-containing amino acids and mixed with DNA from λ phage, which contained the *lac* O^+ section of DNA. By glycerol gradient centrifugation, it was shown that the labeled repressor protein binds only to DNA that contained the *lac* O^+ region, thus indicating a specific binding to DNA.

10. (a) Because activated CAP is a component of the cooperative binding of RNA polymerase to the *lac* promoter, absence of a functional *crp* would compromise the positive control exhibited by CAP.

(b) Without a CAP binding site, there would be a reduction in the inducibility of the *lac* operon.

11. Since the four genes for erythritol catabolism are closely spaced and appear to be under coordinate control, an operon is likely to be involved. The product of the *eryD* gene is probably involved in repressing a promoter site. The system is induced when erythritol interrupts the action of the *eryD* repressor. These data are consistent with an inducible system of regulation.

12. Attenuation functions to reduce the synthesis of tryptophan when it is in full supply. It does so by reducing transcription of the *tryptophan* operon. The same phenomenon is observed when tryptophan activates the repressor to shut off transcription of the *tryptophan* operon.

13. It is likely that attenuation evolved as yet another means to regulate gene output. It provides a fine level of control over gene expression and attests to the complex measures that organisms have taken to effectively regulate their genomes. Attenuation can be achieved in a rather straightforward manner with amino acids, since their availability determines the availability of corresponding charged tRNAs. It is the availability of, or lack of, those charged tRNAs that regulates transcription. Overall, then, attenuation provides a direct route for amino acids to control gene expression.

14. Neelaredoxin appears to be a protein that defends anaerobic and perhaps aerobic organisms from oxidative stress brought on by the metabolism of oxygen. The generation of oxygen free radicals (creates the oxidative stress) is dependent on several molecular species including O_2 and H_2O_2. Apparently, relatively high levels of neelaredoxin are produced at all times (*constitutively expressed*) even when potential inducers of gene expression are not added to the system. Additional neelaredoxin gene expression is not responsive (*induced*) as a result of O_2 and H_2O_2 treatment.

15. Since selection was for rapid fermentation of lactose, one would expect that the operon is in the "on" or constitutive state because lactose must be converted to glucose and galactose for lactic acid to be formed through fermentation. Several types of mutations could cause the constitutive state: a mutation in the operator such that it may not recognize the repressor protein or a mutation in the repressor gene such that an ineffective (or no) repressor protein is made. In both cases, the term "mutation" would include not only base alterations, but also larger scale changes such as deletions, duplications, or insertions.

16. When arabinose is present in the medium, the structural genes for the *arabinose* operon are transcribed. If the structural genes for the *lac* operon replaced the structural genes for the *ara* operon, then in the presence of arabinose, the *lac* structural genes would be transcribed and β-galactosidase would be produced at induced levels.

17. Attenuation of the *trp* operon in *E. coli* involves the amino acid tryptophan and the leader region of mRNA to form a termination configuration for transcription. Riboswitches, on the other hand, encompass a variety of mechanisms that both terminate and allow transcription, depending on the particular metabolic requirements of the organism. In both cases, conformational changes are induced in the leader regions of mRNA and gene regulation is achieved.

18. Because a repressor stops transcription, one would consider this system, as described here, as being under negative control.

19. Since a substance supplied in the medium (the antibiotic) causes the synthesis of the efflux pump components, two situations seem appropriate. Under a *negative control* system, the antibiotic would interrupt the repressor to bring about induction (this would be an inducible system). Under *positive control*, the antibiotic would activate an activator (this again would be an inducible system).

20. First, notice that in the first row of data, the presence of tm in the medium causes the production of active enzyme from the wild-type arrangement of genes. From this, one would conclude that the system is *inducible*. To determine which gene is the structural gene, look for the *IE* function and see that it is related to *C*. Therefore, *C* codes for the **structural gene**. Because when *B* is mutant, no enzyme is produced, *B* must be the **promoter**. Notice that when genes *A* and *D* are mutant, constitutive synthesis occurs; therefore, one must be the operator and the other gene codes for the repressor protein. To distinguish these functions, one must remember that the repressor operates as a diffusible substance and can be on the host chromosome or the F factor (functioning in *trans*). However, the operator can operate only in *cis*. In addition, in *cis*, the constitutive operator is dominant to its wild-type allele, whereas the mutant repressor is recessive to its wild-type allele. Notice that the mutant *A* gene is dominant to its wild-type allele, whereas the mutant *d* allele is recessive (behaving as wild-type in the first row). Therefore, the *A* locus is the **operator** and the *D* locus is the **repressor** gene.

21. Because the deletion of the regulatory gene causes a loss of synthesis of the enzymes, the regulatory gene product can be viewed as one exerting *positive control*. When tis is present, no enzymes are made; therefore, tis must inactivate the positive regulatory protein. When tis is absent, the regulatory protein is free to exert its positive influence on transcription. Mutations in the operator negate the positive action of the regulator. On the next page (F16.3) is a model that illustrates these points.

F16.3 Model of regulatory system described in problem #21. This is an example of *positive* control.

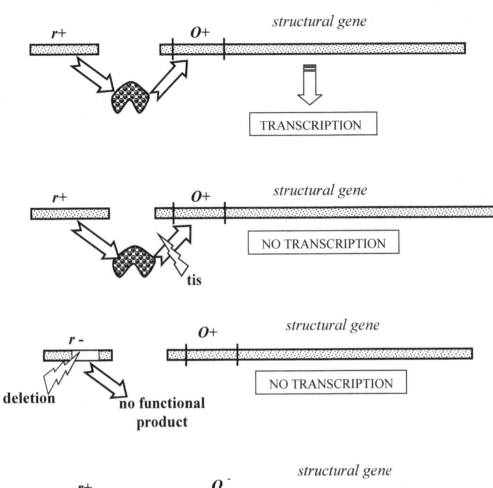

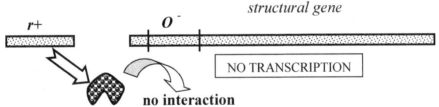

22. The first two sentences in the problem indicate an inducible system in which oil stimulates the production of a protein, which turns on (positive control) genes to metabolize oil. The different results in strains #2 and #4 suggest a *cis*-acting system. Because the operon by itself (when mutant as in strain #3) gives constitutive synthesis of the structural genes, the *cis*-acting system is also supported. The *cis*-acting element is most likely part of the operon.

23. (a) Call one constitutive mutation *lexA⁻* (mutation in the repressor gene product) and the other O^{uvrA-} (mutation in the operator).

(b) One can make partial diploid strains using F'. O^{uvrA-} will (given the other genes brought in by the F' element) be dominant to O^{uvrA+} and *lexA⁻* will be recessive to *lexA⁺*. O^{uvrA-} will act in *cis*.

24. If one could develop an assay for the other gene products under SOS control, with a *lexA⁻* strain, the other gene products should be present at induced levels.

25. You will need to identify the complementary regions. This is one of the rare cases in this handbook where the entire answer will not be directly given. You will find four regions that "fit." To get started, find the CACUUCC sequence. It pairs, with one mismatch, with a second region. Hint: The third region is composed of seven bases and starts with an AG.

26. (a) The simplest model for the action of R and D in *Chlamydia* would be to have the repressor element (R) become ineffective in binding the *cis*-acting element (D) when heat-shocked. This could happen in two ways. Either the supercoiled DNA alters its conformation and becomes ineffective at binding R or the D-binding efficiency of the R protein is altered by heat. In either case, the genes for infectivity are transcribed in the presence of the heat shock. **(b)** The most straightforward comparison between the heat-shock R and D system in *Chlamydia* and the heat-shock sigma factor in *E. coli* would be where the R-D system is inactivated in *Chlamydia*, and a sigma factor is activated by heat in *E. coli*.

27. Since all the regulatory elements are present in the engineered plasmid, one must consider the influence of glucose, through CAP, on the production of structural genes. With glucose present, there will be limited (considered here as no) synthesis of the structural genes regardless of the presence of lactose. I^s will act as a dominant to I^+ because, being insensitive to lactose, once it binds to an operator it will shut it off. O^c will act only in *cis* and allow production of its structural genes regardless of the presence or absence of lactose unless there is glucose in the medium. With glucose in the medium, an operon with O^c will be shut off because of catabolite repression. Expected results are presented below:

	Medium Condition			
Genotype	**Lactose**	**Glucose**	**β-galactosidase**	**Green Colonies**
$I^+O^+Z^+/p-I^+O^+GFP$	−	+	−	−
	+	+	−	−
	+	−	+	+
$I^+O^+Z^-/p-I^+O^cGFP$	−	+	−	−
	+	−	−	+
$I^+ O^+ Z^+/p-I^sO^cGFP$	−	+	−	−
	+	−	−	+
$I^+O^cZ^+/p-I^sO^+GFP$	−	+	−	−
	+	−	+	−

Chapter 17: Regulation of Gene Expression in Eukaryotes

Concept Areas	Corresponding Problems
Overview	1, 2, 3
Nuclear Organization	5, 22
Chromatin Structure	4, 6, 8, 15, 17, 19, 20, 23, 25
Chromosomal Proteins	6, 7, 18
Regulatory Elements	1, 10, 28, 29
Transcription Factors	1, 11, 12, 30
Promoters, Enhancers, Silencers	9, 13, 16, 21, 30
Posttranscriptional Regulation	2, 24, 26, 27, 28
RNA regulatory molecules	1, 14, 27

Concepts and Processes Checklist

(Check topic when mastered – provide examples where appropriate – understand the context of each entry)

○ **Eukaryotic Gene Regulation...**

  ○ tightly controlled

  ○ multiple cell types

  ○ many different levels

  ○ more DNA than prokaryotes

  ○ histones and other proteins

  ○ chromatin structural changes

  ○ mRNAs spliced, capped

  ○ polyadenylation

  ○ presence of nuclear membrane

  ○ RNA transport/regulation

  ○ different half-lives of mRNAs

  ○ modulation of translation

  ○ RNA polymerase II

  ○ DNA amplifications

○ **Eukaryotic Gene Expression...**

  ○ chromatin structure

  ○ histones and nonhistone proteins

○ **Chromosome Territories...**

  ○ chromosome painting

  ○ chromosome territory

  ○ interchromosomal domain

  ○ transcription factory

  ○ open chromatin

  ○ closed chromatin

  ○ nucleosome associations

○ **Histone Modifications...**

  ○ changes to nucleosomes

  ○ DNA modifications

  ○ H2A and H3

  ○ H2A.Z and H3.3

  ○ histone acetyltransferase (HATs)

  ○ histone tail

  ○ histone deacetylase (HDACs)

  ○ repositioned nucleosomes

  ○ SWI/SNF

- DNA methylation
- 5-methylcytosine
- CG doublet
- CpG island
- 5-azacytidine

- **Eukaryotic Transcription Initiation...**
  - *cis*-acting sequence
  - *trans*-acting factors
  - promoter elements
  - core promoter
  - proximal promoter elements
  - focused promoters
  - transcription start site
  - dispersed promoters
  - Initiator (Inr)
  - TATA box
  - TFIIB recognition element (BRE)
  - downstream promoter element (DPE)
  - motif ten element (MTE)
  - CAAT box
  - GC box
  - GGGCGG element
  - enhancers and silencers
  - need not be fixed
  - variable orientation
  - position independent
  - silencer
  - tissue- or temporal-specificity

- **Eukaryotic Transcription Initiation...**
  - transcription factors
  - activators

- repressors
- tissue- or temporal-specificity
- metallothionein IIA
- multiple *cis*-acting elements
- *hMTIIA*
- BLE
- ARE
- various *cis*-elements
- GRE
- MTF1
- DNA-binding domain
- *trans*-activating
- *trans*-repression
- helix-turn-helix (HTH)
- zinc-finger
- basic leucine zipper (bZIP)

- **Activators and Repressors Interact...**
  - RNA polymerase II
  - transcription initiation complex
  - pre-initiation complex (PIC)
  - RNA polymerase platform
  - general transcription factors
  - TFIID, TFIIB, TFIIA, etc.
  - TBP (TATA binding protein)
  - TAFs (TBP associated factors)
  - unwinding of promoter DNA
  - elongation complex
  - chromatin remodeling
  - PIC assembly
  - RNAP II
  - coactivators
  - enhanceosome

- **Gene Regulation in a Model…**

  - *GAL* gene system in yeast

  - structural genes

  - regulatory genes

  - inducible

  - null mutations

  - positive control

  - DNase hypersensitive

  - UAS elements

  - Gal4p, Gal3p

  - SAGA

  - various transcription factors

  - PIC

  - SWI/SNF

- **Posttranscriptional Gene Regulation…**

  - removal of introns

  - splicing

  - poly-A tail

  - 5' cap

  - alternative splicing

  - *CT/CGRP*

  - polyadenylation signal

  - proteome

  - *Dscam*

  - RNA editing

  - myotonic dystrophy

  - DM1, DM2

  - *DMPK*

  - trinucleotide repeat

  - *ZNF9*

  - spliceopathies

- sex determination

- *Drosophila*

- *Sex lethal* (*Sxl*)

- *transformer* (*tra*)

- *doublesex* (*dsx*)

- 2X:2A and other ratios

- DSX-M, DSX-F

- mRNA stability

- half life, $t_{1/2}$

- poly-A binding protein

- decapping enzymes

- nonsense-mediated decay

- adenosine-uracil rich element

- translational regulation

- posttranslational regulation

- p53, DNA damage

- Mdm2

- ubiquitin

- RNA interference (RNAi)

- RNA-induced gene silencing

- *unc-22*

- small interfering RNAs (siRNAs)

- microRNAs (miRNAs)

- Dicer

- RNA-induced silencing complex

- RISC

- RITS

- therapeutic RNAi

- **The Immune System and Antibody…**

  - antigen

  - antigen recognition

- ○ humoral immunity
- ○ immunoglobulin
- ○ antibody
- ○ B lymphocyte
- ○ B cell
- ○ light (L) chains
- ○ heavy (H) chains
- ○ constant region
- ○ variable region
- ○ **Gene Rearrangements in the K…**
  - ○ κ light-chain gene

- ○ C exon
- ○ LV regions
- ○ J region
- ○ hypermutation
- ○ **ENCODE Data Are Transforming…**
  - ○ encyclopedia of DNA elements
  - ○ enhancer RNA
  - ○ "noise"
  - ○ noncoding RNAs

Chapter 17 Regulation of Gene Expression in Eukaryotes

Answers to Now Solve This

17-1. Cancer cells often originate under the influence of mutations in tumor-suppressor genes or proto-oncogenes. Should hypermethylation occur in one of many DNA repair genes, the frequency of mutation would increase because the DNA repair system is compromised. The resulting increase in mutations might occur in tumor-suppressor genes or proto-oncogenes.

17-2. General transcription factors associate with a promoter to stimulate transcription of a specific gene. Some *trans*-acting elements, when bound to enhancers, interact with coactivators to enhance transcription by forming an enhanceosome that stimulates transcription initiation. Transcription can be repressed when certain proteins bind to silencer DNA elements and generate repressive chromatin structures. The same molecule may bind to a different chromosomal regulatory site (enhancer or silencer), depending on the molecular environment of a given tissue type.

17-3. Mutations in the *tra* gene of *Drosophila* can dramatically alter development such that a normal female is produced if the TRA protein is present and a male develops when the TRA protein is absent. A null *tra* allele would produce males because of male-specific splicing, whereas a constitutively active *tra* gene would produce females.

Chapter 17 Regulation of Gene Expression in Eukaryotes
Solutions to Problems and Discussion Questions

1. (a) Mutations within promoters alter transcription efficiencies, whereas deletions alter the initiation point of transcription. Enhancers (and silencers) are chromosomal elements that negatively influence transcription when deleted or altered by mutation. Insertion of an enhancer by recombinant technology increases transcription.

(b) Transcription factors possess a DNA-binding domain that binds to DNA sequences and provides *cis*-regulation. Structural motifs, such as helix-turn-helix, enable DNA binding, and deletions of promoters and surrounding regions suppress such binding.

(c) Scientists determined that injection of certain short double-stranded RNAs in roundworm cells led to the degradation of specific mRNA. This process is called RNA interference (RNAi).

2. Your essay should include an approximation of the percentage of regulatory elements/transcription products in the human genome, the binding sites of regulatory proteins, and the general architecture of regulatory elements within chromatin.

3. There are several reasons for anticipating a variety of different regulatory mechanisms in eukaryotes as compared with prokaryotes. Eukaryotic cells contain greater amounts of DNA, and this DNA is associated with various proteins, including histones and nonhistone chromosomal proteins. *Chromatin* as such does not exist in prokaryotes. In addition, whereas there is usually only one chromosome in prokaryotes, eukaryotes have more than one chromosome all enclosed in a membrane (nuclear membrane). This nuclear membrane separates, both temporally and spatially, the processes of transcription and translation, thus providing an opportunity for post-transcriptional, pre-translational regulation.

While prokaryotes respond genetically to changes in their external environment, cells of multicellular eukaryotes interact with each other as well as the external environment. The structural and functional diversity of cells of a multicellular eukaryote, coupled with the finding that all cells of an organism contain a complete complement of genes, suggests that in some cells certain genes are active that are not active in other cells.

It is often difficult to study eukaryotic gene regulation because of the complexities mentioned above, especially tissue specificity and the various levels at which regulation can occur. Obtaining a homogeneous group of cells from a multicellular organism often requires a significant alteration of the natural environment of the cell. Thus, results from studies on isolated cells must be interpreted with caution. In addition, because of the variety of intracellular components (nuclear and cytoplasmic) it is difficult to isolate, free of contamination, certain molecular species. Even if such isolation is accomplished, it is difficult to interpret the actual behavior of such molecules in an artificial environment.

4. Chromatin is remodeled when there are significant changes in chromatin organization. Such remodeling involves changes in DNA methylation and interaction of DNA with histones in nucleosomes. Nucleosome remodeling complexes alter nucleosome structure and position by a number of processes, including histone modification and the action of enhancers/silencers.

5. Determining the location of individual chromosomes in the interphase nucleus has been made possible by chromosome-painting techniques whereby fluorescent markers attach to specific chromosomes. Each chromosome occupies a discrete domain called a territory, between which are interchromosomal compartments. Transcription factories are nuclear sites where RNA polymerase II is most prevalent.

6. When DNA is transcriptionally active, it is in a less condensed state and, as such, more open to DNase digestion.

7. A major modification of histones involves acetylation by histone acetyltransferase enzymes and deacetylation by histone deacetylases. Histones may be loosened from DNA by the chromatin remodeler SWI/SNF.

8. In general, chromatin is remodeled when there are significant changes in chromatin organization. Such remodeling involves changes in DNA methylation, interaction of DNA with histones in nucleosomes. Nucleosome remodeling complexes alter nucleosome structure and position by a number of processes, including histone modification.

9. *Promoters* are conserved DNA sequences that influence transcription from the "upstream" side (5') of mRNA coding genes. They are usually fixed in position and within 100 base pairs of the initiation site for mRNA synthesis. Examples of such promoter sites are the following: TATA, CAAT, and GC boxes. *Enhancers* are *cis*-acting sequences of DNA that stimulate the transcription from most, if not all, promoters. They are somewhat different from promoters in that the position of the enhancer need not be fixed; it may be significantly upstream, downstream, or within the gene being regulated. The orientation may be inverted without significantly influencing its action. Enhancers can work on different genes; that is, they are not gene specific.

10. In general, activators and repressors change the relationship of RNAP II to the transcription complex. DNA loops are thought to bring distant enhancer or silencer elements into proximity with promoter regions of the genes under their regulation.

11. Basic differences that are known to occur when comparing genetic regulation in prokaryotes and eukaryotes include the following:

– differences in basic chromosome structure
– chromosome remodeling
– histone acetylation
– differences in gene structure
– cell structure (nucleus in eukaryotes)
– levels of potential regulation

    …transcriptional
    …mRNA processing
    …transport
    …selection for processing and translation
    …mRNA stability

– genomic aspects (amplification, etc.)
– biological context in terms of multicellular
   interactions versus single-cell survival

12. Generally, one determines the influence of various regulatory elements by removing necessary elements or adding extra elements. In addition, examining the outcome of mutations within such elements often provides insight as to function.

Assay systems determine the relative levels of gene expression after such alterations.

13. *Focused* promoters appear to define transcription initiation at a single nucleotide, whereas *dispersed* promoters direct initiation from a number of nucleotides covering a relatively large region (50 to 100 nucleotides). Most genes of lower eukaryotes use focused transcription and in general are associated with genes that are highly regulated. Dispersed promoters are more often associated with genes that act constitutively.

14. RNA interference begins with a double-stranded RNA being processed by a protein called Dicer that, in combination with RISC, generates short interfering RNA (siRNA). Unwinding of siRNA produces an antisense strand that combines with a protein to cleave mRNA complementary sequences. Short RNAs called microRNAs pair with the 3'-untranslated regions of mRNAs and block their translation.

15. Recombinational imprecision between any pair of LV and J regions provides variation in amino acid sequence during immunoglobulin formation.

16. Inr, BRE, DPE, and MTE sequences are double-stranded DNA elements located in the transcription start site (Inr), immediately upstream or downstream from the TATA box (BRE), or downstream (DPE, MTE) from the transcription site (+18 to +27 and +28 to +33, respectively).

17. Following is a diagram of a possible mechanism by which supercoiling may positively influence enhancer activity over a relatively long distance.

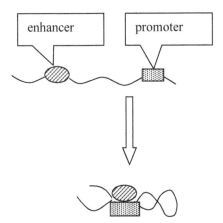

18. Given that DNA methylation plays a role in gene expression in mammals, any change in DNA methylation, plus or minus, can potentially have a negative impact on progeny development. In addition, since $m^5C >>>$ thymine, transitions are likely to cause mutations in coding regions of DNA; when methylation patterns change, new sites for mutation arise. Should mutations occur at a higher rate in previously unmethylated sites (genes), embryonic development is likely to be affected.

19. Assuming that you can identify chromosomes 4 and 10, it should be possible to determine their intimate association and subsequent recombination microscopically. Since formation of a complete heavy chain is dependent on recombination, if such chromosomes are intimately associated, the creature is likely to be at least 13 years of age. If the chromosomes are not associated, the creature is probably younger.

20. Since there are multiple routes that lead to cancer, one would expect complex regulatory systems to be involved. More specifically, whereas in some cases, downregulation of a gene, such as an oncogene, may be a reasonable cancer therapy, downregulation of a tumor-suppressor gene would be undesirable in therapy.

21. **(a)** A deletion within the *GAL4* gene that removes amino acids 1–100 would remove the DNA-binding section and not allow transcriptional activation. **(b)** Without the product of the *GAL3* gene, there would be no disruption of the Gal4p/Gal80p complex and therefore no transcription of the *GAL4* gene. **(c)** If the *GAL80* gene product can't interact with Gal3p, there can be no interaction with the Gal4p/Gal80p complex and therefore no *GAL1* transcription. **(d)** A deletion of one of the four UAS$_G$ elements would reduce transcription of the *GAL1* gene. **(e)** Generally, mutations in the TATA box of a promoter reduce transcription of the relevant gene.

22. Following is a sketch of several RNA polymerase molecules (filled circles) in what might be a transcription factory. In this diagram, eight RNAP II molecules are shown being transcribed. Nascent transcripts are shown projecting from the RNAP II molecules. For simplicity, only one promoter and one structural gene are shown.

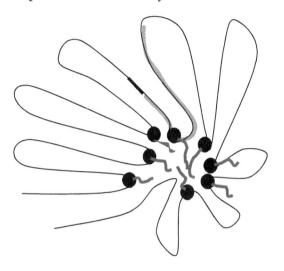

23. 5-azactidine is an analog of cytidine, but it cannot be methylated. When incorporated into DNA, it stimulates the expression of genes. Scientists have determined that cells exposed to 5-azacytidine increase their production of γ chain hemoglobin, which effectively associates with α chains. It is thought that individuals with severe β-thalassemia might benefit from its use; however, because 5-azacytidine is not gene specific, its widespread influence on the genome constitutes a considerable health hazard.

24. Since mRNA stability is directly related to the likelihood of translation, one could use a number of different constructs as shown here and test for luciferase activity in the assay system described in the problem.

5′-cap	3′-tail	mRNA (no cap, no tail)
−	−	+
+	−	+
−	+	+
+	−	−
−	+	−

25. Methylation of CpGs causes a reduction in luciferase expression, which is somewhat proportional to the amount of methylation and patch size. Methylation within the transcription unit more drastically reduces luciferase expression compared with methylation outside the transcription unit. A high degree of methylation outside the transcription unit (593 CpGs) has as great an impact on depressing transcription as the same degree of methylation within the transcription unit.

26. When splice specificity is lost, one might observe several classes of altered RNAs: (1) a variety of nonspecific variants producing RNA pools with many lengths and combinations of exons and introns; (2) incomplete splicing where introns and exons are erroneously included or excluded in the mRNA product; and (3) a variety of nonsense products, which result in premature RNA decay or truncated protein products. It is presently unknown whether cancer-specific splices initiate or result from tumorigenesis. Given the complexity of cancer induction and the maintenance of the transformed cellular state, gene products that are significant in regulating the cell cycle may certainly be influenced by alternative splicing and thus contribute to cancer.

27. One of the targets of the SXL protein is the pre-mRNA encoded by the *tra* gene, which is transcribed in male and female cells. Using RNA-induced silencing, one could specifically alter *tra* pre-mRNA levels in constant genetic backgrounds. Using classical genetics, mutations in the *tra* gene can be isolated by screens to determine the action of *tra* on male/female differentiation. The classical approach is laborious and influenced by different genetic backgrounds of mutant strains. RNA-induced silencing is thought to be relatively specific; however, introduction of double-stranded RNAs into cells produces an artificial environment in which to study gene action.

28. Steroid hormones interact, through receptor molecules, with DNA to regulate genes. In doing so, genes responsible for uncontrolled cell growth may be influenced. If Tamoxifen blocked the pathway by which estrogen influenced DNA, then it might be effective in fighting ER-positive cancer. In fact, Tamoxifen is an antagonist of the estrogen receptor.

29. The most direct way to determine whether the newly discovered GRE (glucocorticoid response element) sequence in the human β-globin is necessary for transcription would be to assemble an assay system that carries the GRE sequence and compare it to one that lacks the sequence. Because GRE is influenced by a glucocorticoid receptor protein only when bound to the glucocorticoid hormone, additional experimental approaches are available. Simply put, is the human β-globin gene responsive to the stimulatory action of the glucocorticoid hormone? If not, it is not likely to be necessary for accurate human β-globin expression. In the *hMTIIA* environment, gene transcription is stimulated when the cytoplasmic receptor binds to the hormone that allows it to enter the nucleus and bind to GRE. Addition of the glucocorticoid hormone to both the human β-globin and *hMTIIA* systems would indicate, in assays, whether each system responded similarly.

30. (1) Devise some way, through enzymatic or RNA action, to eliminate or mask the nuclear location signal. (2) Block the active site of the receptor. (3) Block the interaction of the transcription factor and DNA promoter site.

Chapter 18: Developmental Genetics

Concept Areas	Corresponding Problems
Developmental Concepts	2, 3, 17, 19, 22
Variable Gene Activity Theory	9, 20, 23, 27
Differential Transcription in Development	9, 10, 11, 14, 18, 24, 25
Genetics of Embryonic Development	1, 4, 8, 15
Maternal-Effect Genes and Body Plans	5, 6, 15, 16, 17, 18
Zygotic Genes and Segment Formation	7, 8
Homeotic and Hox Genes	12, 13, 14, 18, 21
Arabidopsis Development	20, 21, 23, 26
Cell-Cell Interactions in C. elegans	1, 22, 23, 24

Concepts and Processes Checklist

(Check topic when mastered – provide examples where appropriate – understand the context of each entry)

- **Differentiated States Develop...**
  - development
  - differentiated state
  - variable gene activity
- **Evolutionary Conservation...**
  - common set of systems
  - conserved DNA sequences
  - homeotic genes
- **Genetic Analysis of Embyronic...**
  - *Drosophila* model organism
  - 10-day development
  - nuclear divisions
  - syncytial blastoderm
  - posterior pole
  - germ cells
  - anterior-posterior
  - dorsal-ventral

- embryogenesis
- maternal effect genes
- zygotic genes
- *gap* genes
- *pair-rule* genes
- *segment-polarity* genes
- segmentation genes
- homeotic selector genes
- runt domain
- *RUNX2*
- cleidocranial dysplasia
- homeotic mutants
- *Antennapedia*
- *Hox* genes
- *bithorax*
- homeobox
- homeodomain

- temporally ordered
- spatially ordered
- cascade
- *Hox* genes and human disorders
- *HOXA, HOXB, HOXC, HOXD*
- synpolydactyly

- **Plants Have Evolved…**

  - *Arabidopsis thaliana*
  - class A, B, and C genes
  - MADS-box proteins

- *C. elegans* **Serves as a Model…**

  - signaling pathways
  - Notch signaling pathway
  - *Caenorhabditis elegans*

- hermaphrodites
- 959 somatic cells
- known cell lineages
- vulval development
- *lin-12*
- gain-of-function

- **Binary Switch Genes…**

  - gene-regulatory networks (GNRs)
  - control of eye formation
  - *twin of eyeless (toy)*
  - *eyeless (ey)*
  - other related genes
  - downstream transcription factors
  - evolutionary conservation

F18.1 Illustration of the relationship between determination and differentiation. Determination sets the program that will later be revealed by differentiation. The variable gene activity hypothesis suggests that different sets of genes are transcriptionally active in differentiated cells.

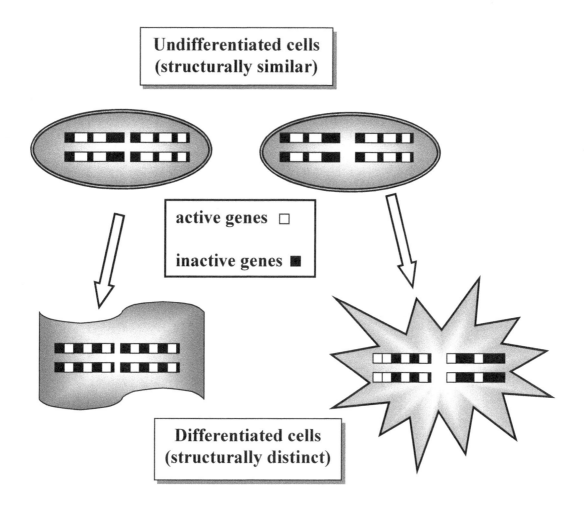

Answers to Now Solve This

18-1. It is possible that your screen was more inclusive; that is, it identified more subtle alterations than the screen of others. In addition, your screen may have included some zygotic effect mutations, which were dependent on the action of maternal effect genes. You may have identified several different mutations (multiple alleles) in some of the same genes.

18-2. Because the engrailed product is absent in *ftz/ftz* embryos, and *ftz* expression is normal in *en/en* embryos, one can conclude that the *ftz* gene product regulates *en*, either directly or indirectly. Because the *ftz* gene is expressed normally in *en/en* embryos, the product of the *engrailed* gene does not regulate expression of *ftz*.

Chapter 18 Developmental Genetics
Solutions to Problems and Discussion Questions

1. (a) In general, mutations provide the window for looking at the structure and function of genes. A number of mutant screens have identified hundreds of genes that influence development. Saturational mutagenesis provides an estimate of the lower limit of genes regulating a particular aspect of development.

(b) Our initial understanding of molecular gradients was based on the discovery of mutations that upset those gradients and alter development. Using a variety of labeling techniques, scientists have described egg gradients at the molecular level.

(c) Mutation analysis and gene replacement methods generally allow one to determine which anatomical structures are formed under their influence.

(d) Mutation analysis using single and multiple defective genes in an organism allowed investigators to determine which genes influenced each portion of vulval development.

(e) When a single gene is responsible for the activation/suppression of a number of developmentally related genes, and its action is one resembling an on/off switch, it is often referred to as a binary switch gene. The *eyeless* gene in *Drosophila* is a highly conserved gene that functions as a binary switch gene.

2. Your essay should include a description and examples of differential gene activity, homeotic genes, vulval development, and a typical signaling pathway such as Notch.

3. *Determination* refers to early developmental and regulatory events that set eventual patterns of gene activity. Determination is not the end result of the regulatory activity; rather, it is the process by which the developmental fate of a particular cell type is fixed. *Differentiation*, on the other hand, follows determination and is the manifestation, in terms of genetic, physiological, and morphological changes, of the determined state.

4. The fact that nuclei from almost any source remain transcriptionally and translationally active substantiates the fact that the genetic code and the ancillary processes of transcription and translation are compatible throughout the animal and plant kingdoms. Because the egg represents an isolated, "closed" system that can be mechanically, environmentally, and to some extent biochemically manipulated, various conditions may develop that allow one to study facets of gene regulation. For instance, the influence of transcriptional enhancers and suppressors may be studied along with factors that impact translational and posttranslational processes. Combinations of injected nuclei may reveal nuclear-nuclear interactions, which could not normally be studied by other methods.

5. The syncytial blasterm is formed as nuclei migrate to the egg's outer margin or cortex, where additional divisions take place. Plasma membranes organize around each of the nuclei at the cortex, thus creating the cellular blastoderm.

6. (a) Genes that control early development are often dependent on the deposition of their products (mRNA, transcription factors, various structural proteins, etc.) in the egg by the mother. When observable, these are maternal-effect genes. **(b)** They are made in the early oocyte or nurse cells during oogenesis. **(c)** Such maternal-effect genes control early developmental events such as defining anterior-posterior polarity. Such products are placed in eggs during oogenesis and are activated immediately after fertilization. **(d)** A variety of phenotypes are possible, and they are often revealed in the offspring of females. Maternal effects reveal the genotype of the mother.

7. (a, b) Zygotic genes are activated or repressed depending on their response to maternal-effect gene products. Three subsets of zygotic genes divide the embryo into segments. These segmentation genes are normally transcribed in the developing embryo and their mutations have embryonic lethal phenotypes. **(c)** The maternal genotype contains zygotic genes, and these are passed to the embryo as with any other gene.

8. The three main classes of zygotic genes are (1) *gap* genes, which specify adjacent segments; (2) *pair-rule* genes, which specify every other segment and a part of each segment; and (3) *segment polarity* genes, which specify homologous parts of each segment.

9. Because the polar cytoplasm contains information to form germ cells, one would expect such a transplantation procedure to generate germ cells in the anterior region. Work done by Illmensee and Mahowald in 1974 verified this expectation.

10. There are several somewhat indirect methods for determining transcriptional activity of a given gene in different cell types. First, if protein products of a given gene are present in different cell types, it can be assumed that the responsible gene is being transcribed. Second, if one is able to actually observe, microscopically, gene activity, as is the case in some specialized chromosomes (polytene chromosomes), gene activity can be inferred by the presence of localized chromosomal puffs. A more direct and common practice to assess transcription of particular genes is to use labeled probes. If a labeled probe can be obtained that contains base sequences that are complementary to the transcribed RNA, then such probes will hybridize to that RNA if present in different tissues. This technique is called *in situ* hybridization and is a powerful tool in the study of gene activity during development.

11. There are a variety of approaches to determine the level of control of a particular gene. First, one may determine whether levels of hnRNA are consistent among various cell types of interest. This is often accomplished by either direct isolation of the RNA and assessment by northern blotting or by use of *in situ* hybridization. If the hnRNA pools for a given gene are consistent in various cell types, then transcriptional control can be eliminated as a possibility. Support for translational control can be achieved directly by determining, in different cell types, the presence of a variety of mRNA species with common sequences. This can be accomplished only when sufficient knowledge exists for specific mRNA trapping or labeling. Clues as to translational control via alternative splicing can sometimes be achieved by examining the amino acid sequence of proteins. Similarities in certain structural/functional motifs may indicate alternative RNA processing.

12. A dominant gain-of-function mutation is one that changes the specificity or expression pattern of a gene or gene product. The "gain-of-function" *Antp* mutation causes the wild-type *Antennapedia* gene to be expressed in the eye-antenna disc and mutant flies to have legs on the head in place of antenna.

13. Many of the appendages of the head, including the mouth parts and the antennae, are evolutionary derivatives of ancestral leg structures. In *spineless aristapedia,* the distal portion of the antenna is replaced by its ancestral counterpart, the distal portion of the leg (tarsal segments). Because the replacement of the arista (end of the antenna) can occur by a mutation in a single gene, one would consider that one "selector" gene distinguishes aristal from tarsal structures. Notice that a "one-step" change is involved in the interchange of leg and antennal structures.

14. Because of the regulatory nature of homeotic genes in fundamental cellular activities of determination and differentiation, it would be difficult to ignore their possible impact on oncogenesis. Homeotic genes encode DNA binding domains, which influence gene expression, and any factor that influences gene expression may, under some circumstances, influence cell-cycle control. However attractive this model, there have been no homeotic transformations noted in mammary glands, so the typical expression of mutant homeotic genes in insects is not revealed in mammary tissue according to Lewis (2000). A substantial number of experiments will be needed to establish a functional link between homeotic gene mutation and cancer induction. Mutagenesis and transgenesis experiments are likely to be most productive in establishing a cause-effect relationship.

15. Two coupled approaches might be used. First, one could make transgenic flies that contain a series of deletions spanning all segments of the *bicoid* mRNA: the coding region and 5' and 3' untranslated regions. Comparison of stabilities of individual, deleted mRNAs with controls would indicate whether a particular segment of the mRNA contains a degradation signal sequence. If a degradation-sensitive region or signal sequence is located by deletion, that same intact region, when ligated to a noninvolved, nondegraded mRNA (like a ribosomal protein or tubulin mRNA) should foster degradation in a manner similar to the *bicoid* mRNA. If the mRNA from the anterior end of the egg is placed in the posterior of another egg, one could ask if the degradation process is comparable.

16. First, it would be interesting to know whether inhibitors of mitochondrial-ribosomal translation would interfere with germ cell formation. Second, one should know what types of mRNAs are being translated with these ribosomes.

17.

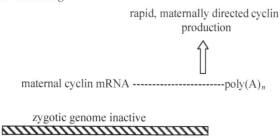

Pre-cell cycle remodeling:

rapid, maternally directed cyclin production

⇑

maternal cyclin mRNA ----------------------poly(A)$_n$

zygotic genome inactive

Post-cell cycle remodeling:

rapid, maternally directed cyclin production

⇑

maternal cyclin mRNA ----------------------poly(A)$_n$

degrade poly(A)

zygotic genome active

cyclins

18. Given the information in the problem, it is likely that this gene normally controls the expression of *BX-C* genes in all body segments. The wild-type product of *esc* stored in the egg may be required to interpret the information correctly stored in the egg cortex.

19. (a) The term "rescued" is often used when the introduction of genes from an outside source (within or among species) restores the wild-type phenotype from a mutant organism. **(b)** Results such as these, and there are many like them, indicate the extreme conservation of protein structure and function across phylogenetically distant organisms. Such results attest to the conservation from a distant common ancestor of fundamental molecular species during development. Failure to adhere to a common developmental theme is rewarded by death.

20. Three classes of flower homeotic genes are known that are activated in an overlapping pattern to specify various floral organs. Class *A* genes give rise to sepals. Expression of *A* and *B* class genes specifies petals, *B* and *C* genes control stamen formation, and expression of *C* genes gives rise to carpels.

21. The *Polycomb* gene family induces changes in chromatin that influence *Hox* gene expression. A gene in *Arabidopsis* has significant homology to the *Polycomb* gene family and also works by altering chromatin structure. The cross reactivity is thus related to the Polycomb product's effect on chromatin. Such parallel functions indicate that mechanisms of regulation are conserved over vast evolutionary distances.

22. Since *her-1⁻* mutations cause males to develop into hermaphrodites, and *tra-1⁻* mutations cause hermaphrodites to develop into males, one may hypothesize that the *her-1⁺* gene produces a product that suppresses hermaphrodite development, whereas the *tra-1⁺* gene product is needed for hermaphrodite development.

23. (a) *let-23* most likely functions earlier than *n300*. **(b)** The double mutant should be vulvaless because both genes block vulva formation.

24. If the *her-1⁺* product acts as a negative regulator, then when the gene is mutant, suppression over *tra-1⁺* is lost and hermaphroditism would be the result. This hypothesis fits the information provided. The double mutant should be male because even though there is no suppression from *her-1⁻*, there is no *tra-1⁺* product to support hermaphrodite development.

25. (a) RNAi allows the potential to knock out the action of a given gene. If successful, such a knockout would be helpful to determine the influence that a particular gene has on development/metabolism.

(b) If there are inefficiencies or off-target effects, then erroneous regulation is likely. At this time, these situations limit the use of RNAi.

26. (a) The patterns somewhat follow expectations in that genes involved in photosynthesis appear to be most active in the leaf and flower. In addition, high levels of protein synthesis in root are expected. Since pollen and seeds would be called upon early in development, it would seem reasonable to have such tissues show strong expression of transcriptional regulators.

(b) Two factors may be driving the expression of photosynthetic gene expression in flowers and seeds. First, since development in plants is more continuous or sequential, genes may not necessarily be shut off when their products are not in demand. Second, perhaps various posttranscriptional modifications redirect the function of photosynthetic gene products. In other words, alternative uses for such gene products may have evolved in plants much like that observed in some animal tissues.

(c) Having a global view of gene expression in an organism and its various tissues and organs allows one to estimate the relative contribution a particular gene may have in development. Since developmental and transcriptional networks are common in development, it is helpful to know the context in which a particular gene may function. Lastly, the only way in which development will be understood at the molecular level is to have a broad view of classes and clusters of gene activity.

27. (a, b) A number of studies indicate that genes in *Drosophila* have evolutionary counterparts (orthologs) in other organisms, including humans. A number of similar genes influence eye development in both insects and vertebrates. Genes that produce eyes are part of a complex network of at least seven genes that constitute the master regulators of eye development. Each gene functions in coordination with others in a conserved network that is used by broad evolutionary groups. Such genes, descended from common ancestral genes that have the same function in different species, are called orthologs.

(c) Since development is dependent on the coordinated output of numerous genes, genetic networks are probably the rule rather than the exception. The fact that a single genetic change (in the case of the mouse homolog of the fly *eyeless* gene) can trigger the formation of ectopic eyes in *Drosophila* shows that major components of developmental networks may be evolutionarily conserved. Another example of a regulatory network involves vulval development in *C. elegans*.

Chapter 19: Cancer and Regulation of the Cell Cycle

Concept Areas	Corresponding Problems
Inherited Cancer	6, 7, 10, 22, 24, 26, 20
Cell Cycle Mechanisms	2, 3, 4, 5
Apoptosis	8
Tumor Suppressors and Oncogenes	1, 9, 10, 11, 12, 13, 14, 24, 27, 28, 30
Chromosome Structure	2, 15, 26
Viruses and Cancer	16, 19
Cancer Biology	1, 12, 17, 18, 20, 21, 23, 27, 29, 31, 32

Concepts and Processes Checklist

(Check topic when mastered – provide examples where appropriate – understand the context of each entry)

- **Cancer Is a Genetic Disease**
  - cellular proliferation
  - metastasis
  - benign
  - malignant
  - clonal origin of cancer
  - Burkitt lymphoma
  - translocation 2/8
  - stem cell hypothesis
  - multistep process
  - multiple mutations
  - carcinogen
  - tumorigenesis
  - adenoma
  - polyp
  - adenomatous polyposis coli
  - *APC*
  - *Kras*
  - clonal expansion
  - carcinoma
  - driver mutation
  - passenger mutation
- **Cancer Cells Contain Genetic…**
  - mutator phenotype
  - genomic instability
  - defective DNA repair
  - chronic myelogenous leukemia
  - Philadelphia chromosome
  - BCR-ABL protein
  - chromosome 9/22
  - xeroderma pigmentosum
  - hereditary nonpolyposis colorectal cancer
  - chromatin modifications
  - cancer epigenetics
- **Cancer Cells Contain Genetic…**
  - differentiated cells
  - cell-cycle defects

- interphase
- G1
- S phase
- G2
- M phase
- G1/S checkpoint
- G2/M checkpoint
- M checkpoint
- signal transduction
- cyclins
- cyclin-dependent kinase
- CDKs
- control of apoptosis
- programmed cell death
- caspase

- **Proto-oncogenes and…**
  - tumor-suppressor genes
  - oncogene
  - *ras* gene family
  - *p53* gene
  - MDM2
  - phosphorylation
  - acetylation
  - CDK4/cyclin D1 complex
  - *RB1* (retinoblastoma 1)
  - retinoblastoma protein (pRB)

- **Cancer Cells Metastasize…**
  - extracellular matrix
  - basal lamina
  - E-cadherin glycoprotein
  - metalloproteinase
  - TIMPs
  - metasis-suppressor genes

- **Predisposition to Some Cancers…**
  - loss of heterozygosity
  - familial adenomatous polyposis
  - FAP
  - *APC* (adenomatous polyposis) gene
  - polyps

- **Viruses Contribute to Cancer…**
  - retroviruses
  - reverse transcriptase
  - provirus
  - acute transforming retrovirus
  - human immunodeficiency virus
  - HIV
  - human T-cell leukemia virus
  - HTLV-1
  - papillomavirus
  - HPV 16, 18
  - hepatitis B Virus
  - human herpesvirus 8
  - Epstein-Barr virus

- **Environmental Agents…**
  - chemicals
  - radiation
  - some viruses
  - chronic infections
  - tobacco smoke
  - red meat
  - animal fat
  - alcohol
  - aflatoxin
  - nitrosamine

Chapter 19 Cancer and Regulation of the Cell Cycle

Answers to Now Solve This

19-1. Several approaches are used to combat CML. One includes the use of a tyrosine kinase inhibitor that binds competitively to the ATP binding site of ABL kinase, thereby inhibiting phosphorylation of BCR-ABL and preventing the activation of additional signaling pathways. In addition, real-time quantitative reverse transcription-polymerase chain reaction (Q-RT-PCR) allows one to monitor drug responses of cell populations in patients so that less toxic and more effective treatments are possible. Being able to distinguish leukemic cells from healthy cells allows one to not only target therapy to specific cell populations, but also to quantify responses to therapy. Because leukemic cells produce a hybrid protein, it may be possible to develop a therapy, perhaps an immunotherapy, based on the uniqueness of the BCR/ABL protein.

19-2. *p53* is a tumor-suppressor gene that protects cells from multiplying with damaged DNA. It is present in its mutant state in more than 50 percent of all tumors. Since the immediate control of a critical and universal cell-cycle checkpoint is mediated by *p53*, mutation will influence a wide range of cell types. The action of *p53* is not limited to specific cell types.

19-3. Cancer is a complex alteration in normal cell-cycle controls. Even if a major "cancer-causing" gene is transmitted, other genes, often new mutations, are usually necessary in order to drive a cell toward tumor formation. Full expression of the cancer phenotype is likely to be the result of interplay among a variety of genes and, therefore, to show variable penetrance and expressivity.

19-4. Unfortunately, it is common to spend enormous amounts of money dealing with diseases after they occur rather than concentrating on disease prevention. Too often, pressure from special interest groups or lack of political will retards advances in education and prevention. Obviously, it is less expensive, in terms of both human suffering and money, to seek preventive measures for as many diseases as possible. However, having gained some understanding of the mechanisms of disease, in this case, cancer, it must also be stated that no matter what preventive measures are taken, it will be impossible to completely eliminate disease from the human population. It is extremely important, however, that we increase efforts to educate and protect the human population from as many hazardous environmental agents as possible. A balanced, multipronged approach seems appropriate.

Chapter 19 Cancer and Regulation of the Cell Cycle

Solutions to Problems and Discussion Questions

1. (a) The clonal origin of cancer cells in a given cancer is supported by findings that mutations, chromosomal or otherwise, are of the same type in all cancerous cells. In addition, the X-chromosome inactivation patterns support the clonal origin of cancer.

(b) The progressive, time- and age-dependent development of tumorigenesis, coupled with the relatively low cancer rate compared to the mutation rate, argues for a multistep mutational model for cancer.

(c) The mutator phenotype, thought by some to be caused by defective DNA repair mechanisms, is characteristic of cancer cells. Numerous cancers, exemplified by xeroderma pigmentosum and hereditary nonpolyposis colorectal cancer, are caused by defective DNA repair systems.

2. Your essay should include describe the general influence of genetics in cancer. Since epigenetic factors alter gene output, it is likely that such factors could cause cancer.

3. The major regulatory points of the cell cycle include the following:

1. late G1 (G1/S)
2. the border between G2 and mitosis (G2/M)
3. in mitosis (M)

4. Kinases regulate other proteins by adding phosphate groups. Cyclins bind to the kinases, switching them on and off. CDK4 binds to cyclin D, moving cells from G1 to S. At the G2/mitosis border, a CDK1 (cyclin-dependent kinase) combines with another cyclin (cyclin B). Phosphorylation occurs, bringing about a series of changes in the nuclear membrane via caldesmon, cytoskeleton, and histone H1.

5. (a) The retinoblastoma gene (*RB1*), located on chromosome 13, encodes a protein designated pRB. Cells progress through the G1/S transition when pRB is phosphorylated and CDK4 binds to cyclin D. In the absence of phosphorylation of pRB, it binds to members of the E2F family of transcription factors, which controls the expression of genes required to move the cell from G1 to S.

(b) When E2F and other regulators are released by pRB, they are free to induce the expression of more than 30 genes whose products are required for the transition from G1 into S phase. After cells traverse S, G2, and M phases, pRB reverts to a nonphosphorylated state, binds to regulatory proteins such as E2F and keeps them sequestered until required for the next cell cycle.

6. To say that a particular trait is inherited conveys the assumption that when a particular genetic circumstance is present, it will be revealed in the phenotype. For instance, albinism is inherited in such a way that individuals who are homozygous recessive express albinism. When one discusses an inherited predisposition, one usually refers to situations in which a particular phenotype is expressed in families in some consistent pattern. However, the phenotype may not always be expressed or may manifest itself in different ways. In retinoblastoma, the gene is inherited as an autosomal dominant, and those who inherit the mutant *RB* allele are predisposed to develop eye tumors. However, approximately 10 percent of the people known to inherit the gene do not actually express it and in some cases expression involves only one eye, rather than two.

7. Familial retinoblastoma is inherited as an autosomal dominant gene with 90 percent penetrance, that is, 90 percent of the individuals who inherit the gene will develop eye tumors. The gene usually expresses itself in youngsters. Because the husband's sister has RB, one of the husband's parents has the gene for RB, and the husband has a 50:50 chance of inheriting that gene. However, because the husband is past the usual age of onset, it is quite likely that he was lucky and did not receive the RB gene. In that case, the chance that a child born to this couple having RB is no higher than the frequency of sporadic occurrence. However, because the gene is 90 percent penetrant, there is a chance that the husband has the gene but does not express it. The probability of that occurrence would be 0.50 (of inheriting the gene) × 0.10 (not expressing the gene) = 0.05. The chance of the husband then passing this nonexpressed gene to his child would be again 0.5, so 0.50 × 0.05 = 0.025 for the child inheriting this gene. If the child inherits the RB gene, he/she has a 90 percent chance of expressing it. Therefore, the overall probability of the child having RB (using this logic) would be 0.025 × 0.9 = 0.0225 or just over 2 percent (or about 1 in 50).

Chapter 19 Cancer and Regulation of the Cell Cycle

To test for the presence of the RB gene in the husband, it is possible in some forms of RB to identify (by molecular probes) a defective or missing DNA segment. Otherwise, one might attempt to assay the RB product in cells to see if it is present and functional at normal levels.

8. Apoptosis, or programmed cell death, is a genetically controlled process that leads to the death of a cell. It is a natural process involved in morphogenesis and a protective mechanism against cancer formation. During apoptosis, nuclear DNA becomes fragmented, cellular structures are disrupted, and the cells are dissolved. Caspases are involved in the initiation and progress of apoptosis.

9. A tumor-suppressor gene is a gene that normally functions to suppress cell division. Since tumors and cancers represent a significant threat to survival and, therefore, Darwinian fitness, strong evolutionary forces would favor a variety of co-evolved and perhaps complex conditions in which mutations in these suppressor genes would be recessive. Looking at it in another way, if a tumor-suppressor gene makes a product that regulates the cell cycle favorably, cellular conditions have evolved in such a way that sufficient quantities of this gene product are made from just one allele (of the two present in each diploid individual) to provide normal function.

10. The nonphosphorylated form of pRB binds to transcription factors such as E2F, causing inactivation and suppression of the cell cycle. Phosphorylation of pRB activates the cell cycle by releasing transcription factors (E2F) to advance the cell cycle. With the phosphorylation site inactivated in the PSM-RB form, phosphorylation cannot occur, thereby leaving the cell cycle in a suppressed state.

11. Imbedded in the plasma membrane, Ras proteins act as molecular switches that transmit molecular signals from outside to inside the cell. Activated Ras proteins transduce a signal, which activates the transcription of genes that start cell division. Mutant Ras proteins are locked into the "on" position, continually signaling cell division.

12. Various kinases can be activated by breaks in DNA. One kinase, called ATM, and/or a kinase called Chk2 phosphorylates BRCA1 and p53. The activated p53 arrests replication during the S phase to facilitate DNA repair. The activated BRCA1 protein, in conjunction with BRCA2, mRAD51, and other nuclear proteins, is involved in repairing the DNA.

13. Oncogenes are genes that induce or maintain uncontrolled cellular proliferation associated with cancer. They are mutant forms of proto-oncogenes, which normally function to regulate cell division. Oncogenes may be formed through point mutations, gene amplification, translocations, repositioning of regulatory sequences, or other mechanisms.

14. Mutations that produce oncogenes alter gene expression either directly or indirectly and act in a dominant capacity. Proto-oncogenes are those that normally function to promote or maintain cell division. In the mutant state (oncogenes), they induce or maintain uncontrolled cell division; that is, there is a gain of function. Generally, this gain of function takes the form of increased or abnormally continuous gene output. On the other hand, loss of function is generally attributed to mutations in tumor-suppressor genes, which function to halt passage through the cell cycle. When such genes are mutant, they have lost their capacity to halt the cell cycle. Such mutations are generally recessive.

15. A translocation involving exchange of genetic material between chromosomes 9 and 22 is responsible for the generation of the "Philadelphia chromosome." Genetic mapping established that certain genes were combined to form a hybrid oncogene (*BCR/ABL*) that encodes a 200-kDa protein that has been implicated in the formation of chronic myelogenous leukemia.

16. Since the evolutionary strategy of a virus is to promote its own replication, and since it does so in a host cell, stimulating cell division in host cells confers an evolutionary advantage. To encourage infected cells to undergo growth and division, viruses often encode genes that stimulate growth and division. Many viruses either inactivate tumor-suppressor genes of the host or bring in genes that stimulate cell growth and division. By inactivating tumor-suppressor genes, the normal breaking mechanism of the cell cycle is destroyed.

17. *Driver mutations* are those that confer a growth advantage to a cancer cell. Other mutations, called *passenger mutations*, increase in cancer cells over time, possibly due to the genomic instability of cancer cells. Such mutations do not appear to contribute directly to the cancerous state of a cell.

18. Normal cells are often capable of withstanding mutational assault because they have checkpoints and DNA repair mechanisms in place. When such mechanisms fail, cancer may be a result. Through mutation, such protective mechanisms are compromised in cancer cells, and as a result they show higher than normal rates of mutation, chromosomal abnormalities, and genomic instability.

19. An acute transforming virus is a retrovirus that carries an oncogene(s), whereas a nonacute virus can induce the activity of cellular genes that bring about tumor formation.

20. Epigenetic effects can be caused by DNA methylation and/or histone modifications, including acetylation and/or phosphorylation. As such, they can silence or activate chromosomes (X chromosome, for example) or certain chromosomal regions and be responsible for parental imprinting or influencing gene activity in heterochromatin. Patterns of nucleotide demethylation and hypermethylation are often different when cancer cells are compared to normal cells.

21. Radiotherapy is often administered externally or internally to damage the cell-cycle machinery, thus shrinking the cancer or killing cells of the cancer. It may be completely or partially effective. Because cells have natural defenses against mutagenic insult, drugs that increase a cell's sensitivity to radiation may be administered. Radiosensitizers and radioprotectors are chemicals that alter a cell's response to radiotherapy. Radiosensitizers make cells more sensitive to therapy, whereas radioprotectors are drugs that protect normal cells from the damage caused by radiation therapy. Radiotherapy kills cells; therefore, side effects are expected.

22. No, she will still have the general population risk of about 10 percent. In addition, it is possible that genetic tests will not detect all breast cancer mutations.

23. Since there are multiple routes that lead to cancer, one would expect complex regulatory systems to be involved. More specifically, whereas in some cases, downregulation of a gene, such as an oncogene, may be a reasonable cancer therapy, downregulation of a tumor-suppressor gene would be undesirable in therapy. Various levels of methylation (hypermethylation and hypomethylation) influence gene activity and, therefore, can cause cancer.

24. Proteases, in general, and serine proteases, specifically, are considered tumor-promoting agents because they degrade proteins, especially those in the extracellular matrix. When such proteolysis occurs, cellular invasion and metastasis are encouraged. Consistent with this observation are numerous observations that metastatic tumor cells are associated with higher than normal amounts of protease expression. Inhibitors of serine proteases are often tested for their anticancer efficacy.

25. When activated, the p53 protein initiates cell-cycle arrest followed by DNA repair and apoptosis. This process involves stimulating transcription of p21, which inhibits the CDK4/cyclin D1 complex. Activated p53 also prevents the cell from initiating the S phase. Through a series of steps, BAX homodimers are formed that lead to apoptosis. Individuals who are heterozygous for p53 need only have a mutation in the existing normal gene to lose the protection of the p53 protein.

26. (a) Since a normal p53 protein is very helpful in preventing cancer, loss of *p53* synthesis through hypermethylation of such a promoter would decrease *p53* concentration and thus be detrimental.

(b) If one has comparison blood from an individual, the origin of a cancer might be detectable through novel DNA present in such blood.

27. Recent evidence indicates that many forms of regulatory RNA are transcribed from noncoding DNA, it is likely that such RNA can influence the output of genes that are related to cancer formation.

28. As with many forms of cancer, a single gene alteration is not the only requirement. The authors (Bose et al.) state "but only infrequently do the cells acquire the additional changes necessary to produce leukemia in humans." Some studies indicate that variations (often deletions) in the region of the breakpoints may influence expression of CML.

29. (a) Because one is working with somatic cells, the usual tests for heterozygosity through crosses are not available. Therefore, one must rely on chemical/physical approaches to answer the question. A genomic library could be constructed of both osteosarcoma cell DNA and noncancerous cells from the same organism. You could then screen the library using labeled probes from the clones carrying the *RB1* gene available to you as stated in the problem. At this point, some indications might emerge because if there is a significant alteration in mutant *RB1* genes, probes may not successfully hybridize to any clones in the cancerous cell DNA library. Assuming that control hybridization occurs in the noncancerous cells, lack of hybridization in the library derived from the osteosarcoma cell line might indicate deletions. However, assuming that hybridization does allow one to identify clones containing putative *RB1* alleles, subcloning into appropriate vectors would allow sequencing to reveal sequence changes in the *RB1* alleles when compared with nonmutant genes. A second approach combines an immunoassay described in part (b) of this problem. Assuming that one can successfully make antibodies to the normal RB1 gene product (pRB), lack of cross-reactivity of the pRB antibodies to proteins from the cancerous cell line would indicate that both *RB1* alleles are mutant.

(b) As indicated in the last portion of part (a) above, one can make antibodies to pRB from the noncancerous cells and test these antibodies for reactivity against proteins from the cancerous cell lines. A pRB-antibody reaction would indicate that the pRB protein is made.

(c) To determine whether addition of a normal *RB1* gene will change the cancer-causing potential of osteosarcoma cells, one could transfer the cloned normal *RB1* gene into the cells by transformation or transfection (often by electroporation or ultrasound). Transformed cells would then be introduced into the cancer-prone mice to determine whether their cancer-causing potential had been altered.

30. (a) The mRNA triplet for Gln is CAG(A). The mRNA triplet that specifies a stop is one of three: UAA, UAG, or UGA. The strand of DNA that codes for the CAG(A) would be the following: 3'-GTC(T)-5'. Therefore, if the G mutated to an A (transition), then the DNA strand would be 3'-ATC(T)-5', which would cause a UAG(A) triplet to be produced, and this would cause the stop.

(b) It is likely to be a tumor-suppressor gene because loss of function causes predisposition to cancer.

(c) Some women may carry genes (perhaps mutant) that "spare" for the *BRCA1* gene product. Some women may have immune systems that recognize and destroy precancerous cells, or they may have mutations in breast signal transduction genes so that cell division suppression occurs in the absence of *BRCA1*.

31. (a, b) Even though there are changes in the *BRCA1* gene, they do not always have physiological consequences. Such neutral polymorphisms make screening difficult in that one cannot always be certain that a mutation will cause problems for the patient.

(c) The polymorphism in PM2 is probably a silent mutation because the third base of the codon is involved.

(d) The polymorphism in PM3 is probably a neutral missense mutation because the first base is involved. However, because there is some first codon position degeneracy, it is possible for the mutation to be silent.

32. Various alterations in gene activity related to hyper- and hypomethylation have been associated with numerous cancers. Hypermethylation usually leads to a suppression of gene activity.

Hormonal response genes often synthesize receptors that respond to a variety of hormones such as androgens, retinoic acid, and estrogens. For example, prostate cancer is often associated with suppressed *ESR1* and *ESR2* activity, both of which are estrogen receptors.

Cell-cycle control genes are involved in both upregulation and downregulation of the cell cycle as they influence cyclins and cyclin-dependent kinases. The cyclin-dependent kinase inhibitor *CDKN2A*, when hypermethylated, fails to inhibit cyclin-dependent kinase and thereby contributes to cancer progression.

A number of *tumor cell invasion genes* have been described, some of which interfere with intercellular adhesion. When such genes are suppressed through hypermethylation, cadherin–catenin adherence mechanisms are compromised, which can influence cell-to-cell contacts.

One of the most common causes of cancer is a breakdown in *DNA repair* mechanisms.

Hypermethylation suppresses the genes that normally supply DNA repair components.

Proper *signal transduction* is required to maintain cell-cell adherence and response to extracellular signals. For example, when *CD44*, an integral membrane protein that is involved in matrix adhesion and signal transduction, is hypermethylated, cells cannot maintain proper cell-cell contact and communication, without which cell-cycle control is compromised.

Chapter 20: Recombinant DNA Technology

Concept Areas	Corresponding Problems
Making DNA Clones	1, 2, 3, 4, 5, 8, 10
Restriction Endonucleases	2, 6, 7, 9, 15, 17, 19, 21, 27
Constructing DNA Libraries	1, 14, 16, 18
Identifying Specific Cloned Sequences	11
Methods of Analysis of Cloned Sequences	13, 19, 26
DNA Sequencing	1, 22, 23
Polymerase Chain Reaction	1, 12, 20, 30, 31, 32, 33, 34
Applications	2, 4, 17, 19, 24, 25, 26, 27, 28, 29, 30, 31

Concepts and Processes Checklist

(Check topic when mastered – provide examples where appropriate – understand the context of each entry)

- ○ **Recombinant DNA Technology...**
  - ○ restriction enzymes
  - ○ DNA cloning vector
  - ○ recognition sequence
  - ○ palindrome
  - ○ cohesive ends
  - ○ blunt-end fragments
  - ○ *Escherichia coli*
  - ○ anneal
  - ○ DNA ligase
  - ○ key properties of vectors
  - ○ several restriction sites
  - ○ independent replication
  - ○ selectable marker gene
  - ○ antibiotic resistance
  - ○ easy to isolate from host
  - ○ plasmid
  - ○ transformation
  - ○ electroporation
  - ○ multiple cloning site
  - ○ *lacZ* gene
  - ○ blue-white selection
  - ○ β-galactosidase
  - ○ *amp*R
  - ○ X-gal
  - ○ insert limitations of plasmids
  - ○ λ (lambda) phage
  - ○ bacterial artificial chromosome
  - ○ BAC
  - ○ yeast artificial chromosome
  - ○ YAC
  - ○ expression vector
  - ○ Ti vectors in plants
  - ○ Ti plasmid
  - ○ *Agrobacterium tumefaciens*

219

- *Rhizobium radiobacter*
- *Saccharomyces cerevisiae*

- **DNA Libraries Are Collections…**

  - genomic library
  - human genome library
  - whole-genome shotgun cloning
  - cDNA library
  - complementary DNA library
  - reverse transcriptase
  - oligo(dT) primer
  - library screening
  - probe, RNA or DNA
  - hybridization
  - detection of probe
  - genomics

- **Polymerase Chain Reaction…**

  - PCR
  - primers
  - DNA polymerase
  - Mg^{2+}
  - denaturation of target
  - 92–95°C
  - annealing of primers
  - 45–65°C
  - extension of primers
  - 65–75°C
  - 25–30 cycles
  - thermostable DNA polymerase
  - *Taq* DNA polymerase
  - *Thermus aquaticus*
  - limitations of PCR
  - applications of PCR

- reverse transcription PCR
- RT-PCR
- quantitative real-time PCR
- qPCR

- **Molecular Techniques…**

  - restriction mapping
  - nucleic acid blotting
  - Southern blot
  - Northern blot
  - Western blot
  - fluorescent *in situ* hybridization
  - FISH
  - spectral karyotypes

- **DNA Sequencing…**

  - dideoxynucleotide chain termination
  - Sanger sequencing
  - dATP, dCTP, dGTP, dTTP
  - dNTP
  - ddNTP
  - gel electrophoresis
  - computer-automated
  - high-throughput DNA sequencing
  - next-generation sequencing
  - NGS
  - pyrosequencing
  - third-generation sequencing
  - gene targeting
  - knockout animal models
  - ES cells
  - *Cre-Lox* system

Chapter 20 Recombinant DNA Technology

Answers to Now Solve This

20-1. (a) Because the *Drosophila* DNA has been cloned into the *Pst*I site in the ampicillin resistance gene of the plasmid, the gene will be mutated, and any bacterium with the recombinant plasmid will be ampicillin sensitive. The tetracycline resistance gene remains active, however. Bacteria that have been transformed with the recombinant plasmid will be resistant to tetracycline; therefore, tetracycline should be added to the medium.

(b) Colonies that grow on a tetracycline medium should contain only the insert. Those bacteria that do not grow on the ampicillin medium probably contain the *Drosophila* DNA insert.

(c) Resistance to both antibiotics by a transformed bacterium could be explained in several ways. First, if cleavage with the *Pst*I was incomplete, then no change in biological properties of the uncut plasmids would be expected. Also, it is possible that the cut ends of the plasmid were ligated together in the original form with no insert.

20-2. The genomic clone probably contained a number of introns that were removed from the mRNA during processing. The cDNA was prepared from mRNA.

20-3 Using the human nucleotide sequence, one can produce a probe to screen the library of the African okapi. Second, one can use the amino acid sequence and the genetic code to generate a complementary DNA probe for screening of the library. The probe is used, through hybridization, to identify the DNA that is complementary to the probe and can allow one to identify the library clone containing the DNA of interest. Cells with the desired clone are then picked from the original plate and the plasmid is isolated from the cells.

Chapter 20 Recombinant DNA Technology
Solutions to Problems and Discussion Questions

1. (a) In general, when DNA fragments of interest have been incorporated into a plasmid, the result is a change in the function of a gene or genes in the plasmid. For instance, if one inserts a piece of DNA into the ampicillin resistance gene, following transformation, the bacterium is no longer resistant to ampicillin. Other techniques involving "insertional mutagenesis" might involve using a medium-driven color change in bacteria that contain a recombinant plasmid.

(b) The choice of method often depends on a variety of circumstances. Sometimes probes are used to screen a library. Such probes may be used to identify particular genes in gels or from membranes containing DNA from lysed bacteria. If appropriate primers are available, PCR can be used to identify particular genes of interest.

(c) Purified genomic DNA is first denatured and then annealed to specific primers. Once primers have annealed, they are extended. The process is repeated to produce many copies of a specific DNA molecule.

(d) Whereas earlier advances relied on single-tube, fluorescent labeling technologies, newer approaches involved solid-phase methodologies in which beads are attached to DNA fragments and amplified by PCR in water droplets in oil. Coupled with pyrosequencing, processes have been greatly accelerated. New trends often involve nanotechnology and solid support systems. The overall goal is to increase the speed and accuracy of sequencing while reducing the per base cost.

2. Your essay should include an appreciation for the relative ease in which sections of DNA can be inserted into various vectors and the amplification and isolation of such DNA. You should also include the possibilities of modifying recombinant molecules.

3. Recombinant DNA technology, also called genetic engineering or gene splicing, involves the creation of associations of DNA that are not typically found in nature. Particular enzymes, called *restriction endonucleases*, cut DNA at specific sites and often yield "sticky" ends for additional interaction with DNA molecules cut with the same class of enzyme. Isolated from bacteria, restriction enzymes fall into several classes, each having peculiarities as to structure and interaction with DNA. A vector may be a plasmid, bacteriophage, or cosmid that receives, through ligation, a piece or pieces of foreign DNA. The recombinant vector can transform (or transfect) a host cell (bacterium, yeast cell, etc.) and be amplified in number. In a DNA cloning experiment, DNA ligase is used to generate the covalent bonds of the phosphodiester backbone to yield an intact double-stranded DNA molecule. Restriction enzymes, on the other hand, break such bonds.

4. Even though the human gene coding for insulin contains a number of introns, a cDNA generated from insulin mRNA is free of introns. Plasmids containing insulin genes (from cDNA) are free of introns, so no processing issue surfaces.

5. Although bacteria are commonly used in cloning, other cell types are also very useful, such as yeast, mammalian, and so on. Bacteria are prokaryotes and as such do not process transcripts as do eukaryotes; therefore, there is often an advantage to using a eukaryotic host. In addition, one might be interested in the influence of a specific DNA segment in a specific host environment, thus necessitating the use of a variety of hosts.

6. This segment contains the palindromic sequence of GGATCC, which is recognized by the restriction enzyme *Bam*HI. The double-stranded sequence is the following:

GGATCC
CCTAGG

7. The simple answer to this question is to assume that one is asking about the advantage to the scientist of having restriction enzyme sites recognize palindromic sites. In this case, the answer would be that single-stranded overhanging ends are often generated, which allow DNA from different sources cut with the same restriction enzyme to generate complementary overhangs, which can anneal to form recombinant molecules.

If one considers the question from a bacterial standpoint, the answer is much more involved. In fact, bacterial chromosomes actually have fewer palindromic sites than expected based on chance. This adaptation stems from the fact that restriction sites cleave at palindromic sequences, and one way to keep them from cleaving the host DNA is to evolve away from such sequences. So why do restriction enzymes often cleave at palindromic sites in the first place? First, the classical Type II restriction enzymes are dimers of identical units that recognize identical sequences. To protect such sequences in the bacterial chromosome from attack, a modification enzyme, a methyltransferase, must fully methylate certain bases on both strands of the DNA at the site of a particular restriction endonuclease attack.

Methyltransferases are typically monomers consistent with the process of methylating newly replicated DNA strands. In order for both strands to be protected by methylation, the sequence must be read the same in both directions on the double helix. So, returning to the original question, the advantage to the bacterium of having palindromic sites for restriction enzymes is more related to the protection of such sites from cleavage.

8. Plasmids were the first to be used as cloning vectors, and they are still routinely used to clone relatively small fragments of DNA. Because of their small size, they are relatively easy to separate from the host bacterial chromosome, and they have relatively few restriction sites. They can be engineered fairly easily (i.e., polylinkers and reporter genes added). For cloning larger pieces of DNA such as entire eukaryotic genes, cosmids are often used. For instance, when modifications are made in the bacterial virus lambda (λ), relatively large inserts of about 20 kb can be cloned. This is an important advantage when one needs to clone a large gene or generate a genomic library from a eukaryote. In addition, some cosmids will accept only inserts of a limited size, which means that small, perhaps less meaningful fragments will not be cloned unnecessarily. Both plasmids and cosmids suffer from the limitation that they can use only bacteria as hosts. BACs are artificial bacterial

chromosomes that can be engineered for certain qualities.

YACs (yeast artificial chromosomes) contain telomeres, an origin of replication, and a centromere and are extensively used to clone DNA in yeast. With selectable markers (TRP1 and URA3) and a cluster of restriction sites, DNA inserts ranging from 100 kb to 1000 kb can be cloned and inserted into yeast. Since yeast, being a eukaryote, undergoes many of the typical RNA and protein processing steps of other, more complex eukaryotes, the advantages are numerous when working with eukaryotic genes.

9. Using a relatively rare recognition site will produce larger fragments that might be desired if one wanted to isolate intact genes or centromeres, and so on. The rarity of a sequence is sometimes related to its length. For example, assuming a random distribution of all four bases, the four-base sequence would occur (on average) every 256 base pairs (4^4), and the six-base sequence would occur every 4096 base pairs (4^6). This is akin to calculating the probability of any particular sequence of bases occurring in a row (of 4 or 6).

10. No. The tumor-inducing plasmid (Ti) that is used to produce genetically modified plants is specific for the bacterium *Agrobacterium tumifaciens,* which causes tumors in many plant species. There is no danger that this tumor-inducing plasmid will cause tumors in humans.

11. A probe is any DNA or RNA that is complementary to some part of a target gene or sequence. Probes are used to identify and/or locate a particular nucleic acid sequence among a pool of sequences.

12. The total number of molecules after 15 cycles would be 16,384, or $(2)^{14}$.

13. Given that there is only one site for the action of *Hind*III, then the following will occur: Cuts will be made such that a four-base single-stranded set of sticky ends will be produced. For the antibiotic resistance to be present, the ligation will reform the plasmid into its original form. However, two of the plasmids can join to form a dimer, as indicated in the diagram that follows.

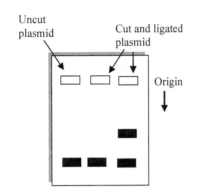

Uncut plasmid

Cut and ligated plasmid

Origin

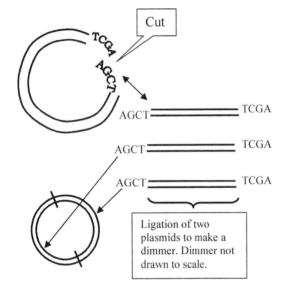

Cut

AGCT ======= TCGA

AGCT ======= TCGA

AGCT ======= TCGA

Ligation of two plasmids to make a dimmer. Dimmer not drawn to scale.

14. A cDNA library provides DNAs from RNA transcripts and is, therefore, useful in identifying what are likely to be functional DNAs. If one desires an examination of noncoding as well as coding regions, a genomic library would be more useful.

15. The problem can be best solved by drawing out the strands and then placing the restriction sites in the appropriate positions as follows:

enzyme I   __350_|____950_____

enzyme II   200|_____1100_____

To determine the orientation of the restriction sites to each other, examine the results of the double-digested DNA and note that there is a 150-bp fragment, meaning that enzyme II cuts within the 350-bp fragment of enzyme I. Therefore, the final map is as follows:

II I
200 _|_|_____950_____
      150

16. There may be several factors contributing to the lack of representation of the 5' end of the mRNA. One has to deal with the possibility that the reverse transcriptase may not completely synthesize the DNA from the RNA template. The other reason may be that the 3' end of the copied DNA tends to fold back on itself, thus providing a primer for the DNA polymerase. Additional preparation of the cDNA requires some digestion at the folded region. Since this folded region corresponds to the 5' end of the mRNA, some of the message is often lost.

17. Option (b) fits the expectation because the thick band in the offspring probably represents the bands at approximately the same position in both parents. The likelihood of such a match is expected to be low in the general population.

18. Assuming that one has knowledge of the amino acid sequence of the protein product or the nucleotide sequence of the target nucleic acid, a degenerate set of DNA strands can be made that can be prepared for cloning into an appropriate vector or amplified by PCR. A variety of labeling techniques can then be used, through hybridization, to identify complementary base sequences contained in the genomic library. One must know at least a portion of the amino acid sequence of the protein product or its nucleic acid sequence in order for the procedure to be applied. Some problems can occur through degeneracy in the genetic code (not allowing construction of an appropriate probe), the possible existence of pseudogenes in the library (hybridizations with inappropriate related fragments in the library), and variability of DNA sequences in the library due to introns (causing poor or background hybridization). To overcome some of these problems, one can construct a variety of relatively small probes of different types that take into account the degeneracy in the code. By varying the conditions of hybridization (salt and temperature), one can reduce undesired hybridizations.

19. Taking the number of bases recognized by *Bam*HI as 6, there would be approximately 4096 base pairs between sites. Given that λ DNA contains approximately 48,500 base pairs, there would be about 11.8 sites (48,500/4096).

20. (a) Heating to 90–95°C denatures the double-stranded DNA so that it dissociates into single strands. It usually takes about five minutes, depending on the length and GC content of the DNA. **(b)** Lowering the temperature to 50–70°C allows the primers to bind to the denatured DNA. **(c)** Bringing the temperature to 70–75°C allows the heat-stable DNA polymerase an opportunity to extend the primers by adding nucleotides to the 3' ends of each growing strand. Each PCR is designed with specific temperatures (not ranges) based on the characteristics of the DNAs (template and primers).

21. *Taq* polymerase is from a bacterium called *Thermus aquaticus*, which typically lives in hot springs. It is heat stable like some other enzymes used in PCR that are isolated from thermal vents in the ocean floor.

22. ddNTPs are analogs of the "normal" deoxyribonucleotide triphosphates (dNTPs), but they lack a 3'-hydroxyl group. As DNA synthesis occurs, the DNA polymerase occasionally inserts a ddNTP into a growing DNA strand. Since there is no 3'-hydroxyl group, chain elongation cannot take place, and resulting fragments are formed, which can be separated by electrophoresis. Where the ddNTP was incorporated, the length of each strand and, therefore, the position of the particular ddNTP are established and used to eventually provide the base sequence of the DNA.

23. It is likely that the DNA that served as the template in the sequencing reaction was not pure so that at the same position (length), more than one type of ddNTP could be incorporated. This could be due to natural polymorphisms, often called single nucleotide polymorphisms (or SNPs) or impure samples.

24. FISH involves the hybridization of a labeled probe to a complementary stretch of DNA in a chromosome. As such, it can be used to locate a specific DNA sequence (often a gene or gene fragment) in a chromosome. Spectral karyotyping uses FISH to detect individual chromosomes, a distinct advantage in identifying chromosomal abnormalities.

25. A knockout animal has a piece of DNA missing, whereas a transgenic animal usually has a piece of DNA added.

26. If a transgene integrates into a coding or regulatory region of the genome, it is likely to alter the function of that sequence. In doing so, a mutational circumstance is possible. Any such random integration may significantly alter the function of the endogenous DNA as well as the transgene.

27. Until the host organism contains the knockout gene in the homozygous state in its sex cells, the knockout gene can not be faithfully transmitted at high frequency.

28. Often, reporter genes are used to indicate a functional transgene, or some surface trait of the recipient organism is indicative of integration of a transgene.

29. (a) The overall size of the fragment is 12 kb. From the A + N digest, sites A and N must be 1 kb apart. N must be 2 kb from an E site. Pattern #5 is the likely choice. Notice that digest A + N breaks up the 6-kb E fragment.

(b) By drawing lines though sections that hybridize to the probe, one can see that the only place of consistent overlap to the probe is the 1-kb fragment between A and N.

30. $T_m(°C) = 81.5 + 0.41(\%GC) - (675/N) = 81.5 + 0.41(33.3) - (675/21) =$ about 63°C. Subtracting 5°C gives us a good starting point of about 58°C for PCR with this primer. Notice that as the percentage of GC and length increase, the $T_m(°C)$ increases. GC pairs contain three hydrogen bonds rather than two as between AT pairs.

31. Applying the formula that follows with the concentrations of Na^+ and formamide in the table gives the following T_m.

$$T_m = 81.5 + 16.6(\log M[Na^+]) + 0.41(\%G + C) - 0.72(\%F)$$

(a)

Na^+	% Formamide (F)	T_m
0.825	20	84.16
0.825	40	69.76
0.165	20	72.56
0.165	40	58.16

(b) Sodium, a monovalent cation, interacts with the negative phosphates that make up the nucleic acid backbone. The repulsive forces between negative phosphates are reduced, and the double helix becomes more stable, thereby requiring a higher temperature for melting. Formamide competes for hydrogen bond locations of the bases and lessens the attractions that hold each double helix together. As the competition for hydrogen bonding increases with increased formamide, the melting temperature lowers.

32. (a) As the percent dT increases, the required annealing temperature correspondingly decreases, given all other parameters being held constant.

(b) Because random sequence primers contain other bases, particularly G, the annealing temperatures need to be adjusted.

(c) At various stages of development, small samples of heart tissue from the right and left side could be collected and compared.

33. (a) Short tandem repeats of the Y chromosome (Y-STRs) vary considerably among individuals and populations. By amplifying Y-STRs by PCR and separating the amplified products by electrophoresis, one can genotypically type an individual as one does with a standard fingerprint. Because tissue samples are often left at the scene of a violent crime, DNA fingerprints are sometimes more available than standard fingerprints. Linking an individual with the time and place of a significant event has multiple forensic applications. Eliminating an individual as a suspect also has important forensic applications.

(b) The nonrecombining region of the Y is maintained strictly in the male population. Of special relevance in forensic applications would be the elimination of half the population (females) from a suspect group.

(c) Because different ethnic groups show different levels of Y-STR polymorphism, different final probabilities occur as products of individual probabilities. Since these probabilities are used to match individuals in forensics, ethnic variations must be taken under consideration.

(d) Although there are many potential uses of DNA samples, generally a "match" is determined by multiplying the occurrence probabilites of each haplotype to arrive at the overall probability (product) of a genotype occurring in a population. If an individual's genotype matches that found in DNA at a crime scene, depending on the frequecies of the haplotypes, one might be able to say that the individual was at the crime scene. However, contamination, inappropriate genotyping, and laboratory expertise may give both false positive and false negative results. Identical twins will have identical DNA fingerprints and may complicate forensic applications.

34. By examining the equations in previous questions it is clear that a variety of factors influence T_m and, therefore, annealing of primers with DNA. Primers with different percentages of GC and/or length will have different annealing temperatures. To factor these variables into a single T_m given a number of other factors (divalent and monovalent cation concentrations, primer and target concentrations) has, to date, been a complex problem that is often unresolvable.

Chapter 21: Genomics, Bioinformatics, and Proteomics

Concept Areas	Corresponding Problems
Genomics Overview	2, 6, 12
Human Genome Project	10, 12, 14, 15, 19, 24
Sequencing	1, 3, 7, 15, 17, 19, 21, 23, 24, 25, 28
Genomic Organization	4, 10, 11, 22, 23,
Bioinformatics	1, 5, 8, 16, 25, 27
Essential Genes, Pseudogenes	9, 26
Proteomics	1, 7, 26
Annotation	13, 20
Microarrays	1, 18

Concepts and Processes Checklist

(Check topic when mastered – provide examples where appropriate – understand the context of each entry)

- **Genomics Overview**
  - genome
  - genomics
  - positional cloning
  - transcriptome analysis

- **Whole-Genome Shotgun Sequencing**
  - structural genomics
  - whole-genome shotgun sequencing
  - shotgun cloning
  - restriction enzymes
  - partial digests of DNA
  - contiguous fragments
  - contigs
  - sequence alignment
  - high-throughput sequencing
  - computer-automated
  - capillary gel

- clone-by-clone approach
- map-based cloning
- BAC
- YAC
- draft sequences
- error checking
- compiling

- **DNA Sequence Analysis...**
  - bioinformatics
  - GenBank
  - accession number
  - NCBI
  - annotation
  - BLAST
  - similarity score
  - identity value
  - E-value
  - exon

227

- ○ intron
- ○ open reading frame (ORF)
- ○ codon bias

- ○ **Genomics Attempts to Identify…**
  - ○ functional genomics
  - ○ homologous genes
  - ○ ortholog
  - ○ paralog
  - ○ protein domains
  - ○ motifs
  - ○ chromatin immunoprecipitation
  - ○ ChIP
  - ○ *ChIP-chip*

- ○ **The Human Genome Project…**
  - ○ HGP
  - ○ establish functional categories
  - ○ analyze genetic variations
  - ○ single-nucleotide polymorphisms
  - ○ SNPs
  - ○ model organisms
  - ○ new sequencing technologies
  - ○ disseminate genome information
  - ○ ELSI program
  - ○ Celera Genomics
  - ○ reference genome
  - ○ 3.1 billion nucleotides
  - ○ genome is dynamic
  - ○ approximately 20,000 genes
  - ○ major features
  - ○ alternative splicing
  - ○ gene clusters
  - ○ deserts

- ○ copy number variations
- ○ CNVs
- ○ HGP on the internet

- ○ **The "Omics" Revolution…**
  - ○ proteomics
  - ○ metabolomics
  - ○ glycomics
  - ○ toxicogenomics
  - ○ metagenomics
  - ○ pharmacogenomics
  - ○ transcriptomics
  - ○ nutrigenomics
  - ○ stone-age genomics
  - ○ Human Epigenome Project
  - ○ International Hap-Map
  - ○ ENCODE
  - ○ "junk DNA"
  - ○ personal genomics
  - ○ Personal Genome Project
  - ○ PGP
  - ○ Charcot-Marie-Tooth disease
  - ○ CMT
  - ○ human microbiome project
  - ○ Genome 10K plan
  - ○ exome sequencing
  - ○ haploid genome
  - ○ mosaicism

- ○ **Comparative Genomics…**
  - ○ yeast
  - ○ roundworm
  - ○ mice
  - ○ zebrafish

- cress plant
- *Drosophila*
- gene density
- intron number
- intron size
- intron distribution
- repetitive sequences
- sea urchin genome
- dog genome
- *Igf1* gene
- body size
- chimpanzee genome
- indels
- Rhesus monkey genome
- pseudogenes
- Neanderthal genome
- Neanderthal mitochondrial genome

- **Comparative Genomics...
  Multigene Families**
  - multigene families
  - superfamily
  - globin gene superfamily
  - myoglobin
  - hemoglobin
  - α-globin
  - β-globin

- **Metagenomics Applies Genomics...**
  - environmental genomics
  - Global Ocean Sampling
    Expedition
  - Venn diagram

- **Transcriptome Analysis...**
  - transcriptomics

- global analysis of gene expression
- DNA microarray analysis
- cDNA
- gene chips
- cluster algorithm
- circadian rhythm

- **Proteomics Identifies...**
  - proteome
  - Protein Structure Initiative
  - PSI
  - two-dimensional gel
    electrophoresis
  - isoelectric focusing
  - sodium dodecyl sulfate
  - polyacrylamide gel
    electrophoresis
  - SDS-PAGE
  - mass spectrometry
  - mass-to-charge ratio (m/z)
  - MALDI
  - time of fight
  - TOF
  - tandem mass spectrometry
  - MS/MS
  - protein microarray
  - *T. rex*
  - *M. americanum*
  - m/z ratios
  - collagen

- **System Biology...**
  - linking genomic studies
  - interactome
  - network maps

Chapter 21 Genomics, Bioinformatics, and Proteomics

Answers to Now Solve This

21-1. (a) To annotate a gene, one identifies gene regulatory sequences found upstream of genes (promoters, enhancers, and silencers), downstream elements (termination sequences), and in-frame triplet nucleotides that are part of the coding region of the gene. In addition, 5' and 3' splice sites that are used to distinguish exons from introns as well as polyadenylation sites are also used in annotation. **(b)** Similarity to other annotated sequences often provides insight as to a sequence's function and may serve to substantiate a particular genetic assignment. Direct sequencing of cDNAs from various tissues and developmental stages aids in verification. **(c)** Taking an average of 20,000 for the estimated number of genes in the human genome and computing the percentage represented by 3,141 gives 15.7 percent. It appears as if chromosome 1 is gene rich.

21-2. Since structural and chemical factors determine the function of a protein, it is likely to have several proteins share a considerable amino acid sequence identity, but not be functionally identical. Since the *in vivo* function of such a protein is determined by secondary and tertiary structures, as well as local surface chemistries in active or functional sites, the nonidentical sequences may have considerable influence on function. Note that the query matches to different site positions within the target proteins. A number of other factors suggesting different functions include associations with other molecules (cytoplasmic, membrane, or extracellular), chemical nature and position of binding domains, posttranslational modification, signal sequences, and so on.

21-3. Because blood is relatively easy to obtain in a pure state, its components can be analyzed without fear of tissue-site contamination. Second, blood is intimately exposed to virtually all cells of the body and may, therefore, carry chemical markers to certain abnormal cells it represents, theoretically, an ideal probe into the human body. However, when blood is removed from the body, its proteome changes and those changes are dependent on a number of environmental factors. Thus, what might be a valid diagnostic for one condition might not be so under others. In addition, the serum proteome is subject to change depending on the genetic, physiologic, and environmental state of the patient. Age and sex are additional variables that must be considered. Validation of a plasma proteome for a particular cancer would be strengthened by demonstrating that the stage of development of the cancer correlates with a commensurate change in the proteome in a relatively large, statistically significant pool of patients. Second, the types of changes in the proteome should be reproducible and, at least until complexities are clarified, involve tumorigenic proteins. It would be helpful to have comparisons with archived samples of each individual at a disease-free time.

Chapter 21 Genomics, Bioinformatics, and Proteomics

Solutions to Problems and Discussion Questions

1. (a) Generally, contigs are suspected to be part of the same chromosome in that their end sequences overlap.

(b) Identification of a protein-coding region is suspected if similar sequences are conserved in other species and various upstream, downstream, splicing, and punctuation sequences are present and in the proper reading frames.

(c) Comparisons of base sequence data with other organisms indicate conservation of a considerable number of sequences. Because of such conservation, functional relationships are strongly supported. Adding additional support are comparative mutation analyses indicating similar function.

(d) Proteomics is the identification and analysis of proteins in cells, tissues, and organisms. Genome annotation provides an estimate of the number of protein coding genes, whereas a number of sophisticated techniques including electrophoresis, chromatography, spectrophotometry, and microarrays indicate the number of proteins actually produced. The finding that there are many more types of proteins than genes in the genome has generated a number of explanations.

(e) By comparing the amino acid sequences of proteins, the base sequences of genes, and intron/exon architecture, researchers have determined that many genes originated by duplication. Sequence divergence often alters duplicated genes, thus providing the raw material for the evolution of new genes.

(f) Microarrays provide a method for identifying active genes by the hybridization of complementary gene products to stretches of DNA. Different hybridization patterns indicate that although some genes are expressed in almost all cells, others show cell- and tissue-specific expression.

2. Your essay should include a description of traditional recombinant DNA technology involving cutting and splicing genes, as well as modern methods of synthesizing genes of interest, PCR amplification, microarray analysis, etc.

3. Functional genomics seeks to understand functional components within the genome and similarities of genomes across phylogenetic and evolutionary distances. Comparative genomics analyzes the arrangement and organization of families of genes within and among genomes.

4. Whole-genome shotgun sequencing involves randomly cutting the genome into numerous smaller segments. Overlapping sequences are used to identify segments that were once contiguous, eventually producing the entire sequence. Difficulties in alignment often occur in repetitive regions of the genome. Map-based sequencing relies on known landmarks (genes, nucleotide polymorphisms, etc.) to orient the alignment of cloned fragments that have been sequenced. Compared to whole-genome sequencing, the map-based approach is somewhat cumbersome and time consuming. Whole-genome sequencing has become the most common method for assembling genomes, with map-based cloning being used to resolve the problems often encountered during whole-genome sequencing.

5. Understanding the genome is dependent on the field of bioinformatics, in which computer and mathematics applications are used to organize, share, and analyze data generated by sequencing data. World access to such data is dependent on the ability to store, efficiently share, and obtain the maximum amount of information from protein and DNA sequences. As genomics emerged, bioinformatics became a significant player and today occupies an intellectual enterprise that fuses biological data with information technology, mathematics, and statistical analysis. Most applications, such as the identification of informational content in the genome and DNA sequencing, rely on sequence alignments in nucleic acids and proteins.

6. The main goals of the Human Genome Project are to establish, categorize, and analyze functions for human genes. As stated in the text:

> To analyze genetic variations between humans, including the identification of single-nucleotide polymorphisms (SNPs)

> To map and sequence the genomes of several model organisms used in experimental genetics, including *E. coli*, *S. cerevisiae*, *C. elegans*, *D. melanogaster*, and *M. musculus* (the mouse)

To develop new sequencing technologies, such as high-throughput computer-automated sequencers, to facilitate genome analysis

To disseminate genome information, among both scientists and the general public

7. High-throughput technologies allow comprehensive analyses of a number of labor-intensive tasks that would normally take days or weeks to be reduced to half-day activities. By shortening sequencing times, numerous organisms can be sequenced to yield highly informative comparative sequences (comparative genomics). Applied to both genomics and proteomics, high-throughput technologies allow rapid analyses and deployment of genomic information.

8. One initial approach to annotating a sequence is to compare the newly sequenced genomic DNA to the known sequences already stored in various databases. The National Center for Biotechnology Information (NCBI) provides access to BLAST (Basic Local Alignment Search Tool) software, which directs searches through databanks of DNA and protein sequences. A segment of DNA can be compared to sequences in major databases such as GenBank to identify matches that align in whole or in part. One might seek similarities to a sequence on chromosome 11 in a mouse and find that or similar sequences in a number of taxa. BLAST will compute a similarity score or identity value to indicate the degree to which two sequences are similar. BLAST is one of many sequence alignment algorithms (RNA-RNA, protein-protein, etc.) that may sacrifice sensitivity for speed.

9. Pseudogenes are nonfunctional versions of genes that resemble gene sequences but contain significant nucleotide changes, which prevent their expression. They are formed by gene duplication and subsequent mutation.

10. The human genome is composed of more than 3 billion nucleotides in which about 2 percent code for genes. Genes are unevenly distributed over chromosomes, with clusters of gene-rich regions separated by gene-poor ones (deserts). Human genes tend to be larger and contain more and larger introns than in invertebrates such as *Drosophila*. It is estimated that at least half of the genes generate products by alternative splicing. Hundreds of genes have been transferred from bacteria into

vertebrates. Duplicated regions are common, which may facilitate chromosomal rearrangement. The human genome appears to contain approximately 20,000 protein-coding genes; however, there is still uncertainty as to the total number.

11. ChIP analysis allows geneticists to assess the relationships between DNA and proteins, such as transcription factors. In doing so, it is often possible to estimate the functional results of such interactions.

12. Because many repetitive regions of the genome are not directly involved in production of a phenotype, they tend to be isolated from selection and show considerable variation in redundancy. Length variation in such repeats is unique among individuals (except for identical twins) and, with various detection methods, provides the basis for DNA fingerprinting. Single nucleotide polymorphisms also occur frequently in the genome and can be used to distinguish individuals.

13. One usually begins to annotate a sequence by comparing it, often using BLAST, to the known sequences already stored in various databases. Similarity to other annotated sequences often provides insight as to a sequences function. Hallmarks to annotation are the identification of gene regulatory sequences found upstream of genes (promoters, enhancers, and silencers), downstream elements (termination sequences), and triplet nucleotides that are part of the coding region of the gene. In addition, 5' and 3' splice sites that are used to distinguish exons from introns and polyadenylation sites are also used in annotation. Similar hallmarks are used to annotate prokaryotic genes; however, because prokaryotic genes do not contain introns, their annotation is sometimes less complicated. Annotation is an ongoing process and community effort involving scientists worldwide.

14. The PGP provides individual sequences of diploid genomes, and results of such projects indicate that the HGP may underestimate genome variation by as much as fivefold. Genome variation between individuals may be 0.5 percent rather than the 0.1 percent estimated from the HGP. Since the PGP provides sequence information on individuals, fundamental questions about human diversity and evolution may be more answerable.

15. Given the speed, efficiency, and recent cost reductions associated with modern sequencing technologies, some scientists believe it is reasonable to expect that 10,000 (10K) vertebrate genomes can be sequenced in five years. They believe that such a massive pool of sequences would provide insight into genome evolution and speciation, in addition to providing valuable insight to the human genome through comparative genomics.

16. A number of new subdisciplines of molecular biology will provide the infrastructure for major advances in our understanding of living systems. The following terms identify specific areas within that infrastructure:

proteomics: proteins in a cell or tissue
metabolomics: enzymatic pathways
glycomics: carbohydrates of a cell or tissue
toxicogenomics: toxic chemicals
metagenomics: environmental issues
pharmacogenomics: customized medicine
transcriptomics: expressed genes

Many other "-omics" are likely in the future.

17. Metagenomics is a relatively new discipline that examines the genomes from entire communities of microbes in environmental samples of water, air, and soil. Virtually every environment on Earth is being sampled in metagenomics projects. A major initiative is a global expedition called the *Sorcerer II* Global Ocean Sampling (GOS), in which researchers travel the globe by yacht and sample as many microbes as possible. Metagenomics is teaching us more about millions of species of microbes, of which only a few thousand have been well characterized.

18. Most microarrays, known also as gene chips, consist of a glass slide that is coated, using a robotic system, with single-stranded DNA molecules. Some microarrays are coated with single-stranded sequences of expressed sequenced tags or DNA sequences that are complementary to gene transcripts. A single microarray can have as many as 20,000 different spots of DNA, each containing a unique sequence. Researchers use microarrays to compare patterns of gene expression in tissues under different conditions or to compare gene expression patterns in normal and diseased tissues. In addition, microarrays can be used to identify pathogens. Microarray databases allow investigators to compare any given pattern to others worldwide.

19. Aneuploidy in humans occurs for the sex chromosomes (X and Y) and three of the autosomes (13, 18, and 21). Other aneuploids are apparently not compatible with survival. Extra or missing X chromosomes are apparently tolerated because of dosage compensation, whereas Y chromosome aneuploids are most likely compatible with survival because of general paucity of Y-linked genes. Notice that the number of genes on chromosomes 13, 18, and 21 are the lowest for the autosomes. It is probably not coincidental that chromosomes with the fewest genes and no known mechanism for dosage compensation are the only ones that survive as human aneuploids.

20. Increased protein production from approximately 20,000 genes is probably related to alternative splicing and various posttranslational processing schemes. In addition, a particular DNA segment may be read in a variety of ways and in two directions.

21. In general, one would expect certain factors (such as heat or salt) to favor evolution to increase protein stability: distribution of ionic interactions on the surface, density of hydrophobic residues and interactions, and number of hydrogen and disulfide bonds. As seen from examining the codon table, a high GC ratio would favor the amino acids Ala, Gly, Pro, Arg, and Trp and minimize the use of Ile, Phe, Lys, Asn, and Tyr. How codon bias influences actual protein stability is not yet understood. Most genomic sequences change by relatively gradual responses to mild selection over long periods of time. They strongly resemble patterns of common descent; that is, they are conserved. Although the same can be said for organisms adapted to extreme environments, extraordinary physiological demands may dictate unexpected sequence bias.

22. Whereas the β-globin gene family is a relatively large (60 kb) sequence, and restriction analyses show that it is composed of six genes, one is a pseudogene and, therefore, does not produce a product. The five functional genes each contain two similarly sized introns, which, when included with noncoding flanking regions (5' and 3') and spacer DNA between genes, account for the 95 percent mentioned in the question.

23. Any time a DNA sequence is conserved in other species, it is likely that that sequence has an influence on similar phenotypes. The higher the number of species that conserve the sequence, the higher the likelihood of determining its function. Coupled with mutation analysis and physical mapping, comparative genomics provides a powerful method for linking DNA sequences with complex human diseases.

24. (a) arm of human, wing of bird, fin of whale **(b)** It happens that homologous proteins may have similar functions; however, there are many examples where different functions have evolved for homologous proteins. **(c)** If proteins evolved by convergent evolution, they may have similar function, but not share homology. Such proteins may have quite different amino acid sequences, but within general functional groupings and quite different DNA sequences. Code degeneracy may account for some of the DNA sequence variation.

25. Two factors may be significant in causing a similar gene to function one way in one species and another way in a closely related species. Despite the fact that humans and chimps share significant sequence overlap, there are still approximately 35 million single base differences and about 5 million deletion/addition differences. Such changes influence the molecular environment in which a gene is expressed. Second, the external environment, especially in terms of carbohydrate availability and metabolism, has been different during the evolution of these two species. Such environmental differences may engage a different genetic background (therefore, proteome) in which a particular gene is expressed. A protein functioning in one molecular environment may function quite differently in a slightly different environment. Such complexities in gene expression must be addressed when therapies are developed using model organisms.

26. The position of the homologous track is pivotal in determining the 3D structure, which in turn establishes the skeleton for function. Superimposed on the 3D structure will be the particular surface chemistry that emerges as the protein assumes the superstructure. Chaperones are involved in protein 3D maturation.

27. The issue here is whether the organism under consideration is independent and self-reproducing. It appears that the minimum number of genes for a free-living organism is in the range of 250–350. Symbionts can have much smaller genomes and exist with fewer genes because of materials supplied by the host cell. As long as one defines the lifestyle (free-living or symbiont) of the organism in question, it is informative to consider how many genes are needed to accomplish the task of "living."

28. (a) The strength of WES is that one may get lucky and identify a coding issue in a gene that has relevance to the patient's condition. Given the multitude of genetic variances known to exist, this might be akin to looking for a needle in a haystack. Many important regulatory and structural components in the genome are outside the exon pool. Introns are notorious for housing many important sequences. **(b)** You would definitely examine the mitochondrial genome (highly variable between individuals), because a growing list of human conditions are known to involve mitochondrial defects.

Chapter 22: Applications and Ethics of Genetic Engineering and Biotechnology

Concept Areas	Corresponding Problems
Genetically Modified Organisms	1, 2, 3, 5, 6, 25, 26
Use of Genetically Engineered Products	1, 5, 8
Genetic Engineering	4, 9, 16, 24, 25
Diagnosing and Screening Genetic Disorders	1, 10, 11, 12, 14, 21
Gene Therapy	1, 16, 18, 19, 20
Genome Analysis	1, 11
DNA Profiling	10, 15, 21, 26
Ethical Issues	2, 3, 11, 12, 13, 15, 16, 17, 18, 19, 22, 23, 24, 25
Synthetic Genome	7, 25

Concepts and Processes Checklist

(Check topic when mastered – provide examples where appropriate – understand the context of each entry)

- **Genetically Engineered Organisms**
    - recombinant DNA technology
    - biopharmaceutical products
    - therapeutic proteins
    - biopharming
    - insulin production in bacteria
    - Humulin
    - U.S. Food and Drug Administration
    - FDA
    - type I diabetes
    - preproinsulin
    - *A* and *B* chains
    - *lacZ* gene
    - β-galactosidase
    - fusion protein
    - transgenic animal hosts
    - bioreactors
    - biofactories
    - baculovirus
    - α1-antitrypsin
    - anithrombin

- **Recombinant DNA Approaches…**
    - production of vaccines
    - stimulate immune system
    - inactivated vaccine
    - attenuated vaccine
    - subunit vaccine
    - hepatitis B virus
    - Gardasil
    - human papillomavirus
    - HPV
    - DNA-based vaccines

- **Genetic Engineering of Plants…**
    - selective breeding

- increased productivity
- nutritional enhancement
- agricultural biotechnology
- GM crops
- transgenic crops
- herbicide and pest resistance

- **Transgenic Animals…**
  - Chinook salmon
  - mastitis
  - lysostaphin
  - mad cow disease
  - enviroPig
  - phytase
  - GloFish

- **Synthetic Genomes…**
  - *Mycoplasma genitalium*
  - *Haemophilus influenza*
  - genome transplantation
  - synthetic biology
  - prosthetic genomes
  - synthetic biology for bioengineering
  - Registry of Standard Biological Parts
  - recombinase
  - green fluorescent protein
  - genetically recoded organisms

- **Genetic Engineering…**
  - medical diagnosis
  - DNA-based tests
  - amniocentesis
  - chorionic villus sampling
  - fetal cell sorting

- Materni21
- restriction fragment length polymorphism
- RFLP
- sickle-cell anemia
- allele-specific oligonucleotide
- ASOs
- single-nucleotide polymorphism
- SNP
- preimplantation genetic diagnosis
- PGD
- cystic fibrosis (CF)
- cystic fibrosis transmembrane conductance regulator
- CFTR
- DNA microarray
- field
- genotyping microarray
- genome scanning
- array comparative genomic hybridization
- CGH
- gene-expression microarray
- diffuse large B-cell lymphoma
- DLBCL
- nutrigenomics
- transcriptome analysis

- **Genome-Wide Association Studies**
  - GWAS
  - identify genome variations

- **Genomics Leads to New…**
  - targeted medical treatment

- personalized medicine
- pharmacogenomics
- rational drug design
- Gleevec
- gene therapy
- **Genetic Engineering, Genomics...**
  - ethical, social, legal questions
  - genetic testing
  - Noonan syndrome
  - Genetic Information Nondiscrimination Act
  - ethical dilemmas

- ELSI program
- direct-to-consumer genetic tests
- DTC
- Myriad Genetics
- *BRCA1, BRCA2*
- Genetic Testing Registry
- GTR
- intellectual property
- gene patents
- preconception testing
- 23andMe
- patents and synthetic biology

Answers to Now Solve This

22-1. Digestion involves the process of breaking down foodstuffs for eventual absorption by the small intestine. Antigens are usually quite large molecules, and in the process of digestion, they are sometimes broken down into smaller molecules, thus becoming ineffective in stimulating the immune system. Some individuals are allergic to the food they eat, testifying to the fact that all antigens are not completely degraded or modified by digestion. In some cases, ingested antigens do indeed stimulate the immune system (e.g., oral polio vaccine) and provide a route for immunization. Localized (intestinal) immunity can sometimes be stimulated by oral introduction of antigens, and in some cases, this can offer immunity to ingested pathogens.

22-2. The child in question is a carrier of the deletion in the β-globin gene, just as the parents are carriers. Its genotype is therefore $\beta^A\beta^o$.

22-3. It will hybridize by base complementation to the normal DNA sequence.

Chapter 22 *Applications and Ethics of Genetic Engineering and Biotechnology*

Solutions to Problems and Discussion Questions

1. (a) Physical evidence of gene introduction comes from various forms of analysis, including PCR, RT-PCR, RFLP, Southern blotting, and DNA sequencing. Functional evidence can be obtained from microarray analysis and direct assays of the gene product.

(b) PCR, Southern blot, or similar detection/blotting methods coupled with allele-specific oligonucleotide detection are standard methods to determine the presence of certain genes and their mutations. Coupled with RFLP analysis using *Mst*II and *Cvn*I, it is possible to distinguish sickle-cell from normal hemoglobin DNA.

(c) Microarrays can be used as platforms on which to hybridize DNA or RNA from various tissues. RNA populations from different tissues will give different patterns of hybridization, a so-called transcriptome analysis.

(d) Genome-wide association studies involve scanning the genomes of thousands of unrelated individuals with a particular disease and comparing them with the genomes of individuals who do not have the disease. GWAS attempt to identify genes that influence disease risk.

(e) A number of factors impact the utility of gene therapy. Second, a suitable vector must be selected and properly engineered to carry and deliver the desired product on an appropriate schedule. Second, the vector must be stable yet not trigger an immune response. If the vector is to integrate into the host DNA, it must do so without causing harm.

2. Your essay should include a description of genomic applications that relate to agriculture, health and welfare, scientific exploration and appreciation of the earth's flora and fauna, etc. In addition, areas of patent protection, personal privacy, and potential agricultural and environmental hazards should be addressed.

3. Kleter and Peijnenburg used the BLAST tool from http://www.ncbi.nlm.nih.gov/BLAST to conduct a series of alignment comparisons of transgenic sequences with sequences of known allergenic proteins. Of 33 transgenic proteins screened for identities of at least 6 contiguous amino acids found in allergenic proteins, 22 gave positive results.

4. In general, bacteria do not process eukaryotic proteins in the same manner as eukaryotes. Transgenic eukaryotes are more likely to correctly process eukaryotic proteins, thus increasing the likelihood of their normal biological activity.

5. From a purely scientific viewpoint, there will be no added danger to consuming cow's milk from cloned animals. However, some individuals may have an aversion to organismic cloning, and supporting such activities through consumption of products of cloned organisms may be viewed negatively on moral grounds. It is likely that public sentiment will pressure for labeling of "cloned products" on the grounds that consumers should be able to make an informed choice as to the origin of such products.

6. (a) Both the saline and column extracts of Lkt50 appear to be capable of inducing at least 50 percent neutralization of toxicity when injected into rabbits. **(b)** In order for a successful edible vaccine to be developed, numerous hurdles must be overcome. The immunogen must be stably incorporated into the host plant hereditary material, and the host must express only that immunogen. During feeding, the immunogen must be transported across the intestinal wall unaltered or altered in such a way as to stimulate the desired immune response. There must be guarantees that potentially harmful by-products of transgenesis have not been produced. In other words, broad ecological and environmental issues must be addressed to prevent a transgenic plant from becoming an unintended vector for harm to the environment or any organisms feeding on the plant (directly or indirectly).

7. The Venter team compared a number of genomes each with a small number of genes and identified 256 genes that may represent the minimum number of genes for life. The team also used transposon-based mutations to determine the number of genes essential for life. Finally, it synthesized short DNA segments and assembled them into a synthetic genome that possessed characteristics of living systems.

8. Even though you have developed a method for screening seven of the mutations described, it is possible that negative results can occur when the person carries the gene for CF. In other words, the specific probes (or allele-specific oligonucleotides) that have been developed will not necessarily be useful for screening all mutant alleles. In addition, the cost-effectiveness of such a screening proposal would need to be considered.

9. A microarray is a solid support containing an orderly arrangement of DNA samples. A typical array contains thousands of DNA spots that may be small oligonucleotides, cDNAs, or short genomic sequences. Labeled sequences hybridize to the immobilized DNAs by standard base pairing. Such technology allows a method for monitoring RNA expression levels of thousands of genes in virtually any cell population. Using microarray technology, researchers can observe the overall behavior of the genome in cancer and normal cells and, by comparison, determine which genes are active or inactive under various circumstances. It is possible to identify the set of genes whose expression or lack thereof defines the properties of each tumor type. This application can, therefore, lead to precise diagnosis and refine possible therapies. In addition, microarray profiling can be used to determine the efficacy of particular therapies. For instance, one can monitor responses to radiation and/ or chemotherapy to determine the degree to which cells are responding to a particular cancer treatment.

10. Since both mutations occur in the CF gene, children who possess both alleles will suffer from CF. With both parents heterozygous, each child born will have a 25 percent chance of developing CF.

11. At this point, there is considerable reluctance to allow the open sharing of genetic information among institutions. In general, the establishment of governmental databases containing our most intimate information is viewed with skepticism. It is likely that considerable time and discussion will elapse before such databases are established.

12. Using restriction enzyme analysis to detect point mutations in humans is a tedious trial-and-error process. Given the size of the human genome in terms of base sequences and the relatively low number of unique restriction enzymes, the likelihood of matching a specific point mutation, separate from other normal sequence variations, to a desired gene is low.

13. Such widespread screening of newborns would allow the identification of a virtually infinite number of variables associated with the human genome that might be of scientific and personal interest. Some basis for certain disease states might be identified. However, disadvantages would be the likely stigmatizing of certain individuals and numerous issues of privacy invasion.

14. Genome-wide association studies involve scanning the genomes of thousands of unrelated individuals with a particular disease and comparing them with the genomes of individuals who do not

have the disease. GWAS attempt to identify genes that influence disease risk.

15. There are over 2,000 variations of the CFTR, and many different expression of symptoms. Bacteria can be harbored in one individual that are harmful to other CF individuals. In this case, the school wished to protect the other CF students at the school because of the possibility of bacterial contamination.

16. In the case of haplo-insufficient mutations, gene therapy holds promise; however, in "gain-of-function" mutations, in all probability, the mutant gene's activity or product must be compromised. RNAi strategies may apply more effectively. Addition of a normal gene probably will not help unless it can compete out the mutant gene product.

17. Each person must decide to make use of genetic information in a complex informational, societal, and personal environment. What is a sound decision for one individual may not be appropriate for another. Hopefully, those individuals making such life-altering decisions will do so with sound information from the scientific community and sufficient understanding of the ramifications of such decisions.

18. Certainly, information provided to physicians and patients about genetic testing is a strong point in favor of wide distribution. It would probably be helpful for companies involved in genetic testing to also participate by providing information peculiar to their operations. It would be necessary, however, that any individual results from tests would be held in strict confidence. It would be helpful if pooled statistical data would be available to the public in terms of frequencies of false positives and negatives, as well as population and or geographical distributions.

19. Given the use to which genetic tests are put and their extreme personal nature, it would seem that FDA regulation is one way to decrease the distribution of misinformation that may be vital to individuals and families.

20. It is a personal decision to have one's genome sequenced. However, doing so may identify variations that may be alarming, but have no consequences. Such "false positives" may have a negative impact on an individual. In addition, one must consider a variety of consequences associated with a publicly available genome sequence: employment bias, personal relationships, etc.

21. Given the present state of understanding of behavioral genetics, it is unlikely that any definitive conclusions can be reached by such an analysis.

22. Raw genomic information is difficult to interpret, and regulation of such companies has fallen behind the technology. 23andMe provides ancestry information but has stopped giving disease-related results. Recently (November 2013) the FDA warned 23andMe to stop marketing its genomic service.

23. There are numerous methods for generating transgenic mammals using retroviral vectors. One method involves injection of an engineered retroviral RNA into embryonic (pronuclear) cells directly. Another scheme uses cultured embryonic stem cells (ES) and is presented in the mouse example that follows.

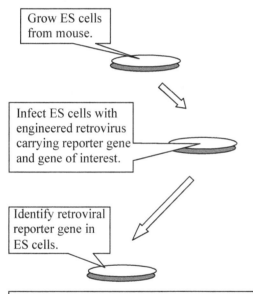

Grow ES cells from mouse.

Infect ES cells with engineered retrovirus carrying reporter gene and gene of interest.

Identify retroviral reporter gene in ES cells.

Inject engineered ES cells into blastocysts of mouse. Introduce injected blastocysts into pseudopregnant female by ovaductal transplantation.

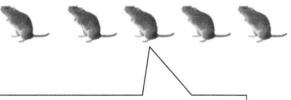

Examine progeny for reporter gene and gene of interest. Select for crosses that, through Mendelian inheritance, may allow establishment of a strain containing the reporter gene and the gene of interest.

24. Sample size: Is the sample size sufficiently robust to minimize spurious correlations? Epigenetic factors: Since the genome is strongly influenced by epigenetic factors, how might this influence a study based on SNPs? Environmental factors: Have samples been compiled in such a way as to negate significant differences in environmental exposure? Genetic background: Since the entire genome is not compared, what suppressors and/or modifiers that mask or enhance the expression of certain genes are present, but missed? What emergent properties are present in the entire allelic architecture? Population stratification: Might there be allelic frequency differences peculiar to the case population as compared with the control group? Such population frequency differences may result from differences in ancestry, depending on the composition of the cases and the controls.

25. (a) Since a gene is a product of the natural world, it does not conform to section 101 of U.S. patent laws, which govern patentable matter. **(b)** Since both the direct-to-consumer test for the *BRCA1* and *BRCA2* genes and Venter's "first-ever human-made life form" are original in their process or development, they should be patentable. However, the *BRCA1* and *BRCA2* genes are works of nature, and the genes themselves should not be patentable.

26. There are several reasons that CF mice do not exhibit airway symptoms similar to those in humans with CF. First, the distribution of cell types, CFTR presence, and chloride/sodium handling differ in the upper and lower airways of mice and humans. Second, mice tend not to suffer from airway bacterial infections that severely influence human pathology. A complete review of this topic is available in Grubb and Boucher, 1999, *Physiological Reviews*, vol. 71, 5193–5214.

Chapter 23: Quantitative Genetics and Multifactorial Traits

Concept Areas	Corresponding Problems
Phenotypic Expression	1, 3, 5, 10, 21, 23, 24, 28, 29
Continuous Variation and Polygenes	1, 2, 4, 5, 6, 7, 22, 23, 25
Genetic Basis	1, 5, 6, 7, 25, 26
Heritability	3, 9, 12, 13, 14, 15, 16, 17, 18, 19, 26, 27
Mapping	3, 20
Statistics	11, 27, 29
Twin Studies	1, 3, 8

Concepts and Processes Checklist

(Check topic when mastered – provide examples where appropriate – understand the context of each entry)

- **Quantitative Inheritance**
  - polygenic
  - multifactorial
  - complex traits
- **Not All Polygenic Traits...**
  - meristic traits
  - threshold traits
  - Type II diabetes
- **Quantitative Traits Can Be...**
  - multiple-factor hypothesis
  - multiple-gene hypothesis
  - additive alleles
  - nonadditive allele
  - calculate number of polygenes
  - $1/4^n$
  - $(2n + 1)$
- **The Study of Polygenic Traits...**
  - normal distribution

- mean
- variance
- standard deviation
- standard error of the mean
- covariance
- correlation coefficient
- analysis of quantitative character
- **Heritability Values Estimate...**
  - heritability
  - phenotypic variance (V_P)
  - genotypic variance (V_G)
  - environmental variance (V_E)
  - genotype-by-environment interaction variance ($V_{G \times E}$)
  - broad-sense heritability (H^2)
  - narrow-sense heritability (h^2)
  - additive variance (V_A)

- dominance variance (V_D)
- interactive variance (V_I)
- artificial selection
- selection response
- selection differential
- realized heritability

- **Twin Studies Allow...**
  - monozygotic twins (MZ)
  - identical twins
  - dizygotic twins (DZ)
  - fraternal twins
  - concordant
  - discordant

- limitations of twin studies
- epigenetics

- **Quantitative Trait Loci...**
  - QTL
  - QTL mapping
  - RFLP
  - microsatellites
  - SNPs
  - expression QTLs
  - eQTLs
  - *ORFX*
  - protein QTLs
  - pQTLs

Chapter 23 Quantitative Genetics and Multifactorial Traits

Answers to Now Solve This

23-1 (a) Since 1/256 of the F_2 plants are 20 cm and 1/256 are 40 cm, there must be four gene pairs involved in determining flower size.

(b) Since there are nine size classes, one can conduct the following backcross: $AaBbCcDd \times AABBCCDD$

The frequency distribution in the backcross would be:

1/16	=	40 cm
4/16	=	37.5 cm
6/16	=	35 cm
4/16	=	32.5 cm
1/16	=	30 cm

23-2. (a) Taking the sum of the values and dividing by the number in the sample gives the following means:

mean sheep fiber length = 7.7 cm   *mean fleece weight* = 6.4 kg

The variance for each is: *variance sheep fiber length* = 6.097   *variance fleece weight* = 3.12

The standard deviation is the square root of the variance: *sheep fiber length* = 2.469
fleece weight = 1.766

(b, c) The covariance for the two traits is 30.36/7, or 4.34; the correlation coefficient is +0.998.

(d) There is a very high correlation between fleece weight and fiber length, and it is likely that this correlation is not by chance. Even though correlation does not mean cause and effect, it would seem logical that as you increased fiber length, you would also increase fleece weight. It is probably safe to say that the increase in fleece weight is directly related to an increase in fiber length.

23-3. *Monozygotic twins* are derived from a single fertilized egg and are thus genetically identical. They provide a method for determining the influence of genetics and environment on certain traits. *Dizygotic twins* arise from two eggs fertilized by two sperm cells. They have the same genetic relationship as siblings. The role of genetics and the role of the environment can be studied by comparing the expression of traits in monozygotic and dizygotic twins. The higher concordance value for monozygotic twins indicates a significant genetic component, for a given trait. Notice that for traits including blood type, eye color, and mental retardation, there is a fairly significant difference between MZ and DZ groups. However, for measles, the difference is not as significant, indicating a greater role of the environment. Hair color has a significant genetic component, as do idiopathic epilepsy, schizophrenia, diabetes, allergies, cleft lip, and club foot. The genetic component to mammary cancer is present but minimal according to these data.

Solutions to Problems and Discussion Questions

1. In general, polygenic conditions involving thresholds occur if a range of expression is possible, but the trait is either expressed or not expressed. In addition, with polygenic systems (including those with thresholds), environmental factors carry considerable impact. **(b)** The number of polygenes involved in a polygenic trait can often be estimated by solving for n in the formula if the ratio of F_2 individuals resembling either of the two extreme P_1 phenotypes can be determined:

$$1/4^n$$

It is also possible to estimate the number of polygenes using the $(2n + 1)$ rule, where $(2n + 1)$ is the number of possible phenotypes, and n equals the number of additive loci. **(c)** The multiple-factor hypothesis was originally based on experiment results involving pigmentation in wheat. Such results showed that a number of additive alleles acting in Mendelian fashion could explain continuous variation. **(d)** When a number of parameters are known, environmental impact on a quantitatively inherited trait is often assessed by heritability estimates (broad and narrow sense). Using highly inbred strains of plants and animals, reared under varying conditions, and twin studies in humans is helpful in determining the environmental impact on traits. **(e)** Differences in inherited disease states indicate that copy number variation and epigenetics alter the genotypes of all individuals, including monozygotic twins.

2. Your essay should include a description of various ratios typical of Mendelian genetics as compared with the more blending, continuously varying expressions of neo-Mendelian modes of inheritance. It should contrast discontinuous inheritance and continuous patterns.

3. (a) *Polygenes* are those genes that are involved in determining continuously varying or multiple factor traits.

(b) *Additive alleles* are those alleles that account for the hereditary influence on the phenotype in an additive way.

(c) *Correlation* is a statistic that varies from -1 to $+1$ and describes the extent to which variation in one trait is associated with variation in another. It does not imply that a cause-and-effect relationship exists between two traits.

(d) *Monozygotic twins* are derived from a single fertilized egg and are thus genetically identical. They provide a method for determining the influence of genetics and environment on certain traits. *Dizygotic twins* arise from two eggs fertilized by two sperm cells. They have the same genetic relationship as siblings. The role of genetics and the role of the environment can be studied by comparing the expression of traits in monozygotic and dizygotic twins. The higher concordance value for monozygotic twins indicates a significant genetic component for a given trait.

(e) *Heritability* is a measure of the degree to which the phenotypic variation of a given trait is due to genetic factors. A high heritability indicates that genetic factors are major contributors to phenotypic variation, whereas environmental factors have little impact.

(f) QTL stands for quantitative trait loci, which are situations in which multiple genes contribute to a quantitative trait.

(g) Continuous variation results from the interaction of a number of gene loci specifying a given trait. Rather than stepwise inheritance patterns, phenotypic distributions are more curve-like.

4. If you add the numbers given for the ratio, you obtain the value of 16, which is indicative of a dihybrid cross. The distribution is that of a dihybrid cross with additive effects.

(a) Because a dihybrid result has been identified, two loci are involved in the production of color. There are two alleles at each locus, for a total of four alleles.

(b, c) Because the description of red, medium red, and so on gives us no indication of a *quantity* of color in any form of units, we would not be able to actually quantify a unit amount for each change in color. We can say that each gene (additive allele) provides an equal unit amount to the phenotype, and the colors differ from one another in multiples of that unit amount. The number of additive alleles needed to produce each phenotype follows:

1/16	=	dark red	=	*AABB*
4/16	=	medium-dark red	=	*2AABb* *2AaBB*
6/16	=	medium red	=	*AAbb* *4AaBb* *aaBB*
4/16	=	light red	=	*2aaBb* *2Aabb*
1/16	=	white	=	*aabb*

(d)

F₁ = all light red
F₂ = 1/4 medium red
2/4 light red
1/4 white

5. (a) It is *possible* that two parents of moderate height can produce offspring that are much taller or shorter than either parent because segregation can produce a variety of gametes, as illustrated here:

rrSsTtuu × *RrSsTtUu*
(moderate)   (moderate)

Offspring from this cross can range from the very tall *RrSSTTUu* (14 "tall" units) to the very short *rrssttuu* (8 "small" units).

(b) If the individual with a minimum height, *rrssttuu*, is married to an individual of intermediate height, *RrSsTtUu*, the offspring can be no taller than the height of the taller parent. Notice that there is no way of having more than four uppercase alleles in the offspring.

6. As you read this question, notice that the strains are inbred and therefore homozygous and that approximately 1/250 represents the shortest and tallest groups in the F₂ generation. See the ¼ⁿ formula in the text.

(a, b) Referring to the text, see that where four gene pairs act additively, the proportion of one of the extreme phenotypes to the total number of offspring is 1/256. The same may be said for the other extreme type. The extreme types in this problem are the 12-cm and 36-cm plants. From this observation one would suggest that four gene pairs are involved.

(c) If there are four gene pairs, there are nine $(2n + 1)$ phenotypic categories and eight increments between

these categories. Since there is a difference of 24 cm between the extremes, 24 cm/8 = 3 cm for each increment (each of the additive alleles).

(d) A typical F₁ cross that produces a "typical" F₂ distribution would occur when all gene pairs are heterozygous (*AaBbCcDd*), independently assorting, and additive. There are many possible sets of parents that would give an F₁ of this type. The limitation is that each parent has genotypes that give a height of 24 cm as stated in the problem. Because the parents are inbred, it is expected that they are fully homozygous. An example follows:

AABBccdd × *aabbCCDD*

(e) Since the *aabbccdd* genotype gives a height of 12 cm, and each uppercase allele adds 3 cm to the height, there are many possibilities for an 18 cm plant:

AAbbccdd,
AaBbccdd,
aaBbCcdd, and so on.

Any plant with seven uppercase letters will be 33 cm tall:

AABBCCDd,
AABBCcDD,
AABbCCDD, for example

7. (a) There is a fairly continuous range of "quantitative" phenotypes in the F₂ and an F₁ that is between the phenotypes of the two parents; therefore, one can conclude that some phenotypic blending is occurring that is probably the result of several gene pairs acting in an additive fashion. Because the extreme phenotypes (6 cm and 30 cm) each represent 1/64 of the total, it is likely that there are three gene pairs in this cross. Remember that trihybrid crosses that show independent assortment of genes have a denominator (4^3) of 64 in ratios and the fact that there are seven categories of phenotypes, which, because of the relationship $2n + 1 = 7$, would give the number of gene pairs (n) of 3. The genotypes of the parents would be combinations of alleles that would produce a 6-cm *(aabbcc)* tail and a 30-cm *(AABBCC)* tail, whereas the 18-cm offspring would have a genotype of *AaBbCc*.

(b) A mating of an *AaBbCc* (for example) pig with the 6-cm *aabbcc* pig would result in the following offspring:

Gametes (18-cm tail)	Gamete (6 cm-tail)	Offspring
ABC		AaBbCc (18 cm)
ABc		AaBbcc (14 cm)
AbC		AabbCc (14 cm)
Abc	abc	Aabbcc (10 cm)
aBC		aaBbCc (14 cm)
aBc		aaBbcc (10 cm)
abC		aabbCc (10 cm)
abc		aabbcc (6 cm)

In this example, a 1:3:3:1 ratio is the result. However, had a different 18-cm tail pig been selected, a different ratio would occur:

$$AABbcc \times aabbcc$$

Gametes (18-cm tail)	Gamete (6-cm tail)	Offspring
ABc	abc	AaBbcc (14 cm)
Abc		Aabbcc (10 cm)

8. For height, notice that average differences between MZ twins reared together (1.7 cm) and those MZ twins reared apart (1.8 cm) are similar (meaning little environmental influence) and considerably less than differences of DZ twins (4.4 cm) or sibs (4.5 cm) reared together. These data indicate that genetics play a major role in determining height.

However, for weight, notice that MZ twins reared together have a much smaller (1.9 kg) difference than MZ twins reared apart, indicating that the environment has a considerable impact on weight. By comparing the weight differences of MZ twins reared apart with DZ twins and sibs reared together, one can conclude that the environment has almost as much an influence on weight as genetics.

For ridge count, the differences between MZ twins reared together and those reared apart are small. For the data in the table, it would appear that ridge count and height have the highest heritability values.

9. Comparison of phenotypic variances between monozygotic and dizygotic traits provides an estimate of broad-sense heritability (H^2).

10. Many traits, especially those we view as quantitative, are likely to be determined by a polygenic mode with possible environmental influences. The following are some common examples: height, general body structure, skin color, and perhaps most common behavioral traits, including intelligence.

11. At first glance, this problem looks as if it will be an arithmetic headache; however, the problem can be simplified.

(a) The mean is computed by adding the measurements of all of the individuals and then dividing by the number of individuals. In this case, there are 760 corn plants. To keep from having to add 760 numbers, merely multiply each height group by the number of individuals in each group. Add all the products and then divide by n (760). This gives a value for the mean of 140 cm.

(b) For the variance, use the formula given below (as in the text):

$$s^2 = V = n\Sigma f(x^2) - (\Sigma fx)^2 / n(n - 1)$$

To simplify the calculations, determine the square of each height group (100 cm, for example); then multiply the value by the number in each group.

For the first group (100 cm), we would have

$$100 \times 100 \times 20 = 200,000$$

The rest of the groups is as follows:

$$
\begin{aligned}
110 \times 110 \times 60 &= 726,000 \\
120 \times 120 \times 90 &= 1,296,000 \\
130 \times 130 \times 130 &= 2,197,000 \\
140 \times 140 \times 180 &= 3,528,000 \\
150 \times 150 \times 120 &= 2,700,000 \\
160 \times 160 \times 70 &= 1,792,000 \\
170 \times 170 \times 50 &= 1,445,000 \\
180 \times 180 \times 40 &= 1,296,000 \\
&= 15,180,000
\end{aligned}
$$

Now, the mean squared, multiplied by n, is as follows:

$$140 \times 140 \times 760 = 14,896,000$$

Completing the calculations gives the following:

$$(15,180,000 - 14,896,000)/759$$
$$= 284,000/759$$
$$s^2 = V = 374.18$$

(c) The *standard deviation* is the square root of the variance, or 19.34.

(d) The *standard error of the mean* is the standard deviation divided by the square root of *n*, or about 0.70. The plot approximates a normal distribution. Variation is continuous.

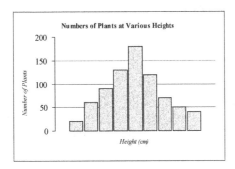

12. (a) Using the following equations, H^2 and h^2 can be calculated as follows:

For back fat:

Broad-sense heritability $= H^2 = 12.2/30.6 = 0.398$
Narrow-sense heritability $= h^2 = 8.44/30.6 = 0.276$

For body length:

Broad-sense heritability $= H^2 = 26.4/52.4 = 0.504$
Narrow-sense heritability $= h^2 = 11.7/52.4 = 0.223$

(b) For a trait that is quantitatively measured, the relative importance of genetic versus environmental factors may be formally assessed by examining the heritability index (H^2 or broad heritability). In animal and plant breeding, a measure of potential response to selection based on additive variance and dominance variance is termed narrow-sense heritability (h^2). A relatively high narrow-sense heritability is a prediction of the impact selection may have in altering an initial randomly breeding population. Therefore, of the two traits, selection for back fat would produce more response.

13. The formula for estimating heritability is

$$H^2 = V_G/V_P$$

where V_G and V_P are the genetic and phenotypic components of variation, respectively. The main issue in this question is obtaining some estimate of two components of phenotypic variation: genetic and environmental. V_P is the combination of genetic and environmental variance. Because the two parental strains are inbred, they are assumed to be homozygous, and the variances of 4.2 and 3.8 are considered to be the result of environmental influences. The average of these two values is 4.0.

The F_1 is also genetically homogeneous and gives us an additional estimation of the environmental factors.

By averaging with the parents $[(4.0 + 5.6)/2 = 4.8]$ we obtain a relatively good idea of environmental impact on the phenotype. The phenotypic variance in the F_2 is the sum of the genetic (V_G) and environmental (V_E) components. We have estimated the environmental input as 4.8, so 10.3 (V_P) minus 4.8 gives us an estimate of (V_G), which is 5.5. Heritability then becomes 5.5/10.3, or 0.53. This value, when viewed in percentage form, indicates that about 53 percent of the variation in plant height is due to genetic influences.

14. (a) For vitamin A:

$$h_A^2 = V_A/V_P = V_A/(V_E + V_A + V_D) = 0.097$$

For cholesterol: $h_A^2 = 0.223$

(b) Cholesterol content should be influenced to a greater extent by selection.

15. Given that both narrow-sense heritability values are relatively high, it is likely that a farmer would be able to alter both milk protein content and butterfat by selection. The value of 0.91 for the correlation coefficient between protein content and butterfat suggests that if one selects for butterfat, protein content will increase. However, correlation coefficients describe the extent to which variation in one quantitative trait is associated with variation in another and does not reveal the underlying causes of such variation. Assuming that these dairy cows had been selected for high butterfat in the past and increased protein content followed that selection (for butterfat), it is likely that selection for butterfat would continue to correlate with increased protein content. However, there may well be a point at which physiological circumstances change and selection for high butterfat may be at the expense of protein content.

16. $h^2 = (7.5 − 8.5/6.0 − 8.5) = 0.4$
(realized heritability)

17. Given the realized heritability value of 0.4, it is unlikely that selection experiments would cause a rapid and/or significant response to selection. A minor response might result from intense selection.

18. $h^2 = 0.3 = (M2 − 60/80 − 60)$
$M2 = 66$ g

Chapter 23 Quantitative Genetics and Multifactorial Traits

19. Since the rice plants are genetically identical, V_G is zero and $H^2 = V_G/V_P =$ zero. Broad-sense heritability is a measure in which the phenotypic variance is due to genetic factors. In this case, with genetically identical plants, H^2 is zero, and the variance observed in grain yield is due to the environment. Selection would not be effective in this strain of rice.

20. (a, b) In many instances, a trait may be clustered in families; yet, traditional mapping procedures may not be applicable because the trait might be influenced by a number of genes. In general, researchers look for associations to particular DNA sequences (molecular markers). When the trait cosegregates with a particular maker and it statistically associates with that trait above chance, a likely QTL has been identified. Markers such as RFLPs, SNPs, and microsatellites are often used because they are highly variable, relatively easy to assess, and present in all individuals.

21. The best way to approach this problem is to first determine the number of gene pairs involved. Notice that all the F_1 plants are uniform and are in the middle of the extremes of 3 and 15 inches; therefore, the parents must each be homozygous and at the extremes. Notice also that there are 13 classes in the F_2, so there must be six gene pairs. See the text for an explanation of the $2n + 1$ formula.

(a) There are two ways to answer this section: a hard way and an easy way. The hard way would be to take a big sheet of paper, make the cross ($AaBbCcDdEeFf \times AaBbCcDdEeFf$), collect the genotypes, and calculate the ratios. This method would be very laborious and error prone.

The easy way would be to re-read the material on the binomial expansion and note the pattern preceding each expression. Notice that all numbers other than the 1s are equal to the sum of the two numbers directly above them. By enlarging the numbers to include six gene pairs, you can arrive at the 13 classes and their frequencies:

3" = 1	4" = 12	5" = 66
6" = 220	7" = 495	8" = 792
9" = 924	10" = 792	11" = 495
12" = 220	13" = 66	14" = 12
15" = 1		

To check your calculations, be certain that your frequencies total 4096. You will also notice an additional shortcut in that since the distribution is symmetrical, you need only calculate to the center, and the remainder will be in the reverse order.

(b) To determine the outcome of a cross of the F_1 plants in the test cross, apply the formula that allows you to calculate any set of components: $n!/(s!t!)$, where $n =$ total number of events (6), $s =$ number of events of outcome a, and $t =$ number of events of outcome b. For example, to determine how many 6-inch plants would be recovered from the cross $AaBbCcDdEeFf \times aabbccddeeff$, we are really asking how many will have three additive alleles (uppercase) and three non-additive alleles (lowercase).

$$6!/(3!3!) = 20$$

Applying this formula throughout gives the following frequencies:

3" = 1	4" = 6	5" = 15
6" = 20	7" = 15	8" = 6
9" = 1		

The total is 64. You can check your logic by considering that there should be only 1/64 with no additive alleles (3") and 1/64 with all additive alleles (9").

22. The solution to these types of problems rests on determining the ratio of individuals expressing the extreme phenotype to the total number of individuals. In this case, 8:2028 is equal to 1:253, which is close to 1:256. If there are three gene pairs, the ratio is 1:64; four gene pairs, 1:256; or five gene pairs, 1:1024. Therefore, these data indicate that four gene pairs influence size in these guinea pigs.

23. As with many traits that are caused by numerous loci acting additively, some genes have more influence on expression than others. In addition, environmental factors may play a role in the expression of some polygenic traits. In the case of brachydactyly, numerous modifier genes in the genome can influence brachydactyly expression. Examination of OMIM (*Online Mendelian Inheritance of Man*) at http://www.ncbi.nlm.nih.gov/ will illustrate this point.

24. (a, b) Because there are nine phenotypic classes in the F_2, there must be four gene pairs involved. The genotypes of the parents could be symbolized as $AABBCCDD \times aabbccdd$, and the F_1 as $AaBbCcDd$.

25. It is likely that the flies maintained in the *Drosophila* repository are more highly inbred and less heterozygous than those recently obtained from the wild. Response to selection is dependent on genetic variation. The greater the genetic variation in a species, the more likely and dramatic is the response to selection. Therefore, one would expect a greater response to selection in the wild population.

26. $6 \times 5 \times 4 \times 3 \times 2 \times 1/(2 \times 1)(4 \times 3 \times 2 \times 1) = 15$ of a total of 64.

27. Breeders attempt to "select out" this disorder by first maintaining complete and detailed breeding records of afflicted strains. Second, they avoid breeding dogs whose close relatives are afflicted. The molecular-developmental mechanism that causes the "month of birth" effect in canine hip dysplasia is unknown. However, with many, perhaps all, quantitative traits, it is clear that there is a significant environmental influence on both the penetrance and/or expression of the phenotype. With many genes acting in various ways to influence a phenotype, there are opportunities for varied molecular and developmental intraorganismic microenvironments. Stated another way, the longer and more complex the molecular distance from the genome to the phenotype, the greater the likelihood for environmental factors to be involved in expression.

28. (a) The average response to selection (in mm) would be the sum of the differences between the control and offspring, divided by 3: $(2.17 + 3.79 + 4.06)/3 = 3.34$ mm. **(b)** One computes realized heritability by the following formula:

$$h^2 = \frac{M2 - M}{M1 - M}$$

where M represents the mean size (control), $M1$ represents the selected parents, and $M2$ represents the size in offspring.

For 1997:

$$h^2 = (32.21 - 30.04)/(34.13 - 30.04) = 0.53$$

For 1998:

$$h^2 = (31.90 - 28.11)/(31.98 - 28.11) = 0.98$$

For 1999:

$$h^2 = (33.74 - 29.68)/(31.81 - 29.68) = 1.91$$

The overall realized heritability would be the average of all three heritability values, or 1.14.

(b) A key factor in determining response to selection is the genetic variability available to respond to selection. The greater the genetic variability, the greater the response. Another key factor in rapid response to selection often relates to the number of loci involved. If there are few loci, each with large phenotypic effects controlling a trait, response to selection is usually high. Finally, if flower size is not genetically correlated with other floral traits, size alone may not be subject to strong stabilizing selection, which would reduce genetic variation. Therefore, whereas other floral traits may show low response to selection, size alone may be more responsive.

(c) With high heritability, one expects a high genetic contribution to phenotypic variation. Genetic variability that provides rapid adjustments to changing environments is an evolutionary advantage. Therefore, in general, one would expect that high heritability would contribute to high evolutionary potential.

29. (a) The most direct explanation would involve two gene pairs, with each additive gene contributing about 1.2 mm to the phenotype. **(b)** The fit to this backcross supports the original hypothesis. **(c)** These data do not support the simple hypothesis provided in part (a). **(d, e)** With these data, one can see no distinct phenotypic classes, suggesting that the environment may play a role in eye development or that there are more genes involved.

Chapter 24: Neurogenetics

Concept Areas	Corresponding Problems
Methodology of Behavior Genetics	1, 2, 4, 8, 12, 13, 14, 16
Genetic Analysis: Drosophila	1, 10
Genetic Analysis: Humans	1, 3, 4, 7, 11, 12, 13, 14, 15, 16, 17
Genetic Analysis: Caenorhabditis	5, 6, 9, 10

Concepts and Processes Checklist

(Check topic when mastered – provide examples where appropriate – understand the context of each entry)

- **The Central Nervous System...**

  - CNS

  - axon

  - nerve impulse

  - synapses transfer information

  - synaptic cleft

  - neurotransmitter

- **Identification of Genes...**

  - mutant alleles

  - nerve transmission

  - sodium/potassium channels

  - channelopathies

- **Synapses Are Involved...**

  - Huntington disease

  - Alzheimer disease

  - Parkinson disease

  - *MAOA*

  - fragile-X syndrome

- FMRP

- mGluR5 receptor

- **Animal Models Play...**

  - Huntington disease

  - *HD*

  - huntingtin

  - CAG repeats

  - transgenic mouse model

  - mHTT

  - treatment strategies

  - RNAi

  - *Drosophila* animal model

  - learning

  - cAMP

  - short-term memory

  - long-term memory

- **Behavioral Disorders...**

  - schizophrenia

  - twin studies

Chapter 24 Neurogenetics

- RFLP
- SNP
- haplotypes
- GWAS
- CNVs
- autism spectrum disorders

- ADHD
- PGG
- pleiotropy
- epigenetics
- addiction
- alcoholism

Answers to Now Solve This

24-1. One of the easiest ways to determine whether a genetic basis exists for a given abnormality is to cross the abnormal fly to a normal fly. If the trait is determined by a dominant gene, then that trait should appear in the offspring, probably half of them if the gene was in the heterozygous state. If the gene is recessive and homozygous, then one may not see expression in the offspring of the first cross; however, if one crosses the F_1, the trait might appear in approximately 1/4 of the offspring. Such ratios would not be expected if the trait is polygenic, which generates complexities in any study. Modifications of these patterns would be expected if the mode of inheritance is X-linked or shows other modifications of typical Mendelian ratios. One might hypothesize that the trait influences the nervous, cuticular, or muscular system.

24-2. The presence of normal might to some extent soften or dilute the influence of mutant *HD* human genes.

Chapter 24 Neurogenetics

Solutions to Problems and Discussion Questions

1. (a) In general, familial transmission of a trait is indicative of a genetic basis, assuming that the environment is not a strong component. For some species, selection for and against the trait can reveal its genetic basis.

(b) Various stimuli/response experiments indicate that *Drosophila* can learn and remember.

(c) RFLP analysis was used to determine the *HD* gene location on chromosome 4. Trinucleotide repeats appear to be involved in the expression of HD, and various transgenic animal models have indicated the neurodegenerative nature of the disease.

(d) Both twin studies and genomic analyses have helped us understand the nature of schizophrenia. Microarray analysis among schizophrenics identified a cluster of genes involved in myelination that had lower or higher expression levels when compared to nonschizophrenic controls.

2. Your essay should include an overall discussion of the anatomy and chemistry of synapses and neurotransmitters, as well as examples of affected diseases: Alzheimer disease, Angelman syndrome, autism, etc.

3. From the information provided, one can conclude that the tasting trait is determined by a dominant gene. Notice that a 3:1 ratio of tasters to nontasters is obtained in the third cross. This result strongly argues for the *TT* or *Tt* condition providing taste of PTC. Information from other crosses does not contradict the dominant nature of PTC tasting.

4. Concordance for traits such as addictive behavior in monozygotic and dizygotic twins has been applied to many types of behaviors. Monozygotic twins are genetically identical, whereas dizygotic twins are genetically like siblings. Since members of each set of twins are likely to be reared under similar environmental conditions, it is possible to get some estimate of the genetic contribution to a given behavior. A higher rate of concordance for monozygotic twins compared with dizygotic twins often indicates a genetic component to a trait. Although such studies suggest that a genetic component exists, they do not reveal the precise genetic basis of pathological gambling.

5. Because of the rigidity of development in *Caenorhabditis* and the extensive knowledge of cellular fates and connectivity, it represents an excellent experimental organism for the study of development. In addition, because of their fixed fate, cells can be altered, physically and/or genetically, and resulting development and behavior can be studied. However, the behavioral repertoire of *C. elegans* is somewhat narrow. In addition, *C. elegans* has more protein-coding genes than *Drosophila*, another organism whose behavioral genetics has been highly studied. Such an additional number of protein-coding genes coupled with a sparse behavioral repertoire creates a disadvantage when using *C. elegans*.

6. The simplest model would place each component in a linear pathway as shown here:

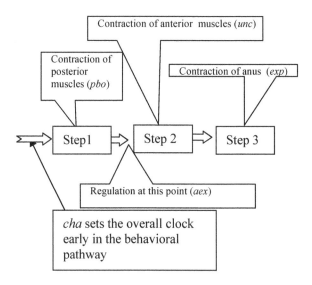

7. A number of issues limit the study of human behavior, including the following:

1. With relatively small numbers of offspring per mating, standard genetic methods are difficult.
2. Records on family illnesses, especially behavioral illnesses, are difficult to obtain.
3. The long generation time makes longitudinal studies difficult.
4. The scientist cannot direct matings.
5. There are limits to the experimental treatments that can be applied.
6. Traits that are interesting to study are often complex and difficult to quantify.

7. Culture and family background may strongly influence behavior.

8. Usually, if traits that are considered to be homozygous (the pure breeds of dogs) fail to breed true, it is likely that the trait is determined by conditioning or complex genetic factors that have minor influences. Such breeds of dogs, although being highly selected, are not homozygous for all genes. Even though the dogs are considered to be pure breeds, it is likely that alleles are segregating and combining in various ways to produce the variations noted. There may also be different interactions with environmental stimuli from subtle genetic variations.

9. Recessive mutations are typically only observed at the phenotypic level when homozygous. Self-fertilization, the ultimate form of inbreeding, greatly enhances the likelihood that recessive genes will become homozygous. Homozygous strains are of considerable advantage when studying complex traits.

10. One might compare gene expression through microarray analysis between space-reared flies with a control population on earth. By comparing behavioral (metabolic, mating, feeding, walking, flying) rituals between the two populations (space and earth), one might be able to correlate genetic expression profiles and determine which genes are most likely to respond to which behavioral alteration. Although there may be a number of parameters that would be interesting to study in this way, one might concentrate the study on genes known to influence muscle and nerve function in flies and humans. A second study might focus on the immune system because it is known that there are surprisingly high genetic correlations between the immune response of flies and mammals (Hoffmann, 2003). Since it is known that microgravity negatively influences the human immune system (reduces mitogenic activity of T cells), a comparison of the gene expression profiles of the immune-response system would also be worthy of study. The behavioral side of the experiment would focus on determining whether changes in gravitational stress alter behavior (inactivity, muscle and nerve use) to a point where the immune response is altered. Coupling the two studies, gene expression profiles associated with behavioral and immune responses might provide insight into a number of significant problems that humans encounter in space flight and thereby be justifiable and relatively inexpensive.

11. (a, b) Schizophrenia is a complex familial brain disorder, with relatives of schizophrenics having a higher incidence than the general population. The closer the relationship to the schizophrenic, the greater is the probability of the disorder occurring. Concordance for schizophrenia is higher in monozygotic twins (~ 50%) than dizygotic twins (~ 17%) and suggests that a genetic component exists along with shared environmental risk factors. Microarrays have been used to identify genes whose expression is altered in schizophrenia. Researchers have isolated RNA from the brains of normal and schizophrenic individuals and used the RNA to prepare cDNA for hybridization to the microarrays. The microarrays carried more than 6000 probes for the human genome. Some of the identified genes have low levels of expression in schizophrenia, whereas others express at high levels. One cluster of genes involved in myelination has lower levels of expression in schizophrenics, whereas some other clusters have increased levels of expression, suggesting that schizophrenia is associated with functional disruption in oligodendrocytes. A variety of genome-wide microarray scans of gene expression in schizophrenia have identified candidate genes whose expression is altered in schizophrenics. Knockout mice missing a myelin-related gene are being studied in order to relate changes in gene expression with specific behavioral phenotypes. From such studies, it is hoped that therapies can be targeted at specific genes involved in schizophrenia. However, gene expression patterns during early development may eventually cause behavioral problems and not be detectable in adult samples regardless of their sophistication.

12. Genome-wide association studies (GWAS) make use of millions of SNPs in an attempt to find associations to a given trait such as schizophrenia. Such studies indicate that no single gene or allele is a defining contributor to this disorder.

13. Some rare mutations and chromosomal aberrations are associated with about 5–15 percent of all cases of autism spectrum disorders (ASD). Genome-wide association studies and copy number variants (CNVs) indicate ASD susceptibility genes, some of which are also risk factors for schizophrenia.

14 . Data in the table indicate that females (*Gasterosteus aculeatus*) spend more time with males having the optimal MHC constitution than with those that do not. As with other organisms, it appears that genetic diversity for the MHC is a selective advantage. Since immunological functions are associated with the MHC complex, mate selection mechanisms that support the maintenance of such diversity seem reasonable from an evolutionary viewpoint.

15. Various genes are known to be involved in mental diseases. In some cases, DNA methylation is correlated with the severity of mental disease. Similar results occur with changes in trinucleotide repeats. Some twin studies show that differences in DNA methylation correlate with mental disease states.

16. DNA hypermethylation generally leads to a downregulation of a given section of DNA. In the case of the *FMR1* gene, such hypermethylation is associated with the expression of the fragile-X syndrome.

17. Most diseases in humans that are known to be caused by CAG repeats behave as gain-of-function because it is the presence of the abnormal protein that causes the disease. Because there are only a few known mechanisms by which repeats are formed and established, it is likely that one of these mechanisms is involved. However, several mechanisms may also be involved.

Chapter 25: Population and Evolutionary Genetics

Concept Areas	Corresponding Problems
Variation	1, 20, 28, 29
Sequence Analysis	1, 3, 5, 22, 31
Hardy–Weinberg Computations	6, 7, 9, 10, 11, 12, 13, 14, 15, 22, 23, 24
Hardy–Weinberg Assumptions	1, 8, 16, 19
Speciation	1, 4, 17, 21, 22, 23, 25, 27
Mutation	2, 7, 17, 18, 19, 30
Gene Therapy	26

Concepts and Processes Checklist

(Check topic when mastered – provide examples where appropriate – understand the context of each entry)

- **Population Genetics**
  - evolutionary aspects
  - speciation
  - microevolution
  - macroevolution
- **Genetic Variation is Present…**
  - population
  - gene pool
  - detecting genetic variation
  - artificial selection
  - nucleotide sequences
  - cystic fibrosis
  - CFTR
  - neutral theory
  - fitness differences
- **Hardy-Weinberg Law**
  - ideal population
  - infinitely large
  - random mating

- no mutation
- no migration
- no selection
- genetic frequencies
- genotypic frequencies
- H-W equation
- genetic variability
- **H-W in Human Populations**
  - examples
  - testing the H-W equilibrium
  - multiple alleles
  - ABO blood groups
  - X-linked traits
- **Natural Selection**
  - genetic variation
  - variations heritable
  - exponential reproduction
  - struggle for survival

Chapter 25 Population and Evolutionary Genetics

- natural selection
- detecting natural selection
- fitness and selection
- types of selection
- directional selection
- stabilizing selection
- disruptive selection
- **Mutation Creates New Alleles...**
    - mutation rates
    - achondroplasia
- **Migration and Gene Flow...**
    - calculations
- **Genetic Drift...**
    - founder effect
    - genetic bottleneck
    - examples
- **Nonrandom Mating...**
    - positive assortive mating
    - negative assortive mating
    - inbreeding
    - coefficient of inbreeding
    - *F*

- **Reduced Gene Flow...**
    - species
    - genetic divergence
    - reproductive isolating mechanisms
    - prezygotic isolating mechanisms
    - postzygotic isolating mechanisms
    - speciation
    - rate of macroevolution
- **Phylogeny...**
    - node
    - phylogenetic trees
    - amino acid sequences
    - cytochrome c
    - genetic equidistance
    - minimal mutational distance
    - molecular clocks
    - genomics
    - molecular evolution
    - genetic divergence
    - Neanderthals and humans
    - our mosaic genome

F25-1 Simple illustration of the relationships among populations, individuals, alleles, and allelic frequencies (*p* and *q*)

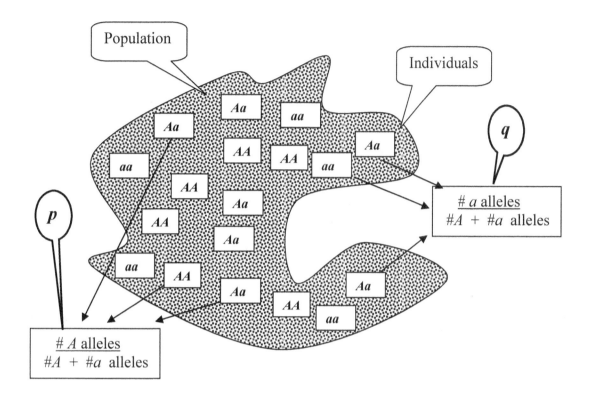

F25-2 Diagram of the relationships among inbreeding, heterosis, and homozygosity. Note that as inbreeding occurs, heterosis decreases and homozygosity increases.

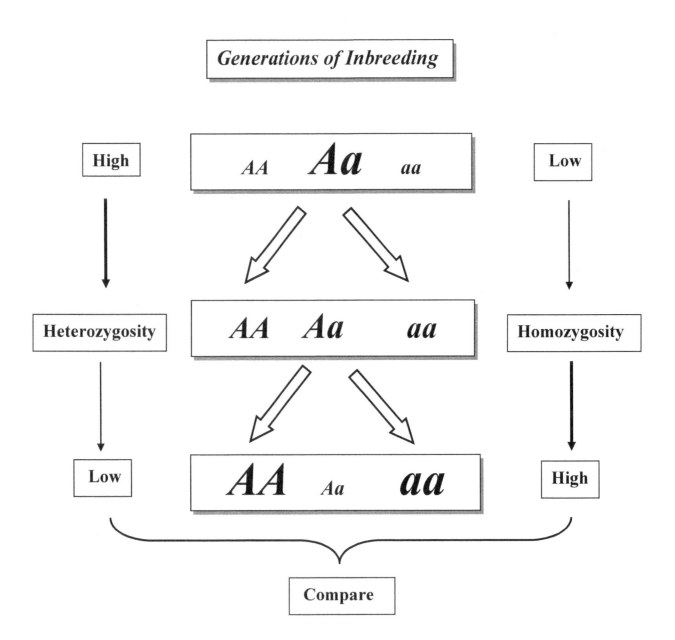

Chapter 25 Population and Evolutionary Genetics

Answers to Now Solve This

25-1. Understanding the Hardy-Weinberg equilibrium allows us to state that if a population is in equilibrium, the genotypic frequencies will not shift from one generation to the next unless there are factors such as selection or migration that alter gene frequencies. Because none of these factors is stated in the problem, we need only to determine whether the initial population is in equilibrium. Calculate p and q, then apply the equation $p^2 + 2pq + q^2$ to determine genotypic frequencies in the next generation.

p = frequency of A
$= 0.2 + 0.3$
$= 0.5$
$q = 1 - p = 0.5$

Frequency of $AA = p^2$
$= (0.5)^2$
$= 0.25$, or 25%

Frequency of $Aa = 2pq$
$= 2(0.5)(0.5)$
$= 0.5$, or 50%

Frequency of $aa = q^2$
$= (0.5)^2$
$= 0.25$, or 25%

The initial population was not in equilibrium; however, after one generation of mating under the Hardy-Weinberg conditions, the population is in equilibrium and will continue to be so (and not change) until one or more of the Hardy-Weinberg conditions are not met. Note that *equilibrium* does not necessarily mean p and q equal 0.5.

25-2. (a) Children: frequency of M allele: $p = 0.25 + 0.25 = 0.5$; frequency of N allele: $q = 0.25 + 0.25 = 0.5$. Adults: frequency of M allele: $p = 0.3 + 0.2 = 0.5$; frequency of N allele: $q = 0.3 + 0.2 = 0.5$. **(b, c)** The allelic frequencies are the same; however, the genotypic frequencies appear to not be in equilibrium for the adult population.

25-3. Given that the recessive allele a is present in the homozygous state (q^2) at a frequency of 0.0001, the value of q is 0.01 and $p = 0.99$.

(a) q is 0.01.

(b) $p = 1 - q$ or 0.99

(c) $2pq = 2(0.01)(0.99) = 0.0198$ (or about 1/50)

(d) $2pq \times 2pq = 0.0198 \times 0.0198 = 0.000392$ (or about 1/255)

25-4. The probability that the woman (with no family history of CF) is heterozygous is $2pq$ or $2(1/50)(49/50)$. The probability that the man is heterozygous is 2/3. The probability that a child with CF will be produced by two heterozygotes is 1/4. Therefore, the overall probability of the couple producing a CF child is $98/2500 \times 2/3 \times 1/4 = 0.00653$, or about 1/153.

Chapter 25 Population and Evolutionary Genetics
Solutions to Problems and Discussion Questions

1. (a) Genetic variation can be assessed in a variety of ways including responses to artificial selection and sequencing of nucleic acids and proteins.

(b) Different alleles will show typical segregation patterns and have similarities in nucleotide and amino acid sequences.

(c) By conducting assays of gene and/or genotypic frequencies over time and space, one can determine whether the genetic structure of a population is changing.

(d) If gene flow between populations becomes sufficiently reduced, divergence may have reached a point where the populations are reproductively isolated. Under this condition, they are usually considered different species.

(e) Various molecular clocks can be used to estimate the time of divergence of two groups of organisms. Such clocks are based on amino acid and/or nucleotide differences and are often validated by comparison with the fossil record.

2. Your essay should include a discussion of the original sources of variation coming from mutation and that migration can cause gene frequencies to change in a population if the immigrants have different gene frequencies compared to the host population. You should also describe selection as resulting from the biased passage of gametes and offspring to the next generation.

3. (a) Missense mutations cause amino acid changes.

(b) Horizontal transfer refers to the process of passing genetic information from one organism to another without producing offspring. In bacteria, plasmid transfer is an example of horizontal transfer.

(c) The fact that none of the isolates shared identical nucleotide changes indicates that there is little genetic exchange among different strains. Each alteration is unique, most likely originating in an ancestral strain and maintained in descendents of that strain only.

4. The classification of organisms into different species is based on evidence (morphological, genetic, ecological, etc.) that they are reproductively isolated.

That is, there must be evidence that gene flow does not occur among the groups being called different species. Classifications above the species level (genus, family, etc.) are not based on such empirical data. Indeed, classification above the species level is somewhat arbitrary and based on traditions that extend far beyond DNA sequence information. In addition, recall that DNA sequence divergence is not always directly proportional to morphological, behavioral, or ecological divergence. While the genus classifications provided in this problem seem to be invalid, other factors, well beyond simple DNA sequence comparison, must be considered in classification practices. As more information is gained on the meaning of DNA sequence differences in comparison to morphological factors, many phylogenetic relationships will be reconsidered, and it is possible that adjustments will be needed in some classification schemes.

5. There are many sections of DNA in a eukaryotic genome that are not reflected in a protein product. Indeed, there are many sections of DNA that are not even transcribed and/or have no apparent physiological role. Such regions are more likely to tolerate nucleotide changes compared with those regions with a necessary physiological impact. Introns, for example, show sequence variation, which is not reflected in a protein product. Exons, on the other hand, code for products that are usually involved in production of a phenotype and, as such, are subject to selection.

6. Because the alleles follow a dominant/recessive mode, one can use the equation $\sqrt{q^2}$ to calculate q, from which all other aspects of the answer depend. The frequency of *aa* types is determined by dividing the number of nontasters (37) by the total number of individuals (125).

$$q^2 = 37/125 = 0.296$$
$$q = 0.544$$
$$p = 1 - q$$
$$p = 0.456$$

The frequencies of the genotypes are determined by applying the formula $p^2 + 2pq + q^2$ as follows:

$$\text{Frequency of } AA = p^2$$
$$= (0.456)^2$$
$$= 0.208, \text{ or } 20.8\%$$

Frequency of $Aa = 2pq$
$$= 2(0.456)(0.544)$$
$$= 0.496, \text{ or } 49.6\%$$

Frequency of $aa = q^2$
$$= (0.544)^2$$
$$= 0.296, \text{ or } 29.6\%$$

When completing such a set of calculations, it is a good practice to add the final percentages to be certain that they total 100 percent. (Note that the calculation requires the assumption that this population is in Hardy-Weinberg equilibrium with respect to the gene for PTC tasting.)

7. For each of these values, one merely takes the square root to determine q, then computes p, then "plugs" the values into the $2pq$ expression.

(a) $q = 0.08$; $2pq = 2(0.92)(0.08)$
$$= 0.1472, \text{ or } 14.72\%$$

(b) $q = 0.009$; $2pq = 2(0.991)(0.009)$
$$= 0.01784, \text{ or } 1.78\%$$

(c) $q = 0.3$; $2pq = 2(0.7)(0.3)$
$$= 0.42, \text{ or } 42\%$$

(d) $q = 0.1$; $2pq = 2(0.9)(0.1)$
$$= 0.18, \text{ or } 18\%$$

(e) $q = 0.316$; $2pq = 2(0.684)(0.316)$
$$= 0.4323, \text{ or } 43.23\%$$

(Depending how one rounds off the decimals, slightly different answers will occur.)

8. In order for the Hardy-Weinberg equations to apply, the population must be in Hardy-Weinberg equilibrium.

9. Assuming that the population is in Hardy-Weinberg equilibrium, if one has the frequency of individuals with the dominant phenotype, the remainder have the recessive phenotype (q^2). With q^2, one can calculate q, and from this value one can arrive at p. Applying the expression $p^2 + 2pq + q^2$ will allow a solution to the question.

10. (a) For the CCR5 analysis, first determine p and q. Since one has the frequencies of all the genotypes, one can add 0.6 and 0.351/2 to provide p ($= 0.7755$); q will be 0.049 and 0.351/2 = 0.2245. The equilibrium values will be as follows:

Frequency of $1/1 = p^2 = (0.7755)^2 = 0.6014$, or 60.14%
Frequency of $1/\Delta 32 = 2pq = 2(0.7755)(0.2245) = 0.3482$, or 34.82%
Frequency of $\Delta 32/\Delta 32 = q^2 = (0.2245)^2 = 0.0504$, or 5.04%

Comparing these equilibrium values with the observed values strongly suggests that the observed values are drawn from a population in Hardy-Weinberg equilibrium.

(b) For the AS (sickle-cell) analysis, first determine p and q. Since one has the frequencies of all the genotypes, one can add 0.756 and 0.242/2 to provide p ($= 0.877$); q will be $1 - 0.877$, or 0.123.

The equilibrium values will be as follows:

Frequency of $AA = p^2 = (0.877)^2 = 0.7691$, or 76.91%
Frequency of $AS = 2pq = 2(0.877)(0.123) = 0.2157$, or 21.57%
Frequency of $SS = q^2 = (0.123)^2 = 0.0151$, or 1.51%

Comparing these equilibrium values with the observed values suggests that the observed values may be drawn from a population that is not in equilibrium. Notice that there are more heterozygotes than predicted, and fewer SS types in the population. Since data are given in percentages, χ^2 values can not be computed.

11. Given that $q^2 = 0.04$, then $q = 0.2$, $2pq = 0.32$, and $p^2 = 0.64$. Of those not expressing the trait, only a mating between heterozygotes can produce an offspring that expresses the trait, and then only at a frequency of 1/4. The different types of matings possible (those without the trait) in the population, with their frequencies, follow:

$AA \times AA = 0.64 \times 0.64 = 0.4096$
$AA \times Aa = 0.64 \times 0.32 = 0.2048$
$Aa \times AA = 0.64 \times 0.32 = 0.2048$
$Aa \times Aa = 0.32 \times 0.32 = 0.1024$
$Aa \times Aa = 0.32 \times 0.32 = 0.1024$

Notice that of the matings of the individuals who do not express the trait, only the last two (about 20 percent) are capable of producing offspring with the trait. Therefore, one would arrive at a final likelihood of $1/4 \times 20$ percent, or 5 percent of the offspring with the trait.

12. The following formula calculates the frequency of an allele in the next generation for any selection scenario, given the frequencies of a and A in this generation and the fitness of all three genotypes:

$$q_{g+1} = [w_{Aa}p_g q_g + w_{aa}q_g^2]/[w_{AA}p_g^2 + w_{Aa}2p_g q_g + w_{aa}q_g^2]$$

where q_{g+1} is the frequency of the a allele in the next generation, q_g is the frequency of the a allele in this generation, p_g is the frequency of the A allele in this generation, and each "w" represents the fitness of its respective genotype.

(a) $q_{g+1} = [0.9(0.7)(0.3) + 0.8(0.3)^2]/[1(0.7)^2$
$+ 0.9(2)(0.7)(0.3) + 0.8(0.3)^2]$

$q_{g+1} = 0.278$ $p_{g+1} = 0.722$

(b) $q_{g+1} = 0.289$ $p_{g+1} = 0.711$

(c) $q_{g+1} = 0.298$ $p_{g+1} = 0.702$

(d) $q_{g+1} = 0.319$ $p_{g+1} = 0.681$

13. The general equation for responding to this question is

$$q_n = q_0/(1 + nq_0)$$

where $n =$ the number of generations, $q_0 =$ the initial gene frequency, and $q_n =$ the new gene frequency.

(a) $n = 1$

$q_n = q_0/(1 + nq_0)$
$q_n = 0.5/[1 + (1 \times 0.5)]$
$q_n = 0.33$ $p_n = 0.67$

(b) $n = 5$

$q_n = q_0/(1 + nq_0)$
$q_n = 0.5/[1 + (5 \times 0.5)]$
$q_n = 0.143$ $p_n = 0.857$

(c) $n = 10$

$q_n = q_0/(1 + nq_0)$
$q_n = 0.5/[1 + (10 \times 0.5)]$
$q_n = 0.083$ $p_n = 0.917$

(d) $n = 25$

$q_n = q_0/(1 + nq_0)$
$q_n = 0.5/[1 + (25 \times 0.5)]$
$q_n = 0.037$ $p_n = 0.963$

(e) $n = 100$

$q_n = q_0/(1 + nq_0)$
$q_n = 0.5/[1 + (100 \times 0.5)]$
$q_n = 0.0098$ $p_n = 0.9902$

(f) $n = 1000$

$q_n = q_0/(1 + nq_0)$
$q_n = 0.5/[1 + (1000 \times 0.5)]$
$q_n = 0.00099$ $p_n = 0.99901$

14. Since a dominant lethal gene is highly selected against, it is unlikely that it will exist at too high a frequency, if at all. However, if the gene shows incomplete penetrance or late age of onset (after reproductive age) it may remain in a population.

15. What one must do is predict the probability of one of the grandparents being heterozygous in this problem. Given the frequency of the disorder in the population as 1 in 10,000 individuals (0.0001), then $q^2 = 0.0001$, and $q = 0.01$. The frequency of heterozygosity is $2pq$, or approximately 0.02, as also stated in the problem. The probability for one of the grandparents to be heterozygous would therefore be $0.02 + 0.02$ or 0.04, or 1/25. (Note: If one considers the probability of both parents being carriers, 0.02×0.02, the answer differs slightly.) If one of the grandparents is a carrier, then the probability of the offspring from a first-cousin mating being homozygous for the recessive gene is 1/16. Multiplying the two probabilities together gives $1/16 \times 1/25 = 1/400$.

Following the same analysis for the second-cousin mating gives $1/64 \times 1/25 = 1/1600$. Notice that the population at large has a frequency of homozygotes of 1/10,000; therefore, one can easily see how inbreeding increases the likelihood of homozygosity.

16. The frequency of an allele is determined by a number of factors, including the fitness it confers, mutation rate, and input from migration. There is no tendency for a gene to reach any artificial frequency such as 0.5. In fact, you have seen that rare alleles tend to remain rare even when they are dominant—unless there is very strong selection for the allele. The distribution of a gene among individuals is determined by mating (population size, inbreeding, etc.) and environmental factors (selection, etc.). A population is in Hardy-Weinberg equilibrium when the distribution of genotypes occurs at or around the $p^2 + 2pq + q^2 = 1$ expression. Equilibrium does not mean 25 percent AA, 50 percent Aa, and 25 percent aa. This confusion often stems from the 1:2:1 (or 3:1) ratio seen in Mendelian crosses.

17. During speciation, individuals or groups of potentially interbreeding organisms become genetically distinct from other members of the species. Members of different populations with substantial genetic divergence are, at first, not reproductively isolated from each other, although gene flow may be restricted. The distinction between such groups is not absolute in that one group may blend with other groups of the species. Any process that favors changes in allele frequencies has the potential of generating substantial genetic differences among different populations.

Factors such as selection, migration, genetic drift, or even mutation may be important in generating significant genetic change. One would certainly include geographic isolation as a major barrier to gene flow and thus an important process in such formation.

Natural selection occurs when there is nonrandom elimination of individuals from a population. Since such selection is a strong force in changing allele frequencies, it should also be considered as a significant factor in subspecies formation.

18. Because three of the affected infants had affected parents, only two "new" alleles, from mutation, enter into the problem. The allele is dominant; therefore, each new case of achondroplasia arose from a single new mutation. There are 50,000 births; therefore, 100,000 gametes (genes) are involved. The frequency of mutation is therefore given as follows: 2/100,000, or 2×10^{-5}.

19. The approximate similarity of mutation rates among genes and lineages should provide more credible estimates of divergence times of species and allow for broader interpretations of sequence comparisons. It also provides for increased understanding of the mutational processes that govern evolution among mammalian genomes. For instance, if the rate of mutation is fairly constant among lineages or cells that have a more rapid turnover, it indicates that replication-related errors do not make a significant contribution to mutation rates.

20. The presence of selectively neutral alleles and genetic adaptations to varied environments contribute significantly to genetic variation in natural populations.

21. Since $r1 = 0.81$ and $r2 = 0.19$, the expected frequency of heterozygotes would be $2pq \times 125$ or $2(0.81 \times 0.19) \times 125 = 38.475$. Given the following equation and substituting the values:

$$F = (H_e - H_o)/H_e$$
$$F = (38.475 - 20)/38.475 = 0.48$$

22. Given that only 10 percent of the sensitive (*bb*) corn borer larvae feeding on Bt corn plants survive, the selection coefficient against them would be 0.9. The *B* allele for resistance exists at an initial frequency of 0.02 (represented as *p*); therefore, $q = 0.98$. The frequency of the *b* allele after one generation of corn borers fed on Bt corn would be computed as follows:

$$q' = q(1 - sq)/1 - sq^2$$
$$q' = 0.98[1 - (0.9)(0.98)]/1 - [(0.9)(0.98)(0.98)]$$
$$q' = 0.852 \text{ and } p' = 0.148$$

23. The following distribution of genotypes occurs among the 50 desert bighorn sheep in which the normal dominant *C* allele produces straight coats.

$CC = 29 =$ straight coats
$Cc = 17 =$ straight coats
$cc = 4 =$ curled coats

Computing, $p = 0.75$, $q = 0.25$, and $2pq = 0.375$ for the expected frequency of heterozygotes. Since 17/50 or 0.34 are observed as heterozygotes, the following equation applies:

$$F = (H_e - H_o)/H_e$$
$$F = (0.375 - 0.34)/0.375 = 0.093$$

This problem could also be solved using the actual numbers of sheep in each category, where there would be 18.75 heterozygotes expected $(2pq)(50)$:

$$F = (18.75 - 17)/18.75 = 0.093.$$

24. The equation for determining the impact of immigration on the gene pool of an existing population is estimated by the following equation:

$$p_i' = (1 - m)p_i + mp_m$$

Substituting in the appropriate values produces the following expression. Note that the value of 0.2 comes from the fact that 10 sheep out of 50 or 20 percent are being introduced and there are no *cc* alleles in the introduced population, so $p_m = 1.0$.

$$p_i' = (1 - 0.2)(0.75) + (0.2)(1.0)$$
$$p_i' = 0.8$$

25. In general, speciation involves the gradual accumulation of genetic changes to a point where reproductive isolation occurs. Depending on environmental or geographic conditions, genetic changes may occur slowly or rapidly. They can involve point mutations or chromosomal changes.

26. Somatic gene therapy, like any therapy, allows some individuals to live more normal lives than those not receiving therapy. As such, the ability of such individuals to contribute to the gene pool increases the likelihood that less fit alleles will enter and be maintained in the gene pool. This is a normal consequence of therapy, genetic or not, and in the face of disease control and prevention, societies have generally accepted this consequence. Germ-line therapy could, if successful, lead to limited, isolated, and infrequent removal of an allele from a gene lineage. However, given the present state of the science, its impact on the course of human evolution will be diluted and negated by a host of other factors that afflict humankind.

27. (a) The gene is most likely recessive because all affected individuals have unaffected parents and the condition clearly runs in families. For the population, since $q^2 = 0.002$, $q = 0.045$, $p = 0.955$, and $2(pq) = 0.086$. For the community, since $q^2 = 0.005$, $q = 0.07$, $p = 0.93$, and $2(pq) = 0.13$.

(b) The "founder effect" is probably operating here. Relatively small, local populations that are relatively isolated in a reproductive sense tend to show differences in gene frequencies when compared with larger populations. In such small populations, homozygosity is increased as a gene has a higher probability of "meeting itself."

28. Reproductive isolating mechanisms are grouped into prezygotic and postzygotic and include the following:

- geographic or ecological
- seasonal or temporal
- behavioral
- mechanical
- physiological
- hybrid inviability or weakness
- developmental hybrid sterility
- segregational hybrid sterility
- F_2 breakdown

29. Reproductive isolating mechanisms are grouped into prezygotic and postzygotic. Prezygotic mechanisms are more efficient because they occur before resources are expended in the processes of mating.

30. In small populations, large fluctuations in gene frequency occur because random gametic sampling may not include all the genetic variation in the parents. The same phenomenon occurs in molecular populations. Two factors can cause the extinction of a particular mutation in small populations. First, sampling error may allow fixation of one form and the elimination of others. If an advantageous mutation occurs, it must be included in the next replicative round in order to be maintained in subsequent generations. If the founding population is small, it is possible that the advantageous mutation might not be represented. Second, although the previous statements also hold for deleterious mutations, if a deleterious mutation becomes fixed, it can lead to extinction of that population.

31. When a population bottleneck occurs and the number of effective breeders is reduced in a population, two phenomena usually follow. First, because the population is small, wide fluctuations in genotypic frequencies occur, thereby revealing deleterious alleles by chance. Second, inbreeding often occurs in small populations, thereby increasing the chance for homozygosity. With increased homozygosity comes an increased likelihood that recessive alleles will be expressed. Since many disease-producing genes are recessive, an increase in genetic diseases is a likely aftermath to a population bottleneck.

32. All of the amino acid substitutions (ala–gly, val–leu, asp–asn, met–leu) require only one nucleotide change. The last change, pro (CC-)–lys (AAA, G), requires two changes (the minimal mutational distance).

33. In general, there are two methods for calibrating molecular data, amino acid and nucleotide substitutions, to absolute times of divergence. First, molecular data are compared with the existing fossil record. Second, major paleontological events such as the Bryophyta/Tracheophyta split during the Ordovician (443–490 Mya) or the Actinopterygii/ Mammalia split during the Devonian (354–417 Mya) can provide some clues for calibration. Both methods are subject to error due to uncertainty of the fossil record and uncertainty of the times of major paleontological events. In addition, different mutation rates, generation times, and population structures occur among different taxa.

34. (a, b) The pattern of genetic distances through time indicates that from the present to about 25,000 years ago, modern humans and Cro-Magnons show an approximately constant number of differences. Conversely, there is an abrupt increase in genetic distance seen in comparing modern humans and Cro-Magnons with Neanderthals. The results indicate a clear discontinuity between modern humans, Cro-Magnons, and Neanderthals with respect to genetic variation in the mitochondrial DNAs sampled.

Review and Discussion Questions (Special Topics #1)

Review Question Answers

1. The major epigenetic alterations of the genome include the following: DNA methylation, histone modification involving acetyl, methyl, and phosphate groups, chromatin remodeling, microRNAs, and long noncoding RNAs. It is likely that additional epigenetic mechanisms await discovery.

2. In general, periodic methylation occurs at CpG-rich regions and promoter sequences. When a gene is imprinted by methylation, it remains transcriptionally silent. In a mammalian embryo, imprinting may silence only the paternal set of chromosomes, for example.

3. Several groups of proteins are involved in histone modification. Some proteins add chemical groups to histones, others interpret modifications, and some proteins remove the added chemical groups to histones. Such modifications influence the structure of chromatin by altering the accessibility of nucleosomes. These chromatin alterations "open" or "close" genes for transcription.

4. Reversible histone modifications influence the structure of chromatin by altering the accessibility of nucleosomes to the transcriptional machinery. These chromatin alterations "open" or "close" genes for transcription.

5. The histone code refers to specific combinations of histone modifications that influence transcription at a particular chromatin region. The sum of many patterns and interactions of histones (histone code) with chromatin brings about changes in gene expression.

6. Imprinting usually involves certain genes, restricted in number, that are altered by passage through meiosis. A maternally derived imprint or a paternally derived imprint may occur. Imprinted alleles are transcriptionally silent in all cells of the organism, whereas epigenetic modifications (methylation) can be reactivated by environmental signals.

7. DNA methylation and histone alterations work in concert. When DNA is unmethylated and histones are acetylated, nucleosomes are spaced in the open configuration and transcription can occur. When DNA is methylated and histones are deacetylated, nucleosomes are relatively close together and transcription is suppressed.

8. In addition to functioning in cellular signaling, microRNAs play a significant role in the developing embryo. miRNAs are involved with RNA silencing through RISCs that act as repressors of gene expression. They do so by making mRNAs less likely to be translated.

9. When mutations occur in imprinted genes, called epimutations, heritable changes in gene activity may occur. Imprinting defects cause Prader-Willi syndrome, Angelman syndrome, Beckwith-Wiedemann syndrome, and several others. In most cases imprinted genes encode growth factors or genes that regulate growth factors.

Discussion Question Answers

1. Historically, demethylation treatments have been applied to human disorders; however, since DNA methylation is a common and significant component of normal genetic regulation, what may be useful for controlling one gene in the genome may have numerous unwanted changes in other parts of the genome. DNA methyltransferase inhibitors such as azacitidine and decitabine have been tested for use in epigenetic cancer therapy.

2. While data are scant, some studies have shown that children born after *in vitro* fertilization are at risk for low to very low birth weight that may have resulted from abnormal imprinting. There also appears to be an increased risk of a child conceived via ART having Beckwith-Wiedemann syndrome. Given these data, it would seem reasonable that such information should be provided to prospective ART users. Each couple would need to reach a decision based on available science and their own value and belief sets.

3. Cancer is a genetic disease that is caused by not only traditional chromosomal and point mutations but also a multitude of other factors that alter gene activity. Epigenetic modifications change gene output and therefore can cause cancer.

4. Plant miRNAs are known to downregulate gene expression, and some foods are the source of miRNAs that circulate in body fluids of humans. Given this information, it has been suggested that as yet poorly understood environmental factors may play a significant role in the regulation of gene function in humans. At this point it might be premature to design a dietary regimen based on such a frail understanding of the role of plant miRNAs in humans.

Review and Discussion Questions (Special Topics #2)

Review Question Answers

1. RNAs, whether single- or double-stranded, play many roles including the transfer of information from DNA to proteins (mRNA, tRNA, rRNA), gene regulation (sncRNA, siRNA, etc.), transposon silencing (piRNA), and epigenetic modifications of DNA (lncRNA).

2. Since RNA can both serve in information storage and transfer and catalyze reactions, it has been hypothesized that RNA was the precursor to molecular life-like events. In addition, RNAs are components of many primitive yet biologically significant reactions.

3. Ribozymes can break and form phosphodiester bonds, which has major implications in support of the RNA World Hypothesis.

4. DNA methylation provides a defense against the integration of foreign DNA into the bacterial chromosome, whereas *CRISPR* loci transcribe crRNAs that guide nucleases to invading complementary DNAs in order to destroy them.

5. Small interferingRNAs (siRNAs) protect cells from exogenous RNAs, while microRNAs (miRNAs) are involved in regulating gene expression. Piwi-interacting RNAs (piRNAs) protect germ cells from the harmful effects of mobile DNA sequences.

6. Through a series of transcriptive and Dicer-related activities, siRNAs are formed that are complementary to centromeric DNA. A RITS silencing complex forms that leads to methylation, thus triggering heterochromatin formation. At this point, the evolution of such a complex process of heterochromatin formation is not well understood.

7. Circular RNA (circRNA) soaks up miRNAs and allows expression of miRNA targets.

8. Interestingly, extracellular RNA is a heterogeneous group composed of mRNAs and miRNAs that, in association with proteins, are secreted from cells in vesicles. These vesicles may serve for protection or signaling.

9. The cytoskeleton plays a major role in the transport and localization of cellular and molecular components. A cell is a regionalized entity that contains a variety of poorly understood molecular gradients, structures, and organelles. Each component is unique and differentiated by a variety of nuclear products. A complex delivery system involving various motor proteins and other poorly understood processes accomplishes such differentiation.

Discussion Question Answers

1. Double-stranded DNA is more stable than RNA and less subject to mutational change. In addition, double-stranded DNA offers a ready template for the manufacture of two daughter DNAs, which, with the exception of mutation, are identical to the parental structure.

2. Negative or positive regulation depends on whether the ribosome binding site is masked or available. When repression occurs, the ribosome binding site (RBS) is masked by sRNA. When positive regulation occurs, sRNA pairing unmasks the RBS.

3. Local translation of proteins is often dependent on mRNAs such as *Drosophila nanos* mRNA, and some human disorders, such as fragile-X syndrome, are dependent on protein localization. Such translocation is essential for many normal cellular functions.

4. In bacteria and Archaea, foreign DNA can be inserted into *CRISPR* loci in the genome, which brings about transcription of crRNAs that guide nucleases to invading complementary DNAs. In addition, foreign DNA can be digested by restriction endonucleases. One form of eukaryotic genome protection involves piRNAs that are pivotal in silencing transposons, mobile DNA sequences that change position. Associated with Piwi proteins, certain proteins (such as RISC) target transposon-derived RNAs and their complementary sequences. This process represses transposon transcription by promoting DNA methylation of transposon DNA.

A broadly functioning protective mechanism involves siRNA in association with RISCs and Dicer, an RNAse III protein.

5. Extracellular species of RNA include mRNAs and miRNAs that are associated with proteins or encapsulated in vesicles. They might function in some form of extracellular signaling by stimulating cell-surface receptors. Perhaps such RNA can be integrated into neighboring cells and bring about the translation of specific proteins.

6. Even though a particular species of mRNA may be fairly uniformly distributed throughout a cell, it does not follow that it is uniformly translated. It is likely that different domains reside in cells that contain different translational signals. Anterior-posterior protein gradients are known to be present in *Drosophila* eggs. If an mRNA finds itself in a particular molecular environment, it may be destined for translation, whereas that same mRNA in another part of a cell may not have the environmental stimulation necessary for translation.

Review and Discussion Questions (Special Topics #3)

Review Question Answers

1. VNTR profiling is a form of DNA profiling that takes advantage of the variable number of tandem repeats (VNTRs) that are located in various regions of the genome. Such repeats are generally made up of DNA sequences between 15 and 100 bp in length. Their use in DNA profiling rests in the fact that the number of repeats varies from person to person. VNTRs can be used to match a DNA sample recovered from a given circumstance (crime, organismic remains, paternity testing, ancient lineage, etc.) with other DNA samples.

2. With the development of the polymerase chain reaction, trace samples of DNA can be used, commonly in forensic applications. STRs are like VNTRs, but the repeat portion is shorter, between two and nine base pairs, repeated from 7 to 40 times. A core set of STR loci, about 13, is most often used in forensic applications.

3. Capillary electrophoresis uses thin glass tubes containing polyacrylamide gel to which amplified DNA is loaded onto the top of the tube. Electrophoresis separates the DNA fragments, and the amount and length of each fragment can be obtained. In addition to the very small amount of original DNA as template, the large amount of fluorescentlylabeled product DNA is easily identified.

4. Since males typically contain a Y chromosome (exceptions include transgender and mosaic individuals), gender separation of a mixed tissue sample is easily achieved by Y chromosome profiling. In addition, STR profiling is possible for over 200 loci; however, because of the relative stability of DNA in the Y chromosome, it is difficult to differentiate DNA from fathers and sons or male siblings.

5. Even though the *AMEL* locus is on both the X and Y chromosome, the X chromosome allele contains a 6-nucleotide deletion that is not found on the Y chromosome.

6. Like Y-chromosome DNA, mtDNA is very stable because it undergoes very little, if any, recombination. Since there is a high copy number of mitochondria in cells, it is especially useful in situations where samples are small, old, or degraded, which is often the case in catastrophes.

7. A profile probability provides a mathematical probability that a sample of DNA taken at random from a population shares the same DNA profile as another sample.

8. The Combined DNA Index System (CODIS) is a collection of DNA databases and analytical tools of both state and federal governments, maintained by the FBI. As of June, 2014 the database contained over 13 million, it contained more than 11 million DNA profiles. DNA profiles are collected from convicted offenders, forensic investigations, and, in some states, those suspected of crimes as well as from unidentified human remains and missing persons (in cases where DNA is available).

9. DNA barcoding is often used in wildlife forensics, where, throughout the world, it is used as one method of cataloging more than 70,000 different species. It is also useful in tracking the smuggling of wildlife and wildlife parts.

10. The prosecutor's fallacy attempts to equate guilt with a numerical probability produced by a single piece of evidence. A match between a crime scene and a suspect does not necessarily mean that the suspect is guilty. Human error, contamination, or evidence tampering all contribute to the complexities of interpreting DNA profiling data.

Discussion Question Answers

1. Generally, natural DNA is contained within cells and is often coupled with various forms of modification (methylation, associated proteins), whereas synthetic DNA is normally free of these factors. Various treatments of DNA with nucleases can often reveal DNA that has been modified.

2. To gain information as to laws and regulations in various states, one could navigate to "Welcome to the DNA Laws Database" within the National Conference of State Legislatures Web site. There, one can select a particular state for its laws and regulations regarding DNA collection and profiling. In general, one will see that most states contain descriptions of the following topics:

(a) Various DNA databases used

(b) Methods of DNA collection

(c) Post-conviction DNA collection of felons

(d) Oversight and advisory committees

(e) Convicted offender statutes

3. In general, the legal profession is charged with seeking the truth regarding a crime. To properly defend a client, it would be absolutely critical that the jury understand the limitations of DNA-based evidence.

4. Somatic mosaicism and chimerism involve a mixture of cell types, the origin of which may involve a variety of embryonic events, some of which are understood. Since a single individual may contain a mixed population of cells, a DNA sample taken from one tissue site may not match a DNA sample taken from another site. This can lead to a conflicted set of results when it comes to matching a DNA sample to a sample of DNA from a crime scene. Taking DNA samples from various sites on an individual may be useful in mitigating such confusion. In addition, in STR DNA profiling mosaicism may present itself at the electrophoresis/analysis stage by additional peaks or peak height imbalances.

Review and Discussion questions (Special Topics #4):

Review Question Answers:

1. Pharmacogenomics is the assessment of an individual's genome in response to a given drug. Pharmacogenetics is more involved with specific genes and their alleles in the design and response to drugs. The focus of pharmacogenetics is related to specific candidate genes.

2. Herceptin is used in the treatment of breast cancer that targets the epidermal growth factor receptor 2 (*HER-2*) gene located on chromosome 17. Overexpression of this gene occurs in about 25 percent of invasive breast cancer cases. Herceptin is a monoclonal antibody that binds specifically to inhibit the HER-2 receptor.

3. The Oncotype DX Assay analyzes the expressionof 21 genes active in breast cancer samples. From information obtained from the assay, a treatment is developed that is more specific than traditional therapies.

4. Cytochrome P450 is composed of a family of enzymes that are encoded by 57 different genes. Certain variants of cytochrome P450 metabolize drugs slowly and can lead to harmful accumulations of a drug. Other variants cause drugs to be eliminated quickly, which can lead to drug ineffectiveness. A pivotal gene, *CYP2D6*, influences the metabolism of approximately 25 percent of all drugs, while *VKORC1* influences the response to warfarin, an anticoagulant drug.

5. Genetic tests are divided into several major groups. Diagnostic tests are designed to test for the presence of genetic alleles that are, or might be, linked to the symptomatic patient. Predictive tests are designed to identify alleles in patients with a family history of a disorder. Carrier tests are used to identify individuals who might carry a mutation that causes a given disorder. Preimplantation tests are performed on early embryos to eliminate potentially harmful conditions, and prenatal tests are available to detect genetic diseases in a fetus.

6. Recently, large-scale genomic sequencing has shown that each tumor is genetically unique. With such information, it is often possible to provide a personalized diagnosis and possibly apply personalized treatments. One such example is the use of Herceptin for the treatment of breast cancer; another is the use of Erbitux and Vectibix to inhibit epidermal growth factor receptors that are commonly expressed in cancer cells.

7. There are many genes in the genome that are not related to cancer, but many are, and those cancer genes that are expressed (or suppressed) can be assayed as to their expressive state. To develop therapies for effective personalized medicine, the activities of those suites of genes peculiar to a particular cancer must be assessed.

8. Using the search function in the PharmGKB database one can find a number of references that discuss the variants of *CYP2D6* and tamoxifen. For example, according to Hertz et al. (Hertz, D., et al. 2012. *The Oncologist*. 17(5): 2011-0418), tamoxifen efficacy is dependent on the highly polymorphic cytochrome P450 gene (*CYP2D6*). Depending on a particular variant genotype, tamoxifen treatment outcome is highly inconsistent. The entire Hertz et al. paper is available through the PharmGKB database and provides a complete and detailed description of the interactions of *CYP2D6* variants and tamoxifen.

Discussion Question Answers:

1. The use of genomic studies to develop personalized disease treatments provides an ever-expanding promise for the enhancement of human health and welfare. At this point in time, genomic information is available for which useful interpretation may be lacking. In other words, one might have information as to a correlation between a genomic profile and a diseased state, but the question of causal relationships may be unanswerable given the present state of knowledge. What does one do with such information?In addition, in some cases, a treatment approach may be obvious, but the treatment itself may not be available. Since personalized, targeted treatments are often very expensive, how does one afford a treatment if it is not covered by insurance and financial relief is not forthcoming?

Review and Discussion questions (Special Topics #4):

2. Given the obvious progress that has occurred in recent years, it is highly likely that more personalized therapies will be developed in the near future. There are several bridges that must be crossed before one can claim universal use and acceptance. First, it will be necessary to close the gap between data collection and interpretation of complex interactions. Second, personalized medicines are dependent on the development of effective therapies that have few side effects and a reasonable cost. Finally, given the complexity of living systems, there will likely be diseases for which therapies will be difficult to develop. In addition, hopefully, incentives will be sufficient for entities to develop therapies for rare, financially less-rewarding diseases.

3. Since it is presently impossible to ensure database security, even though efforts are most sincere, one might conclude that medical records will not be completely secure.

4. At present, genetic discrimination does exist; however, recent developments in health care laws seek to minimize such discrimination by medical insurance companies. It remains to be seen whether genetic discrimination in the workplace will continue.

Review and Discussion Questions (Special Topics #5)

Review Question Answers

1. Traditionally, selective breeding was used to generate strains of organisms that showed favorable traits. With the advent of genetic engineering in the 1970s, recombinant methods were used to modify agriculturally important organisms with more precision and more rapidly. Such methods have increased productivity, reduced pesticide dependence, and enhanced nutrition and flavor.

2. Genetic engineering allows genetic material to be transferred within and between species and to alter expression levels of genes. A transgenic organism is one that involves the transfer of genetic material between different species, whereas the term cisgenic is sometimes used in cases where gene transfers occur within a species.

3. It has recently been determined that GM crops are grown in about 30 countries on about 11 percent of the crop-friendly land on Earth. Five countries account for almost 90 percent of GM crops: the United States, Brazil, Argentina, Canada, and India. The most common GM crops grown in the United States are soybeans and maize, followed by sugar beets, cotton, canola, papaya, and squash.

4. Herbicide-tolerant plants make up approximately 70 percent of all GM plants, the majority of which confer tolerance to the herbicide glyphosate. Glyphosate interferes with the enzyme 5-enolpyruvylshikimate-3-phosphate synthetase, which is present in all plants and is required for the synthesis of the aromatic amino acids phenylalanine, tyrosine, and tryptophan.

5. *Bacillus thuringiensis* (Bt) produces crystal (Cry) proteins that are toxic to certain orders of insects such as Lepidoptera, Diptera, Coleoptera, and Hymenoptera. When ingested by these insects, the Cry proteins bind to receptors in the gut wall, which leads to a breakdown of the gut membranes.

6. The first iteration of Golden Rice involved the introduction of phytoene synthetase originating from the daffodil plant and carotene desaturase from a bacterium engineered into the rice plant.

Resulting rice grains were yellow in color due to the production of beta-carotene. Later versions of Golden Rice 2 involved the introduction of similar genes from maize, thus leading to a much higher production of beta-carotene. At present, Golden Rice 2 is being tested in preparation for use in Bangladesh and the Philippines.

7. Golden Rice 2 involved the introduction of three genes into the T-DNA region of a Ti plasmid. Researchers established embryonic rice cell cultures and employed a positive selection method by growing plant cells on a mannose-containing medium. Surviving cells expressed the *pmi* gene and were stimulated to form calluses that were grown into plants. The desired transgenic constructs were verified using the polymerase chain reaction.

8. The biolistic method of gene introduction achieves DNA transfer by coating the transforming DNA in a heavy metal to form particles that are fired at high speed into plant cells using a gene gun. The introduced DNA may migrate into the cell nucleus and integrate into a plant chromosome.

9. In positive selection, conditions are arranged such that only the organism of interest can grow (mannose selection, for example). In negative selection, a condition is arranged that inhibits the growth of organisms that are of no interest (antibiotic resistance, for example).

10. Roundup-Ready soybeans received market approval almost ten years ago. This GM plant is resistant to the herbicide glyphosate, a broad-spectrum herbicide, because glyphosate interferes with the enzyme 5-enolpyruvylshikimate-3-phosphate synthetase, which is necessary for the plant to synthesize the aromatic amino acids phenylalanine, tyrosine, and tryptophan. The *epsps* gene was cloned from *Agrobacterium* strain CP4 and introduced into soybeans using biolistic bombardment.

Discussion Question Answers

1. In many states, bills have been filed that range from banning GM foods to requiring labeling of such foods. To determine the status of such measures in your state, search for "GM food [your state]" on a major search engine. A comprehensive look at the position the United States takes on GE (genetically engineered, as contrasted with foods modified by traditional selective breeding) can be found at the U.S. Food and Drug Administration Web site (http://www.fda.gov/forconsumers/consumerupdates/ucm352067.htm).

2. There are many positions taken and bills filed in various states to address the question of GM food labeling. Generally, many feel a "right to know" would allow consumers to make educated choices about the food they consume. They would consider it an advantage to be able to judge the safety of a given food if they had information about the possibility that it contains GM components. Others wonder about the usefulness of a GM label if there is little information provided as to how the food has been modified. Of what value would it be

to know that food was genetically modified if the science and specifics about the modifications were not included? How much background knowledge would be needed by the consumer to be able to interpret such information?

3. At this point in time there is probably no "correct" answer that can be given. The person who is completely against GM food consumption might suffer mental anguish to know that there are GM foods "out there" and they may be unwillingly consuming them. Is such anguish harmful to human health even if there is no direct harm done to the physical aspects of human health? If a GM product is tested and found to be safe in animal models and several thousand human volunteers, can one be certain that all individuals who may be exposed to the food will suffer no negative effects? These are but a few of the issues that face consumers as more and more GM products hit the market.

Review and Discussion Questions (Special Topics #6)

Review Question Answers

1. Gene therapy involves the placement of potentially beneficial genes into a person's cells in an effort to correct some faulty genetic state.

2. In *ex vivo* gene therapy, a potential genetic correction takes place in cells that have been removed from the patient. *In vivo* gene therapy treats cells of the body through the introduction of DNA into the patient.

3. In general, integration of the therapeutic DNA into the host genome is advantageous in that more stability of the introduced DNA is enhanced; however, the integration process itself may generate mutations and regulatory alterations. In some cases, integration into the host genome is not necessary; however, the introduced DNA is usually less stable, thus requiring repeated infusions.

4. In many cases, therapeutic DNA hitches a ride with genetically engineered viruses, such as retrovirus or adenovirus vectors. Nonviral delivery methods may use chemical assistance to cross cell membranes, nanoparticles, or cell fusion with artificial vesicles.

5. Viral vectors, such as genetically modified retroviruses or adenoviruses, are often used to deliver therapeutic DNA into host cells. There are several challenges that often attend their use. One problem is that of the viral introduction itself. In some cases, patients mount an immune response to the introduction of such viruses. If the introduced DNA is to be integrated into the host genome, what directs its insertion? Insertion can lead to the creation of mutations and changes in the regulatory machinery of cells. In addition, how will the introduced DNA be regulated? Will proper promoters and enhancers and silencers be in proper alignment to achieve a desired outcome?

6. White blood cells, T cells in this case, were used because they are key players in the mounting of an immune response, which Ashanti was incapable of developing. A normal copy of the *ADA* gene was engineered into a retroviral vector, which then infected many of her T cells. Those cells that expressed the *ADA* gene were then injected into Ashanti's bloodstream, and some of them populated her bone marrow. At the time of Ashanti's treatment, targeted gene therapy was not possible, so integration of the *ADA* gene into Ashanti's genome probably did not replace her defective gene.

7. The treatment of Ashanti DeSilva for SCID was the first successful gene therapy achievement. Ashanti's T cells were treated with genetically engineered retroviral vectors with the goal of inserting a normal copy of the *ADA* gene. Some of the T cells that received the retrovirus integrated the therapeutic DNA. After growing transformed cells in the laboratory, they were injected into Ashanti's bloodstream, and some eventually populated and multiplied in her bone marrow.

8. To some extent, targeted gene therapy is designed to alleviate one of the major pitfalls of gene therapy, random DNA integration. In addition, recent research holds promise for approaches of targeted removal and even the silencing of defective genes. DNA editing makes use of nucleases and zinc-finger arrangements to remove defective genes from the genome.

9. ZFNs, or zinc-finger nucleases, consist of transcription factors that contain two cysteine and two histidine residues that bind zinc atoms and interact with specific DNA sequences. The nuclease portion of a ZFN provides a DNA cutting property that may eventually allow for targeted gene therapy.

10. One method of gene inhibition follows from the use of RNA interference (RNAi) whereby double-stranded RNA molecules are delivered into cells, and the enzyme Dicer cleaves them into relatively short pieces of RNA (siRNA). siRNA can form a complex with enzymes that target mRNA. Another approach to silence genes involves the use of antisense RNA in which RNA is introduced that is complementary to a strand of mRNA, thus blocking its translation.

Discussion Question Answers

1. Because there are many human conditions that result from a number of gene loci, many such diseases will be too complicated to be able to apply present-day approaches for treatment. For less complex genetic conditions, selection of a suitable vector, one that doesn't create a new set of problems (immune response, poor penetration into cells, etc.), will be necessary for widespread use. One major challenge centers on the problem of targeted integration so as not to compromise the normal function of other genes in the genome. In addition, the appropriate regulation of introduced DNA must be achieved before such techniques can become commonplace.

2. Generally, gene therapy is an accepted procedure, given appropriate conditions, for the relief of genetic disease states. Since it is a fairly expensive medical approach, considerable debate attends its use. It remains to be seen whether insurance companies will embrace what might be considered experimental treatments. Use of gene therapy to enhance the competitive status of individuals (genetic enhancement or gene doping) is presently viewed as cheating by most organizations and the public. It is unlikely that germ-line therapy will be viewed favorably by the public or scientific communities; however, this and other issues mentioned here will be the subject of considerable future debate.

3. The widespread use of gene therapy in the future will depend on its success rate, which encompasses the degree to which diseases are treatable, the attending side effects, and the absence of catastrophic failures. Since there are many approaches that are now being studied, ranging from gene replacement to antisense therapies to targeted integration, it is likely that one or more approaches will become viable in treating genetic diseases. Incentives are in place to reward such research should treatments break through the practical and scientific barriers that were discussed in the text.